Managing
Anxiety
Disorders
in primary
care

Managing Anxiety Disorders
in primary care

LEE DAVID

MBBS, BSc, MRCGP, MA in cognitive behavioural therapy
GP and Cognitive Behavioural Therapist

Scion

A CIP catalogue record for this book is available from the British Library.

ISBN 9781911510390

Scion Publishing Limited

The Old Hayloft, Vantage Business Park, Bloxham Road, Banbury OX16 9UX, UK

www.scionpublishing.com

Important Note from the Publisher

The information contained within this book was obtained by Scion Publishing Ltd from sources believed by us to be reliable. However, while every effort has been made to ensure its accuracy, no responsibility for loss or injury whatsoever occasioned to any person acting or refraining from action as a result of information contained herein can be accepted by the authors or publishers.

Readers are reminded that medicine is a constantly evolving science and while the authors and publishers have ensured that all dosages, applications and practices are based on current indications, there may be specific practices which differ between communities. You should always follow the guidelines laid down by the manufacturers of specific products and the relevant authorities in the country in which you are practising.

Although every effort has been made to ensure that all owners of copyright material have been acknowledged in this publication, we would be pleased to acknowledge in subsequent reprints or editions any omissions brought to our attention.

Registered names, trademarks, etc. used in this book, even when not marked as such, are not to be considered unprotected by law.

Cover design by Andrew Magee Design using original artwork by Paul Kessling (www.paulkessling.com)
Typeset by Evolution Design & Digital Ltd (Kent)
Printed in the UK

Last digit is the print number: 10 9 8 7 6 5 4 3 2 1

Contents

Preface

Anxiety disorders are among the commonest mental health conditions and are highly prevalent among patients in primary care. These conditions have a negative impact on people's wellbeing and quality of life and can be disabling and costly to both the patient and the healthcare system. Anxiety can also interfere with the management of people's physical health and may be associated with worsening outcomes for coexisting chronic physical disorders.

Despite the prevalence of anxiety disorders, many patients remain undiagnosed and untreated, although patients with unrecognised anxiety disorders tend to be high users of both primary and secondary care medical services. Individuals experiencing underlying anxiety may present with multiple somatic complaints and co-morbid disorders or may attend recurrently with unexplained physical symptoms. If anxiety remains undetected, they will not receive appropriate treatment and may also undergo unnecessary, potentially dangerous, and costly investigations.

Making a diagnosis of anxiety can be challenging in primary care. But when anxiety disorders are identified, patients can be offered effective treatments, which include self-help, psychological therapy and medication, and this can transform people's lives.

This book aims to improve the recognition and treatment of anxiety disorders in primary care. It provides an overview of the commonest anxiety disorders seen in primary care, including how to recognise each disorder, make the diagnosis, explain the condition to patients, and the different management options. It also includes practical case studies to illustrate how different types of anxiety may present in primary care, and how GPs might begin to assess and manage patients with these conditions.

Cognitive behavioural therapy (CBT) is, in many cases, the most effective treatment for anxiety disorders. This book also includes a brief CBT framework for making sense of each anxiety disorder using a five-areas CBT framework, and an overview of some simple 10 minute CBT strategies for coping with anxiety that can be used to encourage self-care and promote wellbeing.

Further details, including how to access online video-based training and educational DVDs for management of anxiety disorders using 10 minute CBT, can be found on our website: www.10minuteCBT.co.uk.

Lee David

Abbreviations

ACT	acceptance and commitment therapy
ADHD	attention deficit hyperactivity disorder
BDD	body dysmorphic disorder
CBT	cognitive behavioural therapy
COPD	chronic obstructive pulmonary disease
CR	cognitive restructuring
DBT	dialectical behaviour therapy
EMDR	eye movement desensitisation and reprocessing
ERP	exposure and response prevention
GAD	generalised anxiety disorder
GAD-2	two-item GAD assessment
GAD-7	seven-item GAD assessment
HADS	Hospital Anxiety and Depression Scale
LSAS	Liebowitz Social Anxiety Scale
MAOI	monoamine oxidase inhibitor
MBCT	mindfulness-based cognitive therapy
Mini-SPIN	Mini-Social Phobia Inventory
MUS	medically unexplained symptoms
NICE	National Institute for Health and Care Excellence
OCD	obsessive–compulsive disorder
PTSD	post-traumatic stress disorder
SAM	situationally accessible memory
SNRI	selective serotonin and noradrenaline reuptake inhibitor
SSRI	selective serotonin reuptake inhibitor
TCA	tricyclic antidepressant
TSQ	Trauma Screening Questionnaire
VAM	verbally accessible memory
Y-BOCS	Yale–Brown Obsessive Compulsive Scale

Chapter 1
Understanding anxiety disorders

1.1 Introduction

Anxiety is a normal and healthy reaction which arises in everyone when faced with situations that could be dangerous or stressful. The anxiety response involves a series of physiological changes in the body, and in how we think and behave, and enables us to respond rapidly to threat or danger.

However, anxiety can become a problem if it begins to affect people's ability to function and carry out daily activities, or if it interferes with important relationships with other people. If levels of anxiety are significant and persistent, an individual may meet the criteria for the diagnosis of an anxiety disorder. Anxiety disorders place a significant burden on individuals as well as on the healthcare system and society as a whole. The vast majority of anxiety disorders are managed within primary care.

Features that suggest that anxiety is becoming a significant problem include the following:
- Anxiety is frequently triggered when there is not really a significant danger.
- Anxiety arises in situations where it is not usual for people to experience it.
- It continues beyond the point where it is useful, such as after the danger has passed.
- It interferes with people's ability to function in important activities.
- It leads to avoidance of situations in an attempt to minimise or control anxiety and distress.
- Symptoms are persistent or lasting.

1.2 How common are anxiety disorders?

Anxiety disorders are among the most common mental health disorders, with lifetime prevalence rates for experiencing any anxiety disorder ranging from 10.4–28.8% and 12-month prevalence rates of about 18%. The 12-month

Table 1.1 Summary of prevalence rates for common anxiety disorders (NICE, 2011)

Anxiety disorder	12-month prevalence	Lifetime prevalence
Generalised anxiety disorder (GAD)	3.1%	5.7%
Panic disorder	2.7%	4.7%
Agoraphobia without panic disorder	0.8%	1.4%
Phobia (specific)	8.7%	12.5%
Social anxiety disorder	6.8%	12.1%
Obsessive–compulsive disorder (OCD)	1.0%	1.6%
Post-traumatic stress disorder (PTSD)	1.3–3.6%	6.8%

prevalence rates for specific anxiety disorders range from about 1% for obsessive–compulsive disorder (OCD) to 8.7% for specific phobia; however, rates vary widely across different studies depending on the criteria used to determine distress or impairment. *Table 1.1* shows a summary of the 12-month and lifetime prevalence rates for common anxiety disorders.

Anxiety disorders are common and important conditions in primary care, affecting between 1 in 5 and 1 in 12 patients presenting in this setting. Many anxiety disorders, such as health anxiety and generalised anxiety disorder (GAD), are associated with frequent attendances and high use of primary care resources. Conversely, patients with social anxiety may make fewer visits to primary care than those with other anxiety disorders, probably due to attempts to avoid anxiety that arises on visiting health settings.

Common risk factors for anxiety disorders are shown in *Box 1.1*.

Box 1.1   **Risk factors for anxiety disorders**

- Family history of anxiety or other mental health conditions
- Personal history of anxiety in childhood or adolescence, including marked shyness
- Stressful life events or other life difficulties
- Experience of a traumatic event, including abuse
- Female sex
- Co-morbid psychiatric disorder such as depression, substance misuse or another anxiety disorder
- Chronic physical health conditions, such as cardiovascular disease, diabetes, asthma and obesity

1.3 Co-morbid conditions

Mental health conditions

Co-morbid mental health conditions are extremely common in anxiety disorders. Up to 75% of those who are diagnosed with an anxiety disorder have at least one other mental health condition. This can have important implications for diagnosis and treatment. Anxiety disorders co-morbid with other mental health conditions are associated with poorer treatment outcomes, greater severity and chronicity, more impaired functioning and increased health service use.

Physical health conditions

Patients with anxiety disorders also have a higher prevalence and a reduced quality of life associated with a number of physical health conditions, including hypertension and other cardiovascular disorders, gastrointestinal disease, arthritis, thyroid disease, respiratory disease, migraine and allergic conditions.

Box 1.2 | **Mental health conditions which may be co-morbid with anxiety disorders**

- Other anxiety disorders
- Depression
- Alcohol and substance abuse
- Bipolar disorder and psychosis
- Attention deficit hyperactivity disorder (ADHD)
- Personality disorders

1.4 Overview of anxiety

The key features of anxiety disorders include:
- emotional symptoms such as excessive anxiety, fear, worry and panic
- cognitive factors such as excessive focus on feared future outcomes and over-estimation of risk
- physical or somatic symptoms of anxiety, including breathlessness, palpitations, insomnia, headache, pain and gastrointestinal symptoms
- behavioural factors, including avoidance of triggers to anxiety and seeking reassurance through a variety of safety behaviours or rituals.

Anxiety disorders share many common features but also have key differences in both presentation and approaches to treatment. *Table 1.2* contains a brief overview of the characteristics of the most common anxiety disorders.

Table 1.2 Characteristics of anxiety disorders

Anxiety disorder	Characteristics
Generalised anxiety disorder (GAD)	• Uncontrollable, excessive anxiety and worry about multiple different situations or life problems, including 'worry about worry' and difficulty tolerating uncertainty • Often associated with physical symptoms such as fatigue, headache, muscle tension, irritability and insomnia • Repeated loops of worry about potential future problems without planning coping strategies for coping with these difficulties
Panic disorder	• Recurrent unexpected and short-lived episodes of intense fear or discomfort ('panic attacks') lasting around 30–45 minutes • Associated with intense physical symptoms of anxiety including palpitations, breathlessness and chest pain or tightness • Catastrophic misinterpretation of bodily symptoms, such as thoughts about having a heart attack or suffocation, leads to rapidly escalating anxiety symptoms as a vicious cycle • Fear of having further panic attacks
Agoraphobia	• Anxiety and fear of places or situations such as being in a crowd, being outside the home or using public transport • Fears arise from the perception that escape might be difficult or help might not be available in the event of having a panic attack • Avoidance of anxiety-provoking situations typically results in a significant limitation of daily activities • Agoraphobia develops in around two-thirds of patients with panic disorder and only rarely occurs in the absence of panic
Social anxiety	• Fear and avoidance of social or performance situations, such as speaking to unfamiliar people or groups, or eating in public • Fear of being observed or evaluated negatively by other people, often due to anxiety that physical symptoms (such as excessive blushing, sweating, trembling, palpitations and nausea) will be noticeable to others and lead to judgement and rejection • Frequently impacts negatively on educational and work performance
Obsessive–compulsive disorder (OCD)	• Recurrent, unwanted obsessional thoughts and compulsive rituals which cause significant distress and markedly interfere with the individual's daily life • Common obsessional thoughts include a fear of contamination from dirt or germs, concern with order or symmetry, fear of inadvertently harming another person and fear of thinking evil or sinful thoughts • Overwhelming compulsions to repeat certain rituals or behaviours in an attempt to 'neutralise' the thoughts and alleviate the distress, e.g. repeated hand washing, counting, checking or cleaning
Body dysmorphic disorder (BDD)	• Excessive worry about perceived flaws in physical appearance, such as nose shape or a skin condition such as acne • The perceived defect is usually minor or even non-existent, and may not be noticeable to others, but can lead to avoidance of social situations • Sufferers spend vast amounts of time comparing their appearance with other people and checking in mirrors, and go to great lengths to try to conceal the flaw, using hairstyles, make-up and clothing • Sufferers frequently seek cosmetic procedures to treat the perceived defect, although this is rarely successful in alleviating distress

Post-traumatic stress disorder (PTSD)	• PTSD can arise after exposure to an extreme traumatic event that causes intense fear, helplessness or horror, such as acts of violence, severe accidents, natural disasters or military action • Sufferers develop intrusive symptoms such as involuntary re-experiencing of images and other somatic experiences associated with the traumatic event in the form of flashbacks, nightmares and distressing mental imagery • Thoughts or reminders of the traumatic event trigger intense distress, leading to avoidance • Hyperarousal symptoms include hypervigilance for threat, exaggerated startle responses, irritability, difficulty in concentrating and sleep problems • Complex PTSD can arise after severe or multiple traumas and is associated with additional symptoms including a negative self-view, difficulty regulating emotions and problems in relationships with others
Health anxiety	• Preoccupation with an intense fear of having or developing a serious illness • The fear persists despite undergoing appropriate medical evaluation and being reassured that no medical condition is present • Sufferers frequently check their body for signs of illness, browse the internet to look for explanations of their symptoms, and repeatedly attend multiple health professionals seeking investigations, referrals and medical reassurance that nothing serious is wrong • These behaviours may initially alleviate anxiety but lead to an increase in anxiety and repeated attempts for reassurance over the longer term
Specific phobias	• An extreme and unreasonable fear of a specific single object or situation, such as dentists, spiders, lifts, flying or seeing blood, which is out of proportion to the actual danger or threat • Symptoms of anxiety such as nausea, sweating, increased heart rate and shaking occur when the person encounters or thinks about the object or situation • Anxiety leads to avoidance of the source of the phobia

1.5 The purpose of anxiety – the fight or flight response

Anxiety arises when the body prepares to cope with a potential future danger. This is often known as the 'fight or flight' response.

Imagine you are crossing a wide and busy road at a pedestrian crossing. You suddenly notice a truck that has failed to slow down and may not stop in time. It's veering in your direction. You start running for the safety of the pavement a few feet away. How would this feel?

When we feel under threat, our brain becomes aware of the danger. Automatically, our bodies respond rapidly by releasing hormones such as adrenaline and cortisol. These affect the body in a number of ways to help us cope with the potential threat:
• The mind becomes more alert, so we can act faster.
• Our senses sharpen: our field of vision can increase, sometimes causing blurring, and our hearing can become more acute, causing muffling or ringing.

- Our hearts beat faster and harder, quickly sending blood to where it's needed most.
- Blood is diverted to the muscles, which grow tense, ready to fight the danger or run away.
- Sweating increases to help cool the body.
- We breathe more deeply and rapidly, to get more oxygen into our body, which is needed by muscles.
- We may experience an urge to pass urine or empty the bowels or notice a dry mouth as secretions dry up; this is because the lighter we are, the quicker we move.
- Blood is diverted away from our stomach and internal organs and digestion slows down, as it is less important at this time – this can lead to tummy cramps and nausea.
- Nostrils and air passages in lungs open wider to get air in more quickly.

Because of these body changes, you are able to run very quickly to the side of the road and escape being knocked down by the truck.

This series of reactions accounts for the many and varied physical reactions associated with anxiety. These symptoms can be quite unpleasant and include palpitations, over-breathing (which can lead to dizziness and tingling in the hands and around the mouth) and shakiness, as well as tightness and pain in the muscles of the chest and throat. Emotionally, there may be feelings of fear, apprehension, agitation and worry.

The fight or flight response is a very important reaction to keep us safe from dangerous situations. It is also important to note that the symptoms of anxiety are NOT dangerous, even though they may be unpleasant and distressing. They are normal reactions to threat and danger and will gradually fade if the person is able to stay in the feared situation. Understanding this can be the first step in overcoming anxiety.

1.6 CBT model of anxiety

Cognitive behavioural therapy (CBT) offers a helpful framework for understanding anxiety disorders. *Figure 1.1* highlights how an anxious person's thoughts, feelings, physical reactions and behaviour can interact in a vicious cycle.

Feelings and emotions

People with anxiety disorders typically feel fearful, anxious, scared, worried and afraid. They may also become irritable and prone to anger. If anxiety is persistent for long periods, people may also develop secondary low mood and depression.

Physical reactions and body sensations

Common physical reactions relate to the physiological response to the fight or flight reaction described in *Section 1.5*. These include:

- sweating
- shaking and trembling
- feeling tense and on edge
- poor concentration
- hyperventilation – rapid and deep breathing leads to feelings of breathlessness and tightness in the chest, and may also cause numbness and tingling in the hands
- rapid heart rate
- gastrointestinal symptoms including stomach cramps, nausea and symptoms associated with irritable bowel syndrome (IBS)
- feeling dizzy.

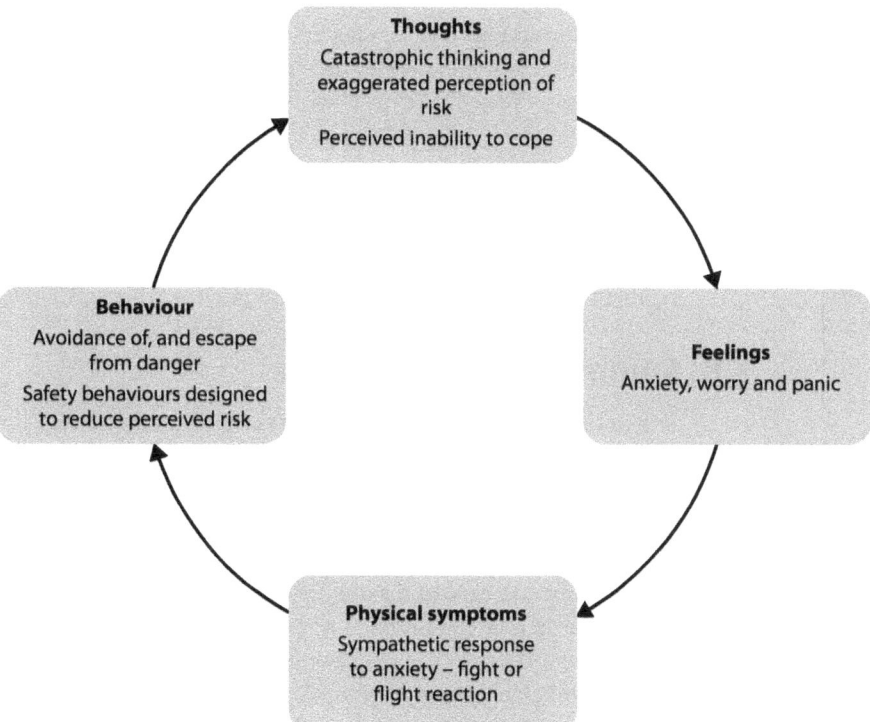

Figure 1.1 Vicious cycles in anxiety.

Thoughts

Certain thoughts and thinking styles are likely to lead to anxiety and to maintain it as a vicious cycle. These include:

- exaggerated perception of the risks and severity of possible dangers
- catastrophic thinking – sufferers focus on the worst possible outcomes
- perceived inability to cope with the danger or to manage their symptoms of anxiety
- lack of problem-solving – sufferers focus on problems rather than solutions.

Typical behaviour in anxiety

Typical behaviour in anxiety disorders involves avoidance of and escape from people, places and activities that might trigger anxiety. People often also carry out 'safety behaviours' which are designed to reduce the risk of future danger. These could include seeking frequent reassurance, repeatedly checking or looking up symptoms on the internet, and staying near other people for security. There is often behaviour associated with physical agitation, such as pacing around, not taking time to relax and being unable to keep still. Some behaviours such as consuming excessive alcohol or taking drugs may be performed in an attempt to 'self-medicate' or mask and control anxiety symptoms.

1.7 Treatment of anxiety

Recognition of anxiety disorders in primary care is important, as there are a variety of effective treatments involving both psychological therapy and medication. These treatments are discussed further in *Chapter 3*.

1.8 Summary and key points

- Anxiety is the body's normal response to potential threat or danger.
- Anxiety symptoms may be unpleasant but are NOT harmful or dangerous.
- Anxiety does not last forever – anxiety symptoms will fade with time.
- Anxiety becomes a problem if it becomes persistent and affects people's ability to carry out daily activities or their relationships with others.
- Avoidance, escape and safety behaviours typically lead to an increase in long-term anxiety as a vicious cycle.
- Anxiety problems are common and can be effectively treated with psychological therapy and medication.

Chapter 2
Initial assessment of anxiety disorders

2.1 Recognition of anxiety

Anxiety disorders are common but under-recognised in primary care. There is also the challenge of differentiating the large number of patients in general practice with mild and transient anxiety, which is likely to resolve without the need for intervention, from those with severe, disabling and persistent symptoms which are likely to benefit from psychological therapy or drug treatment.

Barriers to recognising anxiety disorders

There are a number of barriers to making the diagnosis of an anxiety disorder. Many patients suffering from anxiety disorders do not present directly with anxiety symptoms but instead attend with somatic symptoms such as lethargy, poor sleep, palpitations or muscle tension. Rates of anxiety are also higher in people with co-morbid physical health problems, and health professionals may focus largely on the physical aspects of the presenting complaint. In other cases, GPs may find it hard to raise concerns about potential emotional factors in some individuals who seem resistant to psychological explanations of their symptoms. This is particularly notable in conditions such as health anxiety and BDD, where sufferers may not perceive the condition as psychological in nature and typically attend seeking medical assessments and treatments for a wide spectrum of physical symptoms.

Patient factors, including perceived stigma and avoidance, are also likely to lead to a delay in seeking help for anxiety disorders. Many patients are reluctant to mention psychological symptoms or find it hard to discuss emotional problems. They may fear being unable to cope with the embarrassment of discussing the problem, believe that there is not enough time to address the problem or simply not wish to 'trouble' the doctor. Other patients may hold pessimistic beliefs that doctors can do nothing to help.

When to suspect an anxiety disorder

Individuals at higher risk of anxiety disorders include those:
- with a history of depression or an anxiety disorder
- with a coexisting chronic physical health condition
- with recent or past experience of a traumatic event
- who avoid social or other situations.

Anxiety should also be suspected in people who attend frequently with multiple symptoms. In some cases, the anxiety may be the primary problem, or anxiety may also be associated with a coexisting physical health condition. However, the repeated nature of the presentations offers an opportunity to review psychological factors and ask questions about possible anxiety symptoms.

Some tips for when to suspect anxiety are shown in *Box 2.1*.

Box 2.1	**When should I suspect an anxiety disorder?**

- Do I feel anxious when seeing this patient?
- Does the person come in a lot?
- Do they seek a lot of reassurance which does not appear to have a lasting effect?
- Is there a tendency to catastrophise or focus on the worst-case scenarios?
- Is avoidance having a marked impact on their quality of life?
- Do they have a personal or family history of anxiety?
- Does the person have a substance misuse problem as a strategy for masking symptoms of anxiety?

2.2 Communication skills for identifying and managing anxiety

General communication skills

GPs can improve their skills in recognition of anxiety through increased familiarity with common anxiety disorders and their presentations, and through developing communication skills that facilitate the open discussion of anxiety-related symptoms. Communication skills that can help with recognition of anxiety disorders, as well as other mental health conditions, include:
- establishing a rapport and assuring the patient that you will treat them in a non-judgemental manner and will respect their confidentiality and privacy
- being sensitive to non-verbal cues that are suggestive of anxiety, including the individual's way of responding to questions about their symptoms

- exploration of the person's worries to gain an understanding of how the condition is affecting their life
- using non-verbal cues including making appropriate eye contact
- using shared decision-making and trying to achieve a joint agreement as to the best way to manage the problem.

Explicit discussion of anxiety symptoms

If you do suspect that a person is experiencing anxiety, it is important to explicitly and sensitively raise the issue (*Box 2.2*). This can then lead on to a more formal assessment of anxiety levels, such as initial screening with GAD-2 (see *Chapter 3*).

Further '10 minute CBT' communication skills for identifying and assessing people with anxiety disorders are covered in *Chapter 4*.

Box 2.2   **Raising anxiety with patients**

- *"I've noticed that you seem very anxious about this problem…"*
- *"This really seems to worry you… Do you often worry about your health…?"*
- *"Do you often experience feelings of anxiety…?"*
- *"Have you noticed that anxiety is a problem in other aspects of your life?"*
- *"Are you having to work hard or avoid things to try to stop yourself getting anxious?"*
- Empathetic statement: *"It must be difficult to experience a lot of feelings of anxiety. Anxiety can be very distressing and unpleasant…"*

2.3 Diagnostic and screening tools for anxiety

Routine screening for anxiety disorders is not recommended in primary care; however, there are a number of screening and diagnostic tools that can help to identify anxiety disorders when a clinical suspicion exists.

Two-item Generalised Anxiety Disorder scale (GAD-2)

The two-item Generalised Anxiety Disorder scale (GAD-2) is a very brief two-question screening assessment for anxiety which asks about anxiety symptom over the previous two weeks. GAD-2 seems to have high sensitivity and specificity for GAD and high specificity for panic disorder, social anxiety disorder and PTSD.

A score of 3 or more is suggestive of an anxiety disorder and warrants further assessment.

Box 2.3

Two-item Generalised Anxiety Disorder scale (GAD-2)

Over the last two weeks, how often have you been bothered by the following problems?
- Feeling nervous, anxious or on edge?
- Being unable to stop or control worrying?

Scoring for the GAD-2: Not at all: 0; Several days: 1; More than half the days: 2; Nearly every day: 3.

If a person scores 3 or more, consider a possible anxiety disorder.

If the person scores <3 on the GAD-2, but the health professional is still concerned they may have an anxiety disorder, it can be helpful to ask a third question about avoidance:
- Do you find yourself avoiding places or activities and does this cause you problems?

Generalised Anxiety Disorder assessment (GAD-7)

The Generalised Anxiety Disorder assessment (GAD-7) is a self-administered patient questionnaire which is highly sensitive and specific as a screening tool and severity measure for GAD (see *Box 2.4*). It is also moderately good at screening for other anxiety disorders including panic disorder, social anxiety disorder and PTSD. GAD-7 assesses the patient's anxiety symptoms over the previous two weeks, so cannot be accurately used more frequently than this.

Box 2.4

Generalised Anxiety Disorder assessment (GAD-7)

Over the last two weeks, how often have you been bothered by the following problems?
- Feeling nervous, anxious or on edge?
- Being unable to stop or control worrying?
- Worrying too much about different things?
- Having trouble relaxing?
- Being so restless that it is hard to sit still?
- Becoming easily annoyed or irritable?
- Feeling afraid that something awful may happen?

Scoring for GAD-7: Not at all: 0; Several days: 1; More than half the days: 2; Nearly every day: 3

Interpretation of scores:
- 5–9: mild anxiety
- 10–14: moderate anxiety
- ≥15: severe anxiety

Hospital Anxiety and Depression Scale

The Hospital Anxiety and Depression Scale (HADS) was developed to detect depression, anxiety and emotional distress (see *Box 2.5*). This can be useful for assessing patients with a variety of anxiety disorders as well as to identify co-morbid depression. It is relatively brief and simple to use, taking around 2–5 minutes to complete. Alternate questions relate to depression and anxiety symptoms. The HADS asks the individual to respond as to how they felt in the past week, so the test should not be repeated more frequently than at weekly intervals.

Box 2.5 **Hospital Anxiety and Depression Scale (HADS)**

14 questions (7 anxiety and 7 depression) which involve rating a series of statements about how the individual has felt over the past week, including:

Depression questions
- I feel as if I am slowed down
- I still enjoy the things I used to enjoy
- I can laugh and see the funny side of things
- I feel cheerful
- I can enjoy a good book or radio or TV programme
- I have lost interest in my appearance
- I look forward with enjoyment to things

Anxiety questions
- I feel tense or 'wound up'
- Worrying thoughts go through my mind
- I get sudden feelings of panic
- I feel restless as I have to be on the move
- I can sit at ease and feel relaxed
- I get a sort of frightened feeling like 'butterflies' in the stomach
- I get a sort of frightened feeling as if something awful is about to happen

Each question is scored on a scale from 0 to 3; see bit.ly/HADS14 for more details.

HADS scores are divided into four ranges for both depression and anxiety: normal (0–7), mild (8–10), moderate (11–15) and severe (16–21).

The distress thermometer

For patients with significant communication difficulties such as language barriers, it can be helpful to use the simple concept of a 'distress thermometer' (*Box 2.6*). This question can be asked directly to the individual or to family members and carers.

Box 2.6

Distress thermometer

- How would you rate your level of distress, ranging from 0 (no distress) to 10 (extreme distress)?

Guidelines suggest taking further action if the distress score is rated >4.

Extreme distress — 10
9
8
7
6
5
4
3
2
1
No distress — 0

Disorder-specific screening tools

Information about additional screening tools which may be helpful for the diagnosis of specific anxiety disorders are included within each clinical chapter (*Chapters 5–13*).

2.4 Assessment of anxiety

When you have a strong clinical suspicion that an anxiety disorder is present, the next step is to carry out a thorough assessment. This includes making the diagnosis, followed by a further assessment of the nature, duration and severity of the presenting disorder and associated functional impairment. The assessment should also review any other factors which may have affected the development, course and severity of the disorder.

Identify the specific anxiety disorder

The first step is to identify which specific anxiety disorder an individual is experiencing. This is important, as different disorders have varying explanations and different recommendations for management. It is therefore important to be familiar with each of the anxiety disorders, including the common presentations and features. To help with this, each clinical chapter includes an overview of the key clinical features and diagnostic criteria, and tips for recognising each anxiety disorder. Some questions to help differentiate different anxiety disorders are shown in *Box 2.7*.

Box 2.7

Questions to help differentiate anxiety disorders

Question	Examples of possible answers
What situations, places or objects often trigger your anxiety?	Examples of triggers for anxiety include: • having to talk to a stranger or give a public performance, in social anxiety • reading about health problems on the internet, in health anxiety • looking in the mirror, in BDD • seeing a feared object such as blood or spiders, in specific phobia
Are you avoiding anything to prevent yourself from feeling anxious?	Avoidance is common in a variety of anxiety disorders, e.g.: • Agoraphobia: avoidance of public transport, lifts, crowds and shops • Panic disorder: avoidance of triggers for panic attacks • Social anxiety: avoidance of public speaking, parties or going on a date • PTSD: avoidance of reminders of the traumatic experience
What is the worst thing that might happen if you stayed in the situation?	Thoughts are individual and vary, but may give a clue as to the underlying anxiety disorder, e.g.: • Panic disorder: catastrophic fears about having a heart attack or passing out in public • Health anxiety: recurrent fears about having a serious undiagnosed health problem • Social anxiety: fears of being publicly humiliated and rejected by others
Are you experiencing episodes of severe anxiety or panic attacks?	Panic disorder or agoraphobia commonly involve acute episodes of severe anxiety
Do you worry about lots of different problems? Are you a 'worrier'?	This would be typical in GAD; it may also be co-morbid with other anxiety disorders
Is the anxiety triggered mainly in social or performance situations where you fear being judged negatively by others?	This is typical of social anxiety
Are you carrying out any particular repetitive actions such as continual checking or hand washing to stop yourself feeling anxious?	This is typical of OCD

Box 2.7 – contd	Question	Examples of possible answers
	Do you struggle with unwanted fearful thoughts that come into your mind?	Also common in OCD
	Do you worry about a particular aspect of your physical appearance?	Typical in BDD
	Have you experienced a severe or traumatic event, either recently or in the past, which might be causing distress?	Indicates a risk for developing PTSD
	Do you worry excessively about your health or about developing a particular illness?	Possible health anxiety
	Do you have a discrete phobia about one particular object, animal or situation?	Specific phobias

Differential diagnosis and co-morbidity

It is also important to consider other potential causes of anxiety symptoms including a physical health condition, symptoms arising from medication, or an alternative mental health condition such as depression, substance abuse or psychosis. However, the presence of these conditions does not exclude the diagnosis of an anxiety disorder. Anxiety disorders are frequently co-morbid with other mental health problems, including depression, other anxiety disorders and substance misuse. It is therefore important to carry out a comprehensive assessment which identifies which disorders may be affecting a particular individual.

Initial assessment

The initial assessment of a person with an anxiety disorder should include:
- exploration and evaluation of the anxiety symptoms
- impact of the condition on the person's daily life and functioning and consideration of activities being avoided due to symptoms of anxiety
- review of physical health and associated physical health disorders
- review of prescribed medications and any over-the-counter self-treatments
- use of alcohol and illicit drugs
- general lifestyle factors including sleep, caffeine intake and exercise.

Assessing severity

It is important to determine whether an anxiety disorder is mild, moderate or severe, as this will influence the next steps for treatment. Mild disorders are

| Box 2.8 | Tips for exploring anxiety – ask for a recent typical example of the person's anxiety |

Ask for a recent, typical example of a time that the individual felt anxious. You can explore this in detail, asking about the thoughts, feelings and physical symptoms that arose at the time of the experience. Asking about a specific incident is often easier and more focused than discussing anxiety in general terms, and will help to give more clarity about the type of anxiety that the person is experiencing, as well as helping to manage limited time.

those with relatively few core symptoms, a limited duration, and little impact on day-to-day functioning. The first step in care for mild disorders is usually active monitoring, especially if it is of recent onset and there is no history of moderate to severe problems. Moderate disorders have more marked symptoms and a clear impact on functioning and are likely to require more active intervention. Severe disorders are usually of long duration, have significant symptoms and a marked impact on functioning.

Persistent sub-threshold symptoms that do not meet full diagnostic criteria but have a substantial impact on a person's life, and particularly those that are present for a significant period of time, are also indications for intervention.

Assessment of suicide risk in anxious patients

If an individual is showing signs of severe anxiety, marked functional impairment or co-morbid depression, they may be at increased risk of suicidal thoughts and behaviour. As part of the assessment of people with anxiety disorders, it is therefore important to assess the risk of suicide. Risk factors for increased risk of suicide are shown in *Box 2.9*. Relevant questions when carrying out an assessment of suicide risk include:
- *"Do you feel hopeless about the future?"*
- *"Do you ever think about suicide?"*
- *"Have you made any plans for ending your life?"*
- *"Do you have the means for doing this available to you?"*
- *"What has kept you from acting on these thoughts?"*

If the assessment reveals a risk of self-harm or suicide, then the next steps include:
- assessment of protective factors such as social support networks and family relationships
- giving advice about how to seek further help if things get worse
- making decisions about whether to refer directly to emergency services or specialist mental health services for further assessment.

Box 2.9	**Risk factors that increase the risk of suicide in anxiety disorders**

- Previous attempts at suicide or self-harm
- Concurrent severe depression
- Feelings of hopelessness
- Male gender
- Age <30 years
- Advanced age
- Single or living alone
- History of substance or alcohol abuse
- Family history of suicide
- Recent initiation of antidepressant treatment
- Psychosis
- Concurrent physical illness

Try to regularly reassess the risk of suicide throughout the course of treatment, particularly at high risk periods such as when initiating treatment, during changes in treatment, or at times of increased personal stress.

2.5 Summary and key points

- Anxiety disorders are common but are under-recognised in primary care.
- Many people suffering from anxiety disorders present to primary care with somatic symptoms such as lethargy, poor sleep, palpitations or muscle tension, rather than directly mentioning anxiety symptoms.
- Anxiety should be suspected in people who attend frequently with multiple symptoms.
- Improving health professionals' communication skills can improve the recognition of anxiety disorders.
- Useful diagnostic and screening tools for anxiety include GAD-2, GAD-7 and HADS.
- Asking about a typical day or recent example of the person's anxiety can help to identify which anxiety disorder is present.
- Assessment of anxiety disorders involves reviewing the nature, duration and severity of the presenting disorder and any associated functional impairment, as well as looking for co-morbid mental and physical health conditions and carrying out an assessment of suicide risk if appropriate.

Chapter 3
Management of anxiety disorders

3.1 General principles of management

Aims for managing anxiety disorders

This chapter will give an overview of the management of anxiety disorders. In the UK, the vast majority of this takes place in primary care settings. The main goals for treatment include reducing the frequency and severity of anxiety symptoms, reducing avoidance and other unhelpful anxiety behaviours and enhancing quality of life by improving the person's ability to carry out important daily activities at home, at work and in social situations.

Stepped care approach to treatment

A stepped care model offers a helpful approach to the treatment of most common anxiety disorders. This consists of a treatment ladder which offers the least intrusive effective intervention first and includes explicit criteria for different levels of intervention. Offering stepped care enhances the capacity of mental health services and can increase access to evidence-based psychological interventions when appropriate. *Box 3.1* shows a summary of the NICE stepped approach to management of different anxiety disorders.

Information and education about anxiety disorders

Recognition and assessment of anxiety disorders are covered in *Chapter 2*. The next step is to explain the condition to the patient. This includes explicitly naming the disorder and providing relevant information about it and the available treatment options. Information about treatments should include effectiveness, expected time to onset of therapeutic effects and possible side-effects associated with different treatment choices. The primary care role also involves actively monitoring symptoms and functioning, and signposting and referral to specialist mental health services when appropriate.

Both verbal and written information should be offered in a way that the patient and their family and carers can understand. This should include contact numbers and information about what to do and who should be contacted in a crisis, as well as local and national self-help organisations and support groups. Education about self-care strategies and information on self-help materials such as books or websites may also be helpful.

| Box 3.1 | Stepped care model: a combined summary for anxiety disorders |

Focus of the intervention	Nature of the intervention
Step 1: All disorders – known and suspected presentations of anxiety disorders	**All disorders:** identification, assessment, psychoeducation, active monitoring, referral for further assessment and interventions; this is largely in primary care
Step 2: • GAD • Mild to moderate panic disorder • Mild to moderate OCD • Mild to moderate PTSD	**GAD and panic disorder:** individual non-facilitated and facilitated self-help, psychoeducational groups, self-help groups **OCD:** individual or group CBT, self-help groups **PTSD:** trauma-focused CBT or eye movement desensitisation and reprocessing (EMDR) **All disorders:** support groups, educational and employment support services; referral for further assessment and interventions
Step 3: • GAD with marked functional impairment or that has not responded to a low-intensity intervention • Moderate to severe panic disorder • OCD with moderate or severe functional impairment • PTSD	**GAD:** CBT, applied relaxation, drug treatment, combined interventions, self-help groups **Panic disorder:** CBT, antidepressants, self-help groups **OCD:** CBT, antidepressants, combined interventions and case management, self-help groups **PTSD:** trauma-focused CBT, EMDR, drug treatment **All disorders:** support groups, befriending, rehabilitation programmes, educational and employment support services; referral for further assessment and interventions

Based on NICE (2011, CG123).

When to offer treatment

Many people experiencing mild anxiety symptoms of recent onset, which are associated with stressful life events or problems, will improve without needing specific treatment, and a 'watch and wait' approach can be the most appropriate option (Step one of the stepped care model). However, when an individual's anxiety symptoms fulfil the diagnostic criteria for an anxiety disorder, in terms of severity, duration, distress and impairment, it is likely that they will benefit from some form of treatment and will benefit from discussion and joint decision-making about different treatment options.

Choice of treatment

Treatment options for anxiety disorders include psychological and drug treatments. Recommendations about first-line choices vary between different anxiety disorders and are indicated within each individual chapter. In general terms, the choice of treatment depends on a range of factors, which includes recommendations from guidelines but should also take into account the particular needs and preferences of the individual patient, including:

- patient preference and motivation or ability to engage in treatment
- their past experience of the problem, including any previous treatments and responses to treatment
- severity and duration of the problem
- impact of symptoms on daily life and any relevant social or personal factors
- availability of psychological therapies
- presence of co-morbid disorders such as depression, other forms of anxiety or substance misuse
- presence of physical health conditions and any current concomitant medication.

Managing co-morbid disorders

For people with a co-morbid depressive or other anxiety disorder, it is usually recommended to treat the primary disorder first. This refers to the condition that is more severe and which has the greatest impact on mood and daily functioning. The only exception is that co-morbid substance misuse is usually treated first as this may lead to substantial improvement in the symptoms of an anxiety disorder. The presence of a substance misuse disorder is also likely to reduce the effectiveness of both drug and psychological therapy for anxiety. Drug and alcohol problems may also develop in some people as a strategy of self-medication to cope with distressing symptoms arising from an underlying anxiety disorder. After successful management of drug and alcohol problems, patients should therefore be reassessed for the presence of ongoing or new anxiety symptoms which may require further assessment and treatment.

Relapse prevention

Many anxiety disorders have a chronic relapsing pattern, so strategies to prevent relapse can be very important. People with ongoing psychosocial risk factors or with a history of a recurrent condition may be at higher risk of relapse. Strategies to prevent relapse can include prolonged use of medication, and psychological therapy sessions reviewing strategies for preventing or coping with relapse. Psychological therapies generally have a lower risk of relapse than drug treatments.

3.2 Self-management for anxiety disorders

All patients with an anxiety disorder should be encouraged to adopt self-management strategies as part of their overall treatment plan; these can be used in combination with other treatment choices such as medication. Lifestyle measures such as regular exercise, healthy eating, reducing caffeine and improving sleep patterns are all likely to improve anxiety symptoms.

Self-management can also include the use of self-help approaches such as internet-based educational resources or books ('bibliotherapy') and may be particularly important for patients with mild or recent onset anxiety symptoms. These individuals should be kept under regular review, as they may require more intensive treatment if the symptoms persist or worsen.

Details of useful self-help resources for individual anxiety disorders are included within each chapter.

Self-help organisations and resources

Many patients and families also derive considerable practical and emotional support from local self-help groups and national support organisations and charities. There are a number of UK organisations which offer support for people with anxiety disorders (see *Box 3.2*).

3.3 Psychological therapies for anxiety disorders

Psychological therapies are safe and effective treatments for anxiety disorders and are often the first-line treatment recommendation. They act to reduce symptoms in the short term and are associated with a reduced risk of relapse following successful treatment compared to drug therapies. Cognitive behavioural therapy (CBT) is the most important and widely used approach for anxiety disorders.

Box 3.2   **UK charities supporting people with anxiety disorders**

Anxiety UK: charity offering access to fact sheets, specialist helplines, self-help groups and reduced cost psychological therapies www.anxietyuk.org.uk

Mind: provides advice and support to anyone experiencing a mental health problem, including anxiety disorders www.mind.org.uk

No panic: self-help organisation for anxiety including panic and phobias www.nopanic.org.uk

OCD Action: support for people with OCD; includes information on treatment and online resources www.ocdaction.org.uk

OCD UK: charity run by people with OCD, for people with OCD; includes facts, news and treatments www.ocduk.org

Triumph Over Phobias (TOP UK): network of self-help groups to help overcome phobias and OCD www.topuk.org

---

Cognitive behavioural therapy (CBT)

CBT is the psychological treatment of choice for most anxiety disorders. CBT is a problem-orientated collaborative, brief and time-limited therapy, which typically involves 6–12 sessions. A longer duration of therapy may be needed in complex, severe or long-standing anxiety disorders such as complex PTSD or GAD. CBT is not a 'quick fix' and can take up to 6 weeks for any effect to take place. It can be offered as an individual therapy, but is often also effective in alternative formats, such as in groups, by telephone or via the internet.

CBT should be delivered by qualified practitioners and based on evidence-based treatment manuals for each disorder. Practitioners should be adequately trained and receive regular supervision, as treatment outcomes are strongly related to the expertise and competence of the therapist. The patient's progress through the process of CBT should be measured using outcome measures, such as GAD-7 or HADS scores, and monitoring of adherence to treatment.

As part of the stepped care approach to treatment of anxiety disorders, CBT is usually differentiated into low intensity and high intensity CBT interventions.

Low intensity CBT
Low intensity CBT interventions are usually the first-line psychological approach for mild to moderate anxiety. These typically involve brief treatments and guided self-help with only a limited number of face-to-face sessions. Low intensity CBT practitioners may have undergone less extensive training but still require ongoing supervision. Low intensity CBT interventions include:

- guided self-help based on CBT models for individuals or in groups
- computerised CBT (cCBT)
- CBT group workshops
- behavioural activation groups or guided self-help
- mindfulness group courses.

High intensity CBT

High intensity CBT interventions are generally used for moderate to severe anxiety disorders and when low intensity interventions have been ineffective. These involve more intensive treatment protocols with more experienced CBT therapists and may include:

- individual CBT
- group CBT
- trauma-focused CBT
- EMDR
- applied relaxation
- exposure and response prevention.

Theory of CBT

The CBT model hypothesises that the way people feel is linked to the way they think about or perceive a particular situation, and to how they respond or behave when faced by challenges. CBT for anxiety helps people to identify the thoughts, feelings and behaviours that arise in anxiety-provoking situations, and to make changes in any unhelpful thinking patterns and behaviours that are causing or maintaining anxiety.

CBT is problem-orientated with a focus on 'here and now' problems and difficulties. It involves identifying and achieving the key goals that are likely to improve the person's quality of life, including reducing symptoms of anxiety and improving their ability to function in daily life. For some longer-term or complex conditions, CBT may also involve exploring past experiences to understand how these events may influence current responses to situations.

CBT teaches skills in self-management with the ultimate aim of teaching patients to be their own therapist, by equipping them with the tools to change their unhelpful cognitive and behavioural patterns. This is developed through a strong collaborative, therapeutic relationship, which is developed via skills such as rapport, genuineness, understanding and empathy.

Cognitive elements of CBT include strategies to change unhelpful thoughts and beliefs that are associated with the development of anxiety. Behavioural approaches in anxiety typically involve facing the person's fears through repeated exposure to a stressful situation, leading to an increase in their tolerance for the distressing physical and emotional aspects of the anxiety response, and a gradual decrease in anxiety over time.

Core elements of CBT are shown in *Box 3.3*.

Box 3.3

Core components of CBT

Psychoeducation	The therapist provides education about the nature of anxiety and fear and the rationale of a CBT approach, and illustrates these using examples from the person's own experience.
Guided discovery	Exploring a patient's perspective of a situation, and through wider discussion, helping them to expand their thinking to become aware of their underlying assumptions, and discover alternative perspectives and solutions for themselves.
Self-monitoring	Monitoring and recording thoughts, emotions and physical symptoms in specific situations will help people learn to recognise and change any unhelpful patterns of thinking or behaviour. Self-monitoring may also involve keeping track of activities such as the progress towards a behavioural goal; e.g., by recording the number of walks taken during the past week.
Cognitive restructuring	Identifying and changing inaccurate or unhelpful negative thoughts that contribute to the development of anxiety. This process involves testing ideas for their accuracy and questioning if they are based in absolute fact or represent an unhelpful perception, through a process of guided questioning and written thought recording. Cognitive restructuring addresses beliefs such as an exaggerated perception of threat and may also target self-efficacy and beliefs about coping. The aim is to construct new, balanced, more realistic and helpful beliefs which are less likely to trigger anxiety.
Behavioural experiments	This involves testing out an anxious person's catastrophic predictions about future problems. The patient makes a prediction before completing a feared task and then records whether that prediction came true. Over time, this process helps the person to re-evaluate their fears and provides evidence that catastrophic predictions may not actually happen. Behavioural experiments are also used to help gather evidence to support a reduction in the use of safety behaviours.

Box 3.3 – contd	Exposure	Exposure therapy acts to reduce the fear of particular situations, objects or experiences. Patients learn to face their fears by undertaking imaginal and real-life exposure to feared situations and experiences. With gradual exposure to these fears, the anxiety decreases through a process of habituation. The person also learns that the fears are excessive and irrational. Extinction of fear occurs through repeated exposure.
	Reduce avoidance and unhelpful safety behaviours	This involves a gradual reduction in unhelpful behaviours such as avoidance or other safety behaviours that are maintaining anxiety as a vicious cycle. It is usually carried out in association with exposure and behavioural experiments. The patient faces an anxiety-provoking situation without falling back on safety behaviours such as the presence of a companion or sitting near an exit. Successful coping with anxiety enhances the person's beliefs about their self-efficacy and ability to cope with anxiety.
	Behavioural activation (BA)	Behavioural activation has the aim of enhancing functioning and systematically increasing pleasurable, meaningful or productive experiences. Activity scheduling is used to plan each day in advance. The graded task assignments create manageable steps to help overcome procrastination and avoidance of anxiety-provoking situations. The aim is to stimulate a greater sense of enjoyment in life and change patterns of isolation or procrastination. These techniques help patients re-establish daily routines, increase pleasurable activities and deal with difficult issues through problem-solving.
	Applied relaxation and breathing exercises	Progressive relaxation training and breathing exercises may be used to reduce levels of autonomic arousal related to anxiety.

CBT formulation

A CBT 'formulation' involves creating an individualised map or overview of an individual's problems in terms of cognitive behavioural theory. It is a key element of the therapeutic process in CBT, which helps to make sense of complex problems. The process of developing a formulation is often therapeutic in its own right, by providing a deeper understanding and insight into a patient's problem(s), and also helps to guide the therapy process and decisions about appropriate therapeutic interventions. The formulation would usually include:

- a description of the current problem
- an account of why and how these problems may have developed
- an analysis of the key processes that maintain the problem(s).

A general model of case formulation is illustrated in *Figure 3.1.*

Exposure and response prevention

Exposure and response prevention (ERP) is a form of CBT mainly used for anxiety disorders, particularly OCD and BDD. The therapy involves patients repeatedly testing out their fears and expectations and learning to tolerate anxiety, while being prevented from performing any compulsive rituals or safety behaviours, which are usually carried out in order to reduce distress.

Exposures may be conducted in real life (*in vivo*) or in imagination (imaginal). For example, an OCD sufferer with fears about contamination might carry out ERP by touching a 'contaminated' object such as a door handle without following this by repeated handwashing.

Through the process of repeated ERP, the individual is able to learn that their feared outcomes do not actually happen, even when they fail to perform their rituals. This leads to a reduction in the power of the fears and a reduced desire to carry out compulsive behaviours over time.

ERP can be challenging for patients to participate in, as it is likely to result in an initial increase in the experience of anxiety and internal distress, which gradually decreases over time. Unfortunately, a number of patients are unable to overcome fears about the consequences of not performing compulsive rituals and are unwilling to tolerate the high levels of anxiety that can arise from this process. A significant proportion are likely to refuse to engage in CBT or leave treatment early.

Eye movement desensitisation and reprocessing

Eye movement desensitisation and reprocessing (EMDR) is a psychological therapy developed in the 1980s by Francine Shapiro, which is most commonly used for the treatment of PTSD. The approach involves identifying and working through any distressing trauma-related memories that are leading to 're-experiencing' of the trauma as flashbacks and nightmares. The aim of the therapy is to desensitise and reduce the distress associated with the memory, and to facilitate the reprocessing and integration of these memories within the individual.

The process involves asking the patient to recall the worst aspect of a traumatic memory, which is usually a visual image, along with any associated negative

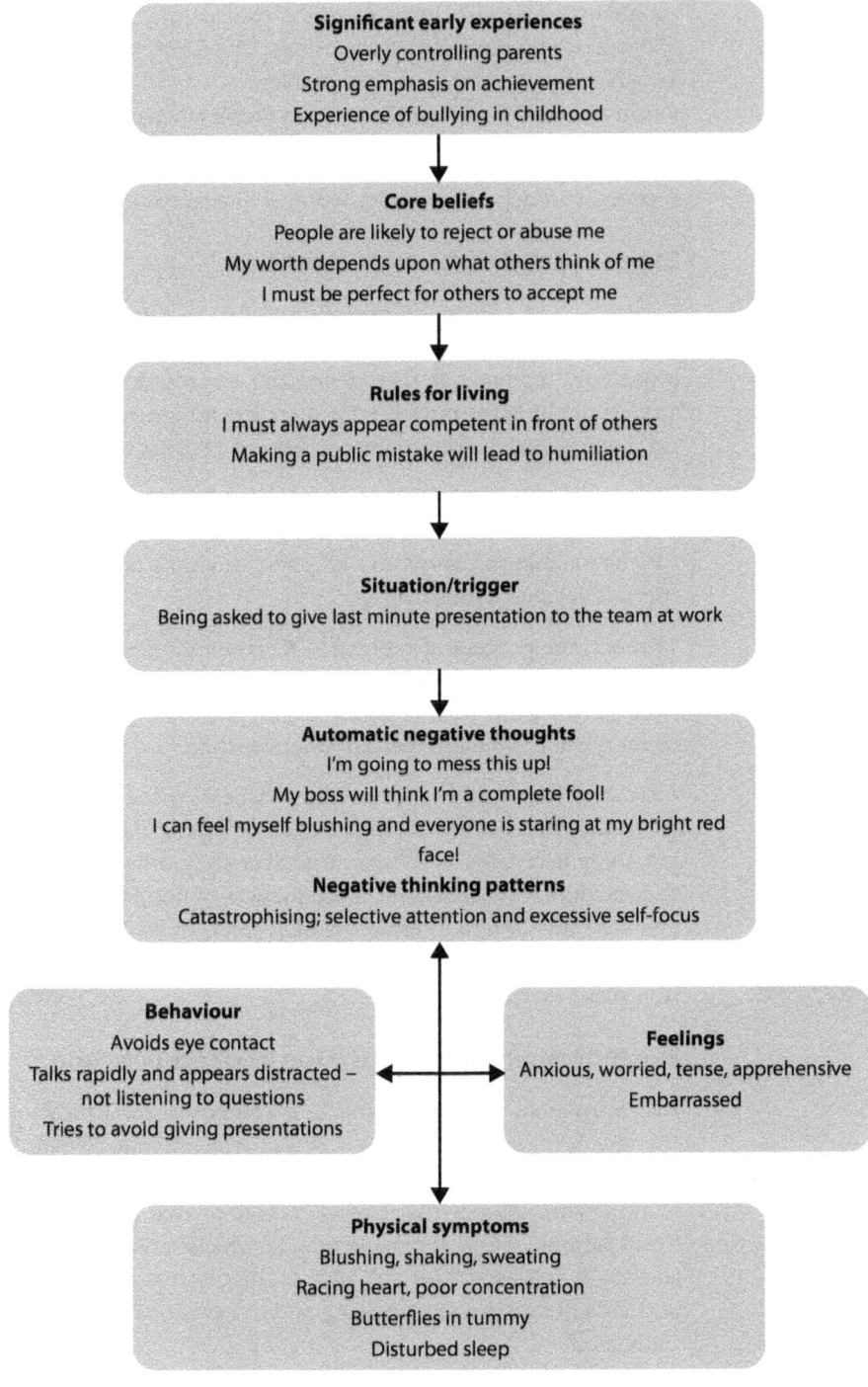

Figure 3.1 Example of case formulation in anxiety.

thoughts and bodily sensations. Simultaneously, they are asked to carry out some form of bilateral stimulation (BLS), which keeps part of their focus on the present moment ('dual attention'). BLS usually involves moving the eyes horizontally from side to side but may also involve bilateral taps or listening to auditory tones. This process is repeated until the memories are no longer distressing.

EMDR is thought to help the brain process the memory and to make sense of the traumatic experience. Normally memories are processed and integrated into the individual's past experiences and understanding of themselves and the world they live in. However, if an experience is traumatic, the information processing system stores the memory in a 'frozen' form without adequately processing it. Sufferers of PTSD continue to re-experience a previous trauma as if it is happening in the present moment, leading to high levels of emotional distress.

EMDR appears to allow the brain to process and assimilate these dysfunctionally stored memories, so that the memories can be recalled verbally without experiencing any of the previously associated distressing emotions and physical sensations. The process also involves developing alternative beliefs about the self, leading to a more positive self-concept.

Third wave or newer approaches to CBT

In recent years, CBT has expanded its focus to include a 'third wave' of psychological therapies which represent an evolution of traditional CBT principles to incorporate concepts such as acceptance, mindfulness, personal values and spirituality. Many of these approaches target the process of thinking rather than the specific content of individual thoughts, to help people become aware of their thoughts and accept them in a non-judgemental way.

Mindfulness-based approaches
Mindfulness-based approaches are designed to train people to cultivate mindfulness and incorporate its practice into daily life. The two components of mindfulness involve paying attention to the present moment and adopting an attitude of non-judgemental openness and acceptance towards inner experiences. This allows people to learn to relate differently to distressing thoughts or emotions that arise, enabling them to respond more effectively to stressful or anxiety-provoking situations. It is also likely to lessen the tendency to adopt experiential avoidance strategies, which are attempts to reduce the intensity or frequency of unwanted internal experiences that contribute to the maintenance of emotional disorders such as anxiety. In addition, the slow and rhythmic breathing involved in mindfulness meditation may alleviate bodily symptoms of distress by balancing sympathetic and parasympathetic responses and reducing hyperventilation.

Mindfulness practices include sitting meditation, mindful movement (including walking meditation and yoga exercises) and using a body scan to mindfully explore bodily sensations, starting with the feet and progressively moving to the head and neck. These exercises focus on paying attention to bodily sensations, emotions and thoughts while embracing a non-judgemental, accepting attitude towards whatever arises until it passes away. Mindfulness programmes also typically include informal practices that aim to integrate mindful awareness in everyday activities, such as mindful eating or brushing of teeth.

Mindfulness approaches vary widely in their format, but two approaches that have been studied more extensively, and which have the highest level of evidence of clinical efficacy, include mindfulness-based stress reduction (MBSR) and mindfulness-based cognitive therapy (MBCT). These usually consist of 8-week 2.5-hour classes in a group format with around twelve participants. Other formats such as retreats, brief interventions, internet-based, and smartphone apps may also have beneficial effects.

Despite the popularity of mindfulness, relatively few clinical trials have specifically examined this treatment in anxiety disorders. However, the limited evidence does suggest that mindfulness approaches do improve symptoms of anxiety and depression across a relatively wide range of severity of these disorders, including when arising in association with other disorders, such as medical problems. MBCT also has good evidence of effectiveness in reducing the risk of relapse in patients with at least three depressive episodes in recurrent depression.

Acceptance and commitment therapy

Acceptance and commitment therapy (ACT) is a behavioural approach which aims to change how a person relates and responds to their internal experiences, including thoughts, emotions, physical sensations and urges, in order to engage more fully in values-based activities and behaviours. ACT uses mindfulness and cognitive 'defusion' techniques to recognise and create a sense of distance from negative or unhelpful thoughts, without getting caught up in them or allowing them to dictate behavioural choices. The therapy also promotes acceptance of distressing internal experiences and reducing the inner struggle to rid ourselves of painful thoughts and sensations. These strategies are used to increase psychological flexibility and allow the development of committed behavioural change to values-based living by engaging more in activities which are in line with core values, and which create a greater sense of meaning and purpose for life.

Dialectical behaviour therapy

Dialectical behaviour therapy (DBT) is a form of CBT which is used to treat intense emotional reactions and relationship difficulties; for example in people with borderline personality disorder. It is usually delivered as a weekly two-hour group programme with regular homework assignments. Some participants may also undergo individual sessions. The therapy process typically lasts for a minimum of one year.

The goal of DBT is to help people develop skills in being able to recognise, accept and regulate intense difficult emotions. As they learn to manage these emotions more effectively, they are able to change long-standing patterns of self-destructive or harmful behaviour. DBT skills include mindfulness, emotion regulation, distress tolerance and interpersonal effectiveness, and are likely to be most relevant for people with long-standing anxiety or trauma in association with emotional dysregulation and high levels of reactivity to challenging life experiences.

Compassion-focused therapy

Compassion-focused therapy (CFT) was developed by Professor Paul Gilbert and uses the development of self-compassion for working with individuals who develop anxiety disorders in association with high levels of shame and self-criticism; for example in complex PTSD. High levels of self-criticism can limit the effectiveness of standard therapies as people may not have developed abilities to experience certain affiliative positive emotions such as safeness, reassurance and compassion. These individuals often come from abusive, bullying, neglectful or highly critical backgrounds.

Metacognitive therapy

Metacognitive therapy focuses on exploring a person's thoughts and beliefs about the content of their thoughts ('metacognitions'), rather than on the specific content of a particular thought.

3.4 Drug treatment for anxiety disorders

General approach to prescribing

Medication can be effective for some anxiety disorders, although often has higher risk of relapse than psychological therapies after treatment is completed. Some factors to consider when prescribing medication are shown in *Box 3.4*.

Over-the-counter medication

Some patients will enquire about the use of herbal preparations or nutritional supplements for managing anxiety. However, the evidence base for such treatments is low, and none are currently recommended treatment options for anxiety disorders. Nevertheless, it is important to ask about self-administered herbal treatments such as St John's wort, which can interact with prescribed medication.

Box 3.4	**Factors to consider before prescribing medication for anxiety disorders**

- Age of the patient
- Diagnosis – the specific anxiety disorder will determine the likely benefits of different drugs
- Previous treatment response
- Risks of deliberate self-harm or accidental overdose
- Potential side-effects and tolerability of each drug
- Possible interactions with existing medications
- Possible discontinuation or withdrawal symptoms
- Likely length of the course of treatment
- The patient's ideas and preferences for treatment
- Local and national treatment guidelines

Initiating medication

New medications should be initiated at low initial doses and gradually increased. This is particularly important for the elderly and in people who are likely to experience increased anxiety associated with any side-effects that might arise whilst starting treatment, such as in health anxiety or generalised anxiety disorder. In some cases, it is helpful to commence with drug doses at half the lowest therapeutic dose.

Always discuss the treatment options and any concerns the person has about taking medication before issuing a prescription. Explain fully the reasons for prescribing and provide written and verbal information on the chosen medication. Important issues to discuss when starting medication are shown in *Box 3.5*.

Monitoring and reviewing treatment

All patients who are prescribed drug treatment should undergo regular review and monitoring to assess the effectiveness of treatment and make any adjustments if needed. Review should take place every 2–4 weeks during the first 3 months of treatment, and monthly thereafter.

The dose of any treatment should be increased gradually at approximately 2-weekly intervals until the optimal effective dose is reached. This is particularly important in certain disorders such as OCD, which typically require higher antidepressant doses for effectiveness. If there is no improvement after a 12-week course, an alternative antidepressant or another form of therapy should be offered.

Box 3.5 **Summary of advice when starting medication**

- Discuss the purpose of the medication and potential benefits of treatment.
- Explore attitudes and expectations about drug treatments and address any concerns that may improve adherence, e.g. explaining that antidepressant treatment is not addictive or associated with craving or tolerance.
- Delayed onset of effect: explain that treatment response is not immediate and is likely to take several weeks before benefit is experienced.
- Possible side-effects or other risks of treatment, including explaining that many side-effects are transient and likely to resolve within the first 2–3 weeks of treatment. The most common side-effects in selective serotonin reuptake inhibitors (SSRIs) include dizziness, numbness and tingling, nausea and vomiting, headache, sweating, anxiety and sleep disturbances.
- Discuss the risk of transient worsening of anxiety symptoms at the start of treatment, particularly in people who are likely to worry about experiencing new physical sensations in the body as the treatment is established. Emphasise that this is likely to resolve after a short period, but if severe the individual should seek medical review.
- The risk of increased suicidal thoughts and behaviour in young adults aged less than 30 years in the early stages of SSRI and selective serotonin and noradrenaline reuptake inhibitor (SNRI) treatment.
- The importance of taking the medication as prescribed, particularly with paroxetine and venlafaxine, to prevent symptoms associated with a discontinuation reaction.
- Likely duration of treatment and the benefits of a prolonged course of treatment after remission to prevent relapse.
- The need to avoid abrupt cessation of treatment and instead have gradual tapering of the dose over an extended period when stopping treatment, to avoid discontinuation reactions.
- Informed consent should be obtained and documented for the off-label use of any medication.
- Provide a clear plan for regular review and monitoring in order to adjust the dose or change the treatment if needed.

People who are at a high risk of suicide should be reviewed more often. This is likely to involve weekly review until there is no indication of increased suicide risk, when the frequency can be gradually reduced.

Review should also address self-management strategies alongside medication, for example by continuing to support them to engage in graduated exposure to feared or avoided social situations.

Antidepressant treatments for anxiety disorders

Antidepressants are the first-line medication for most anxiety disorders, with treatment usually involving an SSRI or SNRI. Treatment with antidepressants usually takes between 2 and 6 weeks to produce an initial response to treatment and full benefit may not be seen for up to 12 weeks.

Selective serotonin reuptake inhibitors

SSRIs are the first-line drug therapy used for anxiety disorders as they are effective for both short-term and long-term treatment and are better tolerated and safer in overdose than other antidepressants. They have evidence of effectiveness for most anxiety disorders, with the exception of specific phobias. SSRIs act by inhibiting the reuptake of serotonin into the presynaptic cell, increasing the levels of serotonin available for binding to postsynaptic receptors and prolonging the effects of serotonin.

SSRIs prescribed in the UK include fluoxetine, citalopram, sertraline, paroxetine and fluvoxamine.

Adverse effects with SSRIs

Side-effects with SSRIs are most common in the first few weeks of treatment, but many will resolve completely with time. The most common side-effects with SSRIs are shown in *Box 3.6*.

Contraindications and cautions

Prescribe SSRIs with caution to people with a history of mania or bipolar disorder, cardiac disease, epilepsy, QT interval prolongation or taking other medication

---

Box 3.6 **Side-effects with SSRIs**

- Gastrointestinal effects including nausea, vomiting, abdominal pain, dyspepsia and increased risk of gastrointestinal bleeding.
- Dizziness, agitation, anxiety, insomnia, headache and tremor.
- Drowsiness – may impair performance of skilled tasks such as driving and operating machinery.
- Sexual dysfunction including diminished sexual interest, erectile dysfunction and anorgasmia.
- Hyponatraemia: other risk factors for this include old age (>80 years), female sex, low body weight, diuretics, diabetes mellitus, hypertension, reduced renal function, volume depletion and chronic obstructive pulmonary disease (COPD). Monitor at-risk individuals for signs of hyponatraemia, which include dizziness, lethargy, nausea, confusion, cramps and seizures.
- Small increased risk of fractures.
- Increased suicide risk – the use of SSRI antidepressants has been linked with suicidal thoughts and behaviour, particularly in young people aged <30 years (see below).

known to prolong the QT interval, or with a history of gastrointestinal bleeding. Consider prescribing a gastroprotective drug in at-risk patients taking a concurrent non-steroidal anti-inflammatory drug (NSAID), particularly in elderly patients.

Serotonin syndrome

Serotonin syndrome is a relatively uncommon adverse drug reaction caused by excessive central and peripheral serotonergic activity. Symptoms can range from mild to life-threatening and typically arise within hours or days following the initiation, dose escalation or overdose of a serotonergic drug. It can also arise when serotonergic drugs are combined or when initiating a new serotonergic drug without allowing a long enough washout period after stopping a previous drug. Severe toxicity is a medical emergency and usually occurs with a combination of serotonergic drugs.

Characteristic symptoms of serotonin syndrome include neuromuscular hyperactivity such as tremor, hyperreflexia, clonus, myoclonus and rigidity. This is associated with autonomic dysfunction including tachycardia, blood pressure changes, hyperthermia, diaphoresis, shivering and diarrhoea, and an altered mental state such as agitation, confusion or mania.

Specialist advice should be sought for possible serotonin syndrome. Treatment consists of withdrawal of the serotonergic medication and supportive care.

Serotonin and noradrenaline reuptake inhibitors

SNRIs are a newer class of antidepressants which act in a similar mechanism to SSRIs, by altering neurotransmitter levels in the brain or prolonging their effects. SNRIs act particularly on serotonin and noradrenaline. SNRIs prescribed in the UK are venlafaxine and duloxetine.

Side-effects of SNRIs. The most common adverse effects for venlafaxine include nausea, insomnia, dry mouth, sleepiness, dizziness, constipation, sweating, nervousness and asthenia.

Common side-effects for duloxetine include nausea, insomnia, dizziness, dry mouth, sleepiness, constipation, anorexia and abnormal dreams.

All SNRIs may also cause sexual dysfunction, increased risk of bleeding and hyponatraemia.

Risks associated with SNRIs. Venlafaxine has a risk of cardiotoxicity, and fatal cardiac arrhythmias have been reported, especially in overdose. It should be avoided in patients with a history of heart disease or electrolyte imbalance, or at high risk of cardiac arrhythmia. Patients taking venlafaxine should be monitored for signs and symptoms of cardiac dysfunction. Venlafaxine can also lead to altered glycaemic control in people with diabetes mellitus, who may require additional blood glucose control monitoring. Venlafaxine should only be prescribed at high dose (300 mg/day or more) under the supervision or advice of a specialist mental health medical practitioner.

Venlafaxine and duloxetine are both associated with dose-related increases in blood pressure and should be avoided in patients with untreated or uncontrolled hypertension. Blood pressure should be checked on initiation and regularly during treatment, particularly during dosage titration. Any hypertension should be well controlled before treatment is initiated, and for people who experience a sustained increase in blood pressure while taking venlafaxine, the dose should be reduced or discontinuation considered.

There is a risk of liver dysfunction associated with duloxetine, particularly during the first months of treatment, and it should be avoided in people with hepatic dysfunction or severe renal impairment.

SNRIs should be prescribed with caution in people with a history of bleeding disorders, mania, glaucoma or increased intraocular pressure, or seizures.

Discontinuation symptoms

SSRIs and SNRIs may be associated with withdrawal reactions on stopping or reducing treatment. The risk of developing discontinuation symptoms is dependent on several factors including the duration and dose of therapy and the rate of dose reduction. Paroxetine and venlafaxine seem to be associated with a greater frequency of withdrawal reactions.

Symptoms usually occur within the first few days of discontinuing treatment and are usually mild to moderate but can sometimes be severe. They are usually self-limiting and normally resolve within 2 weeks, although can occasionally be prolonged for as long as 2–3 months or longer. Common symptoms include dizziness, numbness and tingling, nausea and vomiting, sleep disturbances, sweating, agitation or anxiety, tremor and headache.

To reduce the risk of discontinuation symptoms, treatment can be tapered down gradually over a period of several weeks to months.

SSRIs/SNRIs and the risk of suicidal behaviour

There is a risk of suicidal thoughts and behaviour with the use of any SSRI or SNRI, particularly when used by children, adolescents or young adults under the age of 30. The risk of suicide is greatest in the early stages of SSRI treatment. There are no marked differences in suicidal risk between the different classes and types of antidepressant.

Individuals aged under 30 years starting SSRI/SNRI treatment should be reviewed within one week of initiating treatment and require ongoing weekly monitoring of the risk of suicidal thinking and self-harm for at least the first month.

A suicide risk assessment should be carried out before commencing SSRI/SNRI therapy and the increased risk should be explained to at-risk individuals prior to starting treatment. A suggested way of giving this explanation is shown in *Box 3.7*.

Tricyclic antidepressants

Tricyclic antidepressants (TCAs) block the reuptake of both serotonin and noradrenaline, although to different extents. TCAs have similar efficacy to SSRIs but are more likely to be discontinued because of a worse profile of side-effects. They are therefore generally reserved for use after a lack of response or poor tolerance of initial treatment with an SSRI or SNRI. TCAs are also highly toxic in overdose, potentiate the sedating effects of alcohol, and can prolong the QT interval. TCAs should be avoided in patients considered to be at risk of suicide and in patients with cardiac disease.

The most commonly prescribed TCAs for anxiety disorders are imipramine or clomipramine. They are effective in panic disorder and there is also some evidence for their use in GAD and PTSD. Clomipramine is effective in OCD.

Common side-effects of tricyclics include anxiety, drowsiness, dizziness, agitation and confusion. Anticholinergic effects such as dry mouth, constipation, urinary retention and blurred vision are also common. Cardiovascular effects can include hypotension, tachycardia, arrhythmias and other ECG changes. It may be appropriate to check blood pressure and carry out a baseline ECG for some patients prior to initiating treatment. Other adverse effects include hepatic effects, changes in blood sugar, increased appetite, weight gain and sexual dysfunction.

Monoamine oxidase inhibitors

Monoamine oxidase inhibitors (MAOIs) are effective for panic disorder and social anxiety disorder and are occasionally used for severe, treatment-resistant anxiety disorders. Phenelzine and moclobemide are the most commonly prescribed MAOIs for anxiety. Moclobemide has reduced need for dietary restrictions.

MAOIs have the worst side-effect profile and greatest safety burden of all antidepressants. They interact with tyramine- or dopa-containing foods, including mature cheese, aged meat or liver products and yeast extracts, sympathomimetic drugs, and some alcoholic beverages, which may result in a potentially life-threatening hypertensive crisis. Other side-effects include nausea, postural hypotension, insomnia, anticholinergic symptoms and weight gain. MAOIs are therefore not used routinely and are usually only initiated by mental health specialists.

Trazodone

Trazodone is highly sedating and is occasionally used after non-response to or poor tolerance of SSRI/SNRI treatment in GAD. It is sometimes used to augment SSRI treatment in OCD, and for the treatment of depression with anxiety.

Mirtazapine

There is a small amount of evidence suggesting that mirtazapine may have some benefit in social anxiety disorder, and its sedating effects may be helpful in some highly anxious patients. Adverse effects of mirtazapine include weight gain, excessive sleepiness, lipid abnormalities and leucopenia.

Other drug treatments

Benzodiazepines

Benzodiazepines are effective at reducing the somatic and psychological symptoms of acute anxiety, but should be used with great caution, due to the risk of physical and psychological dependence and withdrawal symptoms, which can develop after only a few weeks of regular treatment. Benzodiazepine use should be at the lowest effective dose for the shortest period of time with a maximum duration of 2–4 weeks. Other side-effects include sedation, dizziness and impaired coordination. A paradoxical increase in hostility, aggression and worsening anxiety can sometimes develop.

Benzodiazepines are occasionally used for their potent, short-term effects, such as to reduce anxiety during the initial weeks of an antidepressant when anxiolytic effects have yet to occur. However, 'as needed' or 'PRN' use of benzodiazepines in anxiety disorders can serve as a safety behaviour which undermines the anxious individual's self-efficacy, powerfully reinforces avoidance of anxiety-provoking situations, encourages longer-term reliance on the drug, and has been associated with a worse response to CBT.

Chronic benzodiazepine use is associated with physiological dependence, cognitive and psychomotor impairment and rebound anxiety upon discontinuation. Patients with a history of substance abuse are at increased risk of benzodiazepine misuse. Benzodiazepine use also increases the risk of lethal overdose when combined with other drugs such as alcohol or opioids. Where clinically indicated, benzodiazepines can be gradually tapered and eventually discontinued over a period of several months. Abrupt withdrawal of benzodiazepines is associated with a risk of confusion, psychosis and convulsions and should be avoided.

Therefore, the use of benzodiazepines should largely be avoided where possible. However, for select individuals with significant residual anxiety despite other treatments, benzodiazepines may help achieve total symptom remission.

Anticonvulsants

Gabapentin and pregabalin act to reduce neuronal excitability and may be effective in reducing anxiety. Pregabalin is licensed for use in GAD and is usually recommended as a second-line approach if SSRIs or SNRIs are not tolerated. Cases of misuse, abuse and dependence have been reported with pregabalin, and it should be avoided in people with a history of drug dependence or misuse. Common side-effects include somnolence and dizziness and discontinuation symptoms may arise, so gradual tapering is recommended when stopping treatment.

Beta blockers
Beta blockers reduce the peripheral physical symptoms of anxiety, such as palpitations and trembling hands. They do not affect the cognitive and emotional symptoms of anxiety. Beta blockers have little evidence to support their use in anxiety disorders, including social anxiety disorder. They may occasionally be useful for performance-related anxiety, but when used in 'as required' dosing regimens, they may act as a safety behaviour which maintains the fear response and worsens anxiety. It is important to check for contraindications to beta blockers, such as asthma.

Buspirone
There is some evidence of efficacy for short-term use of buspirone in managing anxiety. It is occasionally used as an adjunct to an SSRI. Its efficacy is reduced in previous extensive use of benzodiazepines. Common side-effects include nausea and other gastrointestinal symptoms.

Antihistamines
Hydroxyzine may be effective in GAD. It is highly sedating. Other side-effects include anticholinergic effects at high doses, blurred vision and confusion. There is also a risk of QT interval prolongation and torsades de pointes.

Antipsychotics
Atypical antipsychotics such as quetiapine are occasionally used in anxiety disorders such as GAD, OCD and PTSD, usually as an adjunct to other drug therapies in treatment-resistant cases. Most of these uses are unlicensed, and treatment with antipsychotics is usually only initiated within a specialist setting. Side-effects of atypical antipsychotics include sedation, orthostatic hypotension, sexual dysfunctions, metabolic syndrome and extrapyramidal effects.

3.5 Summary and key points

- Most anxiety disorders are managed within primary care.
- Goals for treatment include reducing the frequency and severity of anxiety symptoms, reducing avoidance and other unhelpful anxiety behaviours, and improving functioning and quality of life.
- All patients with an anxiety disorder should be encouraged to adopt self-management strategies as part of their overall treatment plan and this can be used in combination with other treatment choices such as medication.
- Practical and emotional support is available for people experiencing anxiety from local self-help groups and national support organisations and charities.
- Psychological therapies such as CBT are safe and effective treatments for anxiety disorders and are often recommended as first-line treatment.
- Medications such as SSRIs, SNRIs or other antidepressants may be effective for anxiety disorders.
- Drug therapies may have a higher risk of relapse than psychological therapies.
- All patients who are offered drug treatment should undergo regular review every 2–4 weeks during the first 3 months of treatment and subsequently each month.
- People who are at a high risk of suicide should be reviewed more frequently.

Chapter 4
10 minute CBT for anxiety

4.1 What is 10 minute CBT?

10 minute CBT is a flexible way of bringing concepts and strategies derived from CBT into brief 10–30 minute consultations within primary care. There are many 'bite-sized' skills derived from CBT which can be used to improve the management of people with anxiety disorders. 10 minute CBT strategies may be a primary approach for supporting some people with mild to moderate anxiety and can also be used alongside other treatments such as medication or referral for psychological therapy. The strategies are drawn from standard CBT, as well as from behavioural activation, acceptance and commitment therapy, compassion-focused therapy and mindfulness.

10 minute CBT promotes collaborative partnerships between professionals and patients, where individuals are encouraged to understand and take control of managing their own health and their lives. This can help to maximise the use of limited appointment times with health professionals who are working under significant time pressures. Using this approach may act as an investment of time, which can help to reduce emotional distress, reduce repeated attendances, improve relationships with patients, reduce hospital admissions, improve engagement with services and enhance relationships with patients.

4.2 CBT-based communication skills for primary care

In addition to the general communication skills discussed in *Chapter 3*, there are some specific communication skills developed from CBT which can be particularly helpful when seeing patients with an anxiety disorder. These skills form the building blocks for how to effectively implement a 10 minute CBT approach in practice and can be viewed as additional tools to add to the GP toolkit. However, there is no need to feel under pressure to use all the skills in every consultation.

The **Re-FRESHER** model is an approach to bringing CBT communication skills into GP consultations. It consists of a series of brief steps which encourage the patient to reflect on the problem using a CBT framework and emphasises self-efficacy skills and handover of responsibility for managing the problem to the patient. The model includes the following steps:

- **Re**cognise anxiety and **R**aise the issue
- **F**rame the session: manage time effectively
- **Re**cent **E**xample: explore a specific recent example using a CBT framework
- **S**ummarise: reflect back the discussion and highlight any vicious cycles that are present
- **H**andover and **H**omework: strategies to hand over responsibility and encourage self-efficacy and self-management by the patient include setting relevant brief homework tasks
- **E**xplanation: provide an empowering explanation of the problem
- **R**eview and check understanding of the discussion.

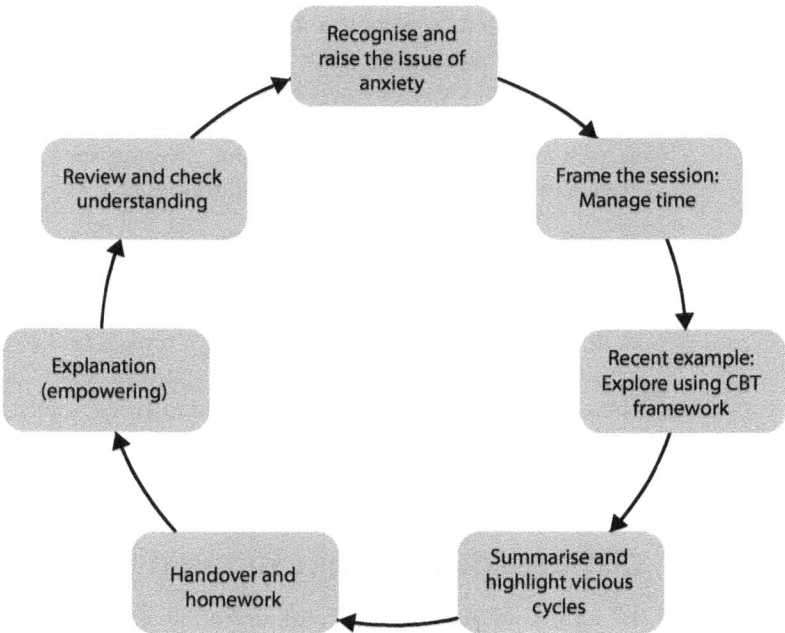

Figure 4.1 10 minute CBT communication skills for anxiety disorders.

Recognise anxiety and raise the issue

Recognition of anxiety is an important skill and the starting point for effective management of anxiety disorders. This is covered in more detail in *Chapter 2*. It is also important to proactively raise the issue of anxiety when you suspect that it might be relevant. Each chapter contains some suggested questions for beginning this discussion.

Frame the session: manage time

This step emphasises the importance of effective time management in primary care. It can be helpful to take a moment at the start of a consultation to think how much time you have available, and how best to use it. Use of CBT strategies does not have to involve a longer consultation and may involve a more effective use of time. Strategies to help manage time include:

- Less is more: don't try to cover too much during a single appointment. Set small and realistic goals. For example, just ask about one or two relevant thoughts, feelings and behaviours or set one small behavioural goal for improving wellbeing.
- Don't take on excessive responsibility for changing a patient's anxiety: this approach is a form of guided self-help, and you can encourage the patient to take the lead in making effective change.
- Use homework to build on your discussion: encourage the patient to actively involve themselves in their own wellbeing using homework tasks between appointments.
- Write down your discussion using a written CBT framework (these can be downloaded from the website www.10minuteCBT.co.uk) and give a copy to the patient to reflect on after the appointment.
- Choose an appropriate patient: begin by choosing patients who are motivated and interested in overcoming their problems using self-help based on CBT, rather than someone complex or lacking motivation to make change.

Recent example: explore using a CBT framework

Next choose a specific and recent example of the patient's difficulty, to explore in more detail. This can be very helpful in managing time, as it keeps the discussion focused and concise. The information gathered can often later be generalised to the person's wider experiences. Useful questions include asking:

- *"Can you give me an example of a recent time that you felt very anxious?"*
- *"When was this?" "Where were you?" "What were you doing?" "Who else was there?"*

This example can then be explored using the five areas of the CBT framework (*Figure 4.2*). There is no need to make this an overly lengthy process. Identifying one or two thoughts, feelings, behaviours and physical symptoms is often enough to get a clearer understanding of the person's experience and may identify some important vicious cycles. Useful general questions for exploring anxiety using a CBT framework are shown in *Box 4.1*.

Box 4.1

Questions for the CBT framework

Thoughts
- What thoughts went through your mind when you were feeling anxious?
- What are your main concerns?
- What does this mean to you/about you?
- What's the most difficult thing about this?
- What's the worst that might happen?
- Did you have any images?

Feelings
- How did you feel emotionally?
- How did that thought make you feel?
- How are you feeling generally?
- You seem quite *[frustrated]* when you say that...

Behaviour
- What did you do when...? What did you do next?
- What's your typical reaction to this situation?
- Is there anything you are avoiding because of your anxiety?
- What do you do to try to stop yourself feeling anxious?
- What would you do differently if you felt better?

Physical symptoms
- Which physical symptoms did you notice?
- How is this affecting you physically?
- Which symptoms concern you the most?
- What was happening in your body?
- How are your other health conditions affecting you physically?

Background/environmental factors
- What else is going on in your life that could be affecting how you feel?
- Is anxiety triggered by specific situations?
- Are there demands at home? Financial difficulties? Do you have someone you can talk to about the problem?
- Are there difficulties at work? Are you unable to work/unemployed?
- Do you recall other family members being anxious?

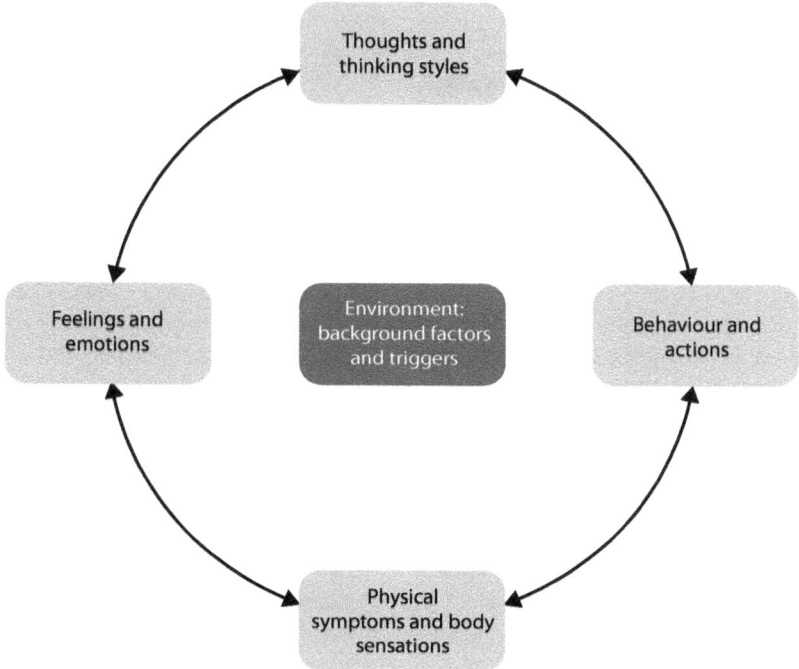

Figure 4.2 CBT framework for understanding anxiety.

Summarise and highlight vicious cycles

The next step is to summarise what you have heard so far using the patient's own words. Summaries help to build in a pause and allow time for both patient and GP to reflect on the discussion and consider what the next steps might be. They help the patient to view their own experiences from an external viewpoint, which may help give a broader perspective on the problem. If you are feeling stuck or unsure what to say next, then giving a mini summary can often help to clarify what the next question might be.

Use the discussion to highlight any obvious links between the five areas of the CBT framework, such as negative thoughts or unhelpful behaviours leading to low mood. Using a written CBT framework which can be annotated with arrows will make this process more effective and will enable a copy to be given to the patient to reflect on after the consultation.

Handover and homework setting

Handover
Handover encourages the patient to reflect on their difficulties and take responsibility for making change. It encourages people to build skills in self-efficacy

Case example 4.1: Emma

Using the CBT framework in anxiety

Emma is 25 and works as a receptionist at a hospital outpatients department. She regularly visits her own GP, Dr Patel, with concerns about her health. Emma experiences a variety of different symptoms and frequently undergoes investigations which have always been normal. She has been seen several times over the past few months with headaches. Dr Patel believes that Emma is experiencing tension-type headaches and that she may also be overusing over-the-counter medication to treat the headaches, leading to medication overuse headache.

Because of Emma's repeated presentations with the same symptom, Dr Patel decides it would be helpful to explore the patient's beliefs about, and behavioural responses to her headaches, using a CBT framework. Because Emma is presenting with headache, the first area that Dr Patel asks about is physical symptoms.

The completed framework is shown below:

Physical symptoms
Frequent headaches
Discomfort in neck and upper back
Tired; general aches and pains

Thoughts
I'm fed up with being in pain
What if it is due to something serious?
Could there be something wrong with my brain?
What if things get worse? I won't be able to cope at work

Feelings
Worried and 'worked up'
Anxious
Frustrated

Behaviour
Take paracetamol most days
Phone my mum and ask her to reassure me there's nothing wrong
Look at health websites on the internet
Visit the GP
Go to bed early instead of seeing friends

Environment and triggers
Work is busy and can be stressful
Things got worse after I had a new boss who can be demanding and impatient
My mum often worries about her health and has a history of depression

The above framework allows Dr Patel to understand and empathise with Emma's anxiety about her headaches. This can help in moving towards the diagnosis of a possible underlying anxiety disorder. At this stage the differential diagnosis includes health anxiety and GAD. The framework also highlights some important vicious cycles of catastrophic negative thinking, feelings of anxiety, and unhelpful behaviour such as reassurance seeking, browsing health websites on the internet, and overuse of paracetamol, which are all likely to be worsening both the headaches and Emma's feelings of anxiety.

Dr Patel can share a written summary of this information with the patient and use it to encourage Emma to self-manage her health more effectively.

and supports them in taking positive steps towards self-management of their health and their lives in general. *Box 4.2* includes some examples of handover questions.

When using 10 minute CBT, an important aim is to stimulate reflection and thought – to encourage people to open up to the possibility of change. There is often insufficient time to systematically work through complex problems, so it may be more realistic to focus on helping people to recognise that change is possible and encouraging them to think more about how they might achieve this themselves.

It is not necessary to have resolved all of the patient's issues before a consultation can finish and it can often be helpful to end a consultation with a handover question. Ending on a 'cliff-hanger' may stimulate the person to reflect on, talk about and take a more active interest in making sense of their own problems after the consultation has ended.

Homework

As part of the handover process you may also wish to set 'homework'. There is evidence that completion of homework predicts better outcomes from CBT, as the patient can generalise what they have learned into daily life. Tasks should be simple, realistic and very easily achievable. They should also be set as a 'no-lose experiment', by saying *"Let's find out what happens if you try something different. We can always learn from it, no matter what the outcome is"*. *Box 4.3* contains some examples of homework tasks that could be used for patients with anxiety disorders.

If you do plan a homework task, always remember to ask about it when you next see the patient (*Box 4.4*). Try to show some enthusiasm and interest in discovering what happened. This will reinforce the importance of homework and encourage them to carry out the agreed tasks. Remember to praise any positive steps or successes, no matter how small these may seem. Where appropriate, homework goals can be re-evaluated and build up in small steps over subsequent consultations.

Box 4.2   **Examples of handover questions**

- What do you make of our discussion today?
- What might you say to a friend in the same situation?
- How might this help you cope better with your health?
- What needs to happen to test out this new idea in your life?
- How might you keep track of the changes and their effects?

Box 4.3	**Examples of homework tasks**

- Think about the discussion and apply it to your own life: the person could review a copy of a CBT framework that was discussed during the consultation and look for ways to apply to their problem(s)
- Complete additional blank CBT frameworks to get a better understanding of situations that trigger anxiety and look for any vicious cycles that might be maintaining anxiety
- Read some self-help information for managing anxiety: including leaflets, books and websites
- Reducing unhelpful anxiety behaviours such as avoidance, reassurance or safety behaviours
- Simple behavioural activation tasks such as increasing exercise or social activities
- Mindfulness-based self-help resources

Box 4.4	**Reviewing homework**

- What had you planned to do? What did you try?
- What happened? What was the short-term effect(s)? What might be the long-term effect(s)?
- What difficulties got in the way? How did you react to these?
- What did you learn from this experience?
- Can you plan your next specific goal? Do you need to make the goal easier, more difficult or the same?
- Do you need to find a way to remind yourself to carry it out or change the focus of the goal?

Explain the problem clearly

Clear and accurate explanations of anxiety can give patients a sense of control over their difficulties and help them to understand, take ownership and find ways to overcome their problems. Where possible, use interactive dialogue and questions to keep the patient actively involved in the discussion and use a CBT framework to break the problem down and make it easier to understand (see *Box 4.5*).

Explanations relating to each anxiety disorder are covered in the individual chapters (*Chapters 5–13*). In general terms, an effective explanation for anxiety should:
- address the patient's specific fears and health beliefs
- emphasise that anxiety symptoms are extremely unpleasant but not dangerous or harmful

Box 4.5 | **Using a CBT framework to explain anxiety**

Thoughts
- In anxiety, our thoughts are focused on what might go wrong in the future
- We tend to look at the worst-case scenario or fear that something terrible might happen
- We think that we will be unable to cope if something does go wrong
- We find it hard to stop thinking about all our problems and difficulties

Feelings
- People with anxiety often feel irritable, worried, fearful, apprehensive, tense or have a sense of dread
- If we are anxious for a long period of time we may start to feel low or depressed as a result

Behaviour
- We often start to avoid activities that might make us anxious
- We might find ways to leave or escape from a situation if we begin to feel anxious
- We do things to try to make ourselves safer, such as staying near other people, holding a railing or sitting near the exit ('safety behaviours')

Physical symptoms
- Acute (short-term, immediate) symptoms of anxiety include rapid breathing, increased heart rate, tense muscles, sweating and shaking
- Longer-term physical reactions include poor sleep, fatigue, reduced appetite, headache and other aches and pains

Next steps after the explanation include:
- talking about how the different areas of the framework are linked and can form a vicious cycle of negative thoughts, feelings and behaviour
- linking the explanation to the patient's own thoughts, feelings and behavioural reactions
- asking a handover question, such as: *"What do you make of this?"* or *"How does this relate to your own experiences?"*
- using a behavioural experiment to demonstrate anxiety symptoms (see *Box 4.6*)

- use positive rather than negative statements, e.g. *"The pain in your chest is due to tightness of the muscles in the chest wall"* rather than *"There is nothing wrong with you"*
- include relevant information about physiological responses to anxiety, e.g. the fight or flight response (see *Chapter 1*)
- reinforce the explanation using practical demonstrations and behavioural experiments (see *Box 4.6*)
- Include a written checklist which has clear explanations for each feared symptom, that the patient can refer to when feeling anxious in future (*Figure 4.3*).

Box 4.6

Using behavioural experiments and practical demonstrations to explain anxiety symptoms

- **Tightness or pain in the chest:** ask the patient to inhale deeply and then immediately take another deep breath, without exhaling between breaths. Notice the tightness in the chest wall that arises. Explain that during hyperventilation, people typically try to breathe in when they have not fully exhaled, leading to a feeling of tightness and eventually pain in the chest wall. Remind the person that pain in the chest does not automatically come from the heart.
- **Dizziness or light-headedness:** asking a patient to breathe deeply 5–6 times will often bring on mild symptoms of hyperventilation such as feeling light-headed, dizzy or getting tingling around the mouth.
- **Tightness in the throat (e.g. associated with a fear of choking):** ask a patient to swallow 5 times rapidly in succession. Notice the tightness that arises very quickly. Having a dry mouth and repeated swallowing as a safety or checking behaviour in anxiety will worsen this sensation.

It's not dangerous to have
a racing heart – my heart
is designed to beat faster
when I do exercise
or get anxious

I've had many panic attacks and
the worst has never happened

If I stay in the situation, the
anxiety will soon pass

Figure 4.3 Checklist for self-reassurance.

Review and check understanding

At the end of the consultation, it is often helpful to briefly review the patient's perception of the discussion. It is not uncommon for patients with anxiety to catastrophise about or misconstrue medical communications, and this process enables you to identify and address any possible misunderstandings. It also ensures that the person fully understands what you have jointly agreed they will try to do for 'homework'. This might involve asking:

- *"Could we finish by checking what you've taken from our discussion today?"*
- *"Can I check what you think are the main causes of your symptoms now?"*
- *"What was the most helpful part of this consultation? Is anything still concerning you?"*
- *"What do you plan to do as a result of our discussion?"*

4.3 10 minute CBT: cognitive skills and strategies

Labelling of thoughts

Cognitive strategies in CBT often involve helping the anxious person to recognise that their fearful or catastrophic thoughts are simply one perspective and may not be entirely accurate. They can learn to view thoughts as opinions open to investigation and evaluation rather than facts.

Identifying and labelling anxiety thoughts as they arise can be a very useful tool for encouraging this process in the limited time available in primary care, which does not require in-depth or lengthy discussion about the accuracy of a particular thought. This represents a form of cognitive defusion, in which the process of recognising and naming thoughts allows the person to distance themselves from the content of the thought.

Writing down anxious thoughts as they arise can be very helpful, perhaps using a diary, or writing on Post-it notes. This helps with recognising that anxiety is arising and enables people to make choices about how to respond.

A GP can facilitate this process in the way that they respond to anxious patients' thoughts and fears. Giving reassurance about health worries on one or two occasions is very appropriate, but for people with an anxiety disorder who present repeatedly about the same symptom, this reassurance is unlikely to be long-lasting and may simply increase anxiety and the desire for further medical reassurance over time. In this situation, some alternative responses might include:

- highlighting and labelling the person's negative thoughts, rather than reassuring or contradicting the worry: *"So, it sounds like you are having some worry thoughts about..."*
- identifying a link between a thought and an emotional response: *"That thought seems to make you feel really anxious..."*
- making an empathetic statement: *"It must be very distressing to be worrying so much..."*
- reflective listening: *"So you are particularly worried that...?"*
- 'ROLLing' with negative thoughts (see *Box 4.7*).

Distraction

Distraction is a useful short-term method of managing negative thoughts by focusing attention on something else. It can help to use distraction when it is difficult to stop thinking or worrying about particular problems. Distraction differs from attempting to suppress or ignore negative thoughts, as it involves trying to actively engage in a different activity.

Distraction should not be used as a way of avoiding problems or situations that need to be dealt with and resolved. If overused, it can develop into a form of safety behaviour which actually reinforces the anxiety loop. Distraction is best viewed as a short-term strategy to use when anxiety is high and to enable the anxious individual to continue with their important daily activities.

Distraction is discussed further in *Chapter 5* with some examples of useful distraction activities.

Building coping strategies

In anxiety it is common to focus on future feared outcomes without planning how to cope with the problem if it did arise. Building the person's coping skills and belief in their ability to deal with future danger is an important method of overcoming anxiety that can be much more effective than simply offering reassurance. This might involve shifting from "What if..." thinking (*"What if something goes wrong...?"*) to "Then what...?" thinking (*"Then what would I do to cope or overcome this problem...?"*) (see *Box 4.8*).

| Box 4.7 | **ROLL with negative thoughts** |

When we experience scary or upsetting thoughts about the future, it is common to try to control these thoughts and get rid of them or stop them from coming. We might try to suppress or avoid thinking these negative thoughts. Unfortunately, trying to control our thoughts in this way is not usually very helpful. Often, the more we try to get rid of unwanted thoughts, the more these thoughts increase in frequency and intensity. Instead of trying to control, reason with, or react to thoughts, we can allow them to enter and leave our mind freely, without engaging with them or getting attached to them.

This process is known as 'ROLLing' with your negative thoughts:

Recognise: when an anxious thought arises, acknowledge and recognise that it is present but that it is just a thought which has popped into your mind: nothing more and nothing less.	*I am having a thought that something really bad is going to happen. I'm thinking about getting ill in the future.*
Observe: watch the thought with kindness and curiosity. Notice its impact on your body and feelings. Just allow it to be, without judging, reacting to, or trying to change it.	*This is another of my worry thoughts. I get these a lot. It's making me feel quite anxious and my chest is getting tight.*
Let go: after recognising and observing your thoughts, you can let them go. You could imagine your thoughts as clouds in the sky, or leaves in a stream, and just watch as they eventually float past and disappear. You don't have to try to push your thoughts away or try to 'get rid' of them, but simply step back and watch them pass by.	*This is a difficult thought, but I don't have to get pulled into it. It's just a thought, not necessarily true. I don't have to respond to it by checking my body or looking on the internet. The thought will pass by if I wait.*

Questions that a GP might ask to help encourage this focus on coping include:
- *"I wonder how you might cope if that really did happen...?"*
- *"I'm wondering what would be a helpful way to look at this situation, which might help you cope with it most effectively...?"*
- *"Have you ever coped successfully with any problems in the past?" "What personal assets or skills have helped you overcome similar difficulties?"*
- *"How might someone else cope with this?" "Could you try that?"*
- *"What help advice and support are available from others?"*

| Box 4.8 | **Moving from "What if…" to "Then what…" thinking** |

James is a 32-year-old salesman who has become increasingly anxious about giving brief presentations, which are an important part of his working role. He tells his GP, Dr White, that he often lies awake the night before the presentation, worrying about what might go wrong. Dr White helps James to identify coping strategies for some of his "what if…" thoughts. He also encourages James to continue this process of planning coping strategies for his worry thoughts during a half-hour period of 'worry time' each day.

"What if…" thoughts and fears	**"Then what…" strategies**
What if my mind goes blank during the presentation?	*I will take a deep breath and look back at my slides. I will try to keep my attention focused on what I want to say rather than on whether I'm doing a good job of presenting.*
What if they ask me a question and I can't think of an answer?	*I can practise beforehand with my colleague and plan what to say in response to any difficult questions. Or I can say that I will find out and come back to them later.*
What if they start looking bored?	*I will try to remember that they might not be bored, maybe just tired or busy. I will keep my concentration on giving the talk as best I can.*
What if I spill something on my suit just before the presentation?	*I will eat breakfast before I leave home and then not eat anything that could damage my suit once I have left the house. I could also take a wet wipe to clean anything that I spill.*
What if my boss thinks it wasn't a very good presentation?	*I can only do my best. He said that he enjoyed the last presentation I gave. Worrying won't make me give a better presentation, probably the opposite! If things are really difficult, I could always look for a job that doesn't involve presentations.*

Problem-solving approaches

Structured problem-solving offers a way of breaking down problems and looking for ways to solve them. This can be helpful in disorders such as GAD, where people tend to focus on worst-case scenarios and don't take time to plan how they might cope with the problems that could arise.

Interestingly, problem-solving therapy does not need to solve all the person's problems to have some effectiveness. Much of the benefit from this process comes from creating a sense of structure and order to problems, which reduces the sense of overwhelm that can arise in many anxiety disorders (see *Box 4.9*). The process of problem-solving also leads to an increased sense of self-efficacy, or the ability to cope with life's difficulties, which can also be important in managing anxiety.

Box 4.9

Problem-solving steps

Make a list of problems	*I don't enjoy my job*
	I'm worried about my finances
	What if we can't pay the rent?
	I keep arguing with my partner
	What if my partner leaves me?
	I forgot my mum's birthday last week
	I'm not seeing my friends very much
	I'm not eating healthily
	I might get ill if I don't have a healthy diet
Is this important? Can it be solved?	*I would like a new job*
For each problem, ask yourself: • Is this an important problem? • Can this problem be solved?	*I want to feel secure in my finances* *I need to pay the rent each month*
In the list above, cross out any problems that are not important and those that cannot be solved.	*I want to argue less with my partner* *I would like to see my friends more often*
Now write a list of only the problems that are <u>both</u> important and can be solved.	*I would like to eat more healthily*
Try to write down what you would like to happen rather than just what is wrong.	
If it can't be solved, let go!	*It's not helpful to keep thinking that my partner will leave me or that I might get ill one day in the future*
For problems that cannot be solved, try to let any worry 'go'. This may be difficult, but it is unhelpful to continually worry about things that we cannot change. If it is hard to let go, try using distraction to focus your mind on something else.	

Box 4.9 – contd		
Choose a problem to solve Pick something that is important and can be solved. Tip: pick an easier problem to think about first!	*I would like to get a new job*	
What's the first step? Break the problem down into the smallest steps you can. Now decide what you need to do first.	*I need to apply for a new job and try to get an interview*	
Think of some solutions Brainstorm at least four possible solutions to the first step. Include ideas that might seem impossible or silly. What are the disadvantages and advantages of each solution? Tip: if you are struggling to find solutions, try breaking the problem down into an even smaller step.	1. *I could ask around if anyone knows about any jobs going* 2. *I could look in the local paper* 3. *I can look on the internet* 4. *I could register with an agency* *The problem is that I don't even have a CV ready yet – I can't apply without one. I think my first step will have to be to get my CV ready.*	
Choose a solution to try out Think about any problems that might arise when you try it and plan some ways for dealing with these.	*I will write my CV and ask a friend to look at it before I give out*	
Plan exactly what you will do What, where, when, how long for, and who with?	*On Saturday, I will spend half an hour straight after breakfast when I've got time and I won't be so tired in the morning*	
Try out the solution!	*I started but I didn't finish*	
What happened? Did any difficulties get in the way? What did you learn from this? Is this still an important problem?	*I spent about 10 minutes on my CV but then I started worrying about whether it was OK, so I stopped and watched TV instead. But it is still important to me to look for a new job.*	
Now plan your next step Do you need to make it easier, more difficult or the same? Do you need to find a way to remind yourself to carry it out or change the focus of the goal?	*I will try again next Saturday. I will ask my friend Estelle to come over and have a look in the afternoon and if it's not finished, she will help and encourage me.*	

Coping with uncertainty

Uncertainty is an aspect of life that cannot be completely avoided. Unfortunately, it is impossible to be 100% certain what will happen in the future, or to be sure that nothing will ever go wrong. However, people with anxiety disorders often find it hard to cope with uncertainty about their health or other potential risks in daily life. Being 'intolerant of uncertainty' means that an individual will tend to experience high levels of anxiety and worry about possible future problems, even if there is only a tiny risk that the event might actually happen. They will often try to plan and prepare for everything as a way of avoiding or eliminating uncertainty.

Common thoughts associated with difficulties tolerating uncertainty include:
- *"I have to be 100% sure that nothing bad is going to happen!"*
- *"I can't tolerate not knowing"*
- *"There's always a risk of something terrible happening"*
- *"The worst could happen".*

Behaviour may include frequent reassurance-seeking from others, excessive list-making, planning and preparation, checking and double-checking, procrastination and avoidance. People may find it hard to delegate tasks to others. There may also be excessive use of distraction techniques in an attempt to block out or avoid worries.

The acronym **ABLE** can be used to help with learning to cope with uncertainty (see *Box 4.10*).

Box 4.10

Learning to tolerate uncertainty: ABLE

Acknowledge and **A**llow what is happening: notice when you are feeling a strong desire for certainty. Notice and give a name to the thoughts and feelings which lie underneath this desire: *"I'm thinking that I couldn't cope if things went wrong"*, *"I'm feeling anxious"* or *"I'm feeling afraid"*. Just allow the thoughts and feelings to be present without resisting or struggling to feel differently.

Breathe: take a deep breath and exhale as slowly as possible. Repeat 3–5 times to create a pause and allow yourself time to decide what to do next.

Let go of the need for certainty: let go of the thought or feeling about needing certainty. It will pass. You don't have to respond to it or act on it. You might imagine it floating away like a bubble or a cloud. Remind yourself that trying to seek certainty is not helpful or necessary and can get in the way of living your life.

Expand your attention and move back to something important. Shift your focus and notice 5 things that you can hear and 5 things that you can see. Then ask yourself: what is most important to you right now? What were you doing before you started to worry? What action is likely to be most helpful in achieving your long-term goals and living a fulfilling and meaning-filled life? Move on to carry out this activity with your full attention.

Managing worry

Several strategies for managing worry are discussed in *Chapter 5* on GAD, including:

- postponing worry during 'worry time': this involves planning to restrict the time spent worrying each day to a regular daily half-hour period of time, and then postponing worries that arise outside this time until later
- using a worry tree: this is a set of simple steps to help with decision-making when worries arise.

Expanding perspective

Expanding perspective can be helpful when an individual is getting stuck in strong negative thoughts or worries about a particular issue and is finding it difficult to see an alternative point of view. This can help to shift out of unhelpful patterns of thinking and can lead to restructuring of negative thoughts. Expanding perspective involves being curious and keeping an open mind, being prepared to break habits and step outside your comfort zone and being willing to see things in a new way. Some questions to help expand perspective are shown in *Box 4.11.*

'Two-tracks' approach

Some patients experiencing problems such as health anxiety and BDD may hold strong beliefs that the cause of their problem is physical, and may find it difficult to accept the diagnosis of an anxiety disorder. It is often counterproductive and stressful for a GP to spend a great deal of time on attempts to persuade or convince the individual that their problem is a mental health one rather than a physical health condition.

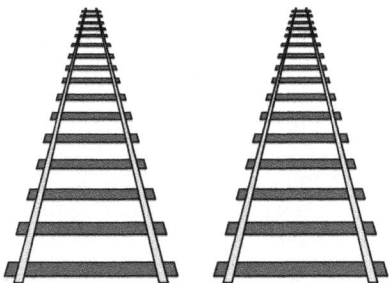

A more helpful strategy may be to take the 'two-tracks' approach, which emphasises that there are two different aspects to the problem, which can be considered separately, although there is likely to be cross-over. This involves balancing the responsibility and importance of caring for physical health, whilst concurrently discussing and addressing psychological and emotional factors which are affecting the individual.

Box 4.11

Expanding perspective

Is this helping me?
- Is the way I'm thinking or looking at the situation helpful? Will it bring about positive change?
- If I let this thought or attitude guide my behaviour, will it help me create a richer and more meaningful life?
- Does thinking this way help me to be the person I want to be and do the things I want to do? If not, where is it taking me?
- What would be a more helpful and accurate way of thinking about this?

Helicopter view: look at the big picture
- If I look at the bigger/smaller picture, does my perspective change?
- SELF: what does this situation mean to me?
- OTHERS: what would it look like to others involved?
- OUTSIDER: how would this seem to someone outside the situation? … someone not emotionally involved?
- FUTURE: will this still be important in one year from now? How about in five years?

Ask my Wise Mind
- What would be the most helpful thought or action (for me and others) in this situation?
- What would I tell a friend in this situation? Can I follow any of this advice?
- Is there anything I can do about this right now? If yes, take appropriate action. If no, accept and move on.
- What's the worst/best/most likely outcome? If the worst did happen, how could I cope with it?

I will take all your physical symptoms seriously and give a thorough medical assessment

Can we also discuss your anxiety and worry about your physical health, which is having a huge impact on your wellbeing?

The two-tracks approach is discussed further in the relevant clinical chapters, including BDD (*Chapter 11*) and health anxiety (*Chapter 13*).

4.4 10 minute CBT: behavioural strategies

Brief graded exposure

Exposure therapy involves helping people to confront their fears, by exposing them to feared objects, activities or situations which have previously been avoided due to anxiety. This process helps reduce anxiety and improve quality of life by enabling people to reduce avoidance and participate more fully in their lives. Graded exposure involves targeting mildly feared stimuli first and gradually progressing to more strongly feared stimuli.

A GP might use principles of brief exposure by jointly creating a simple hierarchy of feared situations and encouraging anxious patients to begin to reduce avoidance and start to take tiny steps towards these (see *Box 4.12*). These steps should be extremely small, to increase the likelihood of success and reduce the risk of triggering excessively high levels of anxiety. It can also help to plan simple coping strategies for managing anxiety symptoms, such as using a breathing technique to prevent hyperventilation and its associated physical sensations.

Box 4.12	**Steps for graded exposure**	
	Step 1: Make a list of situations that trigger anxiety Make a list of situations that are being avoided due to anxiety. Be creative and include lots of examples of situations that would only trigger a small amount of anxiety.	**Example: graded exposure to a dog phobia** • *Talk about dogs* • *Look at cartoon images of dogs* • *Look at a photograph of a dog* • *Watch a video of dogs* • *Look at a dog through a window* • *Watch someone else stroke a dog from a distance* • *Stand at a distance from a dog on a lead* • *Stand right next to a dog on a lead that is sitting quietly* • *Touch or stroke a small dog when it is on a lead* • *Touch or stroke a larger dog on a lead* • *Feed a dog a treat from my hand* • *Be in the park with dogs close by that are off the lead*
	Step 2: Choose a situation to try first Begin by picking one of the easiest or least anxiety-provoking situations from the list.	*I will start by looking at a photograph of a dog*

Box 4.12 – contd		
	Step 3: Plan when and where to face the situation Be specific in choosing a time and place to face the fear. Try to pick a time that will help to achieve this successfully.	*I will do this on Sunday afternoon when I'm not in a rush to get anywhere.*
	Step 4: Face the situation and stick with it! The next step is to face the fear and stay in the situation until anxiety has reduced by at least half. It may take up to 30 minutes to feel comfortable, and even longer as the person progresses up the hierarchy (up to 45 minutes).	*I sat with a book of dogs open on a page with a photograph of a small dog. It made me anxious at first, but it started to fade away after about 10 minutes. After 20 minutes I felt much better, so I closed the book.*
	Step 5: Repeat as often as possible until feeling confident Each exposure should be repeated several times on different days until the person feels comfortable with each step.	*I repeated the process each day for the next week; by the next Saturday I could open the book without feeling anxious at all.*
	Step 6: Cut out safety behaviours If necessary, this step involves removing any safety behaviours such as being with someone else during the anxiety talk. These behaviours stop the person from fully exposing themselves to their fear and learning that they can cope without them.	*The first few times I asked my friend to sit with me while I looked at the photograph of the dog. After that, I asked her to sit in the next room. Finally, I tried it when I was on my own in the house.*
	Step 7: Move up the ladder and repeat the process The next step is to progress to a slightly more challenging situation and repeat the process of exposure to widen the range of activities that the person feels confident to participate in.	*Next, I plan to watch a video about small dogs.*

Reducing other unhelpful anxiety behaviours

It may also be helpful to jointly plan to reduce other unhelpful anxiety behaviours which are maintaining anxiety as a vicious cycle, such as excessive checking, internet searches and reassurance seeking. Family and carers may need to be involved in this process. As with graded exposure, this can be carried out very gradually in small stages or 'micro-steps'. It may be necessary to discuss strategies for managing the anxiety that arises if the safety behaviour is not

Box 4.13 | **Alternatives to reassurance**

- Labelling worries: *"That sounds like another of your worry thoughts..."*
- Empathetic statements: *"It must be very distressing to be worrying so much..."*
- Reflective listening: *"So you are particularly worried that...?"*
- 'Then what ...?' thinking: *"I wonder how you might cope if that really did happen...?"*

carried out. For more severe cases, this process is likely to require the support of an experienced CBT therapist.

Box 4.13 gives some alternatives to try instead of repeatedly offering reassurance.

Activity scheduling and behavioural activation

Behavioural activation is an evidence-based therapy for depression. However, it can also have an important role in patients with anxiety, particularly when this has been present for a long time and is associated with low mood, loss of confidence, fatigue and marked behavioural restriction. Behavioural activation involves taking a structured approach to gradually re-engaging in activities which have been reduced due to low mood and anxiety.

Behavioural changes should be made even in the presence of ongoing low mood and anxiety symptoms by the person behaving 'as if' they feel a little bit brighter or less anxious. This creates the opportunity for positive life experiences and can lead to improvements in energy, mood and self-esteem. Activities that are most likely to lead to positive changes in mood include physical activity and social interaction, and those which are in line with the individual's core values (see *Box 4.14*). Useful questions to encourage positive behavioural changes include:

- What would you do more of if you felt happier or less anxious? How did you previously spend your time?
- What activities are important to you? What direction would you like to take your life?
- What do you care about? Who and what is most important to you? What small activities could you pick that are in line with these values?
- Are you able to take any small steps in this direction? If you only had two minutes to carry out an activity related to this area of your life, what would you do?

Use a 'likelihood ruler' (*Figure 4.4*) to check how likely the person is to actually carry out the planned behaviour, and aim for a score of 8 or higher. Any task that scores below 8 should be broken down into smaller and easier steps.

How likely on a scale of 1 to 10 is it that you will actually
carry out this action within the next two weeks?

| 1 | 2 | 3 | 4 | 5 | 6 | 7 | 8 | 9 | 10 |

Figure 4.4 Likelihood ruler for carrying out a particular behaviour.

Box 4.14

Examples of activities to schedule in behavioural activation

- Physical activity – go for a walk, do 10 minutes of yoga or jogging, or go to the gym
- Social interaction – text, phone or meet a friend or close family member; make eye contact and smile at a neighbour or the local shopkeeper
- Enjoyable activities – restarting hobbies or developing new interests
- Making a start on important work or household tasks – aim for a few minutes or choose a very brief task to get started
- Self-care activities that build a sense of wellbeing ('me time') – read a magazine, have a bath, buy a scented shower gel, paint your nails

---

Activity scheduling involves keeping a diary of current daily activities (see *Box 4.15*), and then taking a structured approach to gradually increasing activities over time. Planned activities should be carried out based on the planned schedule rather than on how the individual feels on a particular day. The choice of activities should largely come from the patient, and should involve a balance of enjoyable, important and meaningful tasks.

Box 4.15

Daily activity diary

Time	Activity	Rate levels of Enjoyment (E) and Importance (I) of each activity from 1–10
7–8 am		
8–9 am		
9–10 am		
10–11 am		
etc.		

Box 4.16

Steps in behavioural activation

Step	What to do	Example
Review your current activity patterns	Use a daily activity diary to monitor current activity patterns or ask yourself: • What activities am I no longer participating in because of anxiety or low mood? • What would I do differently if I felt better or my mood lifted? • What activities or hobbies did I used to enjoy? • What important activities am I postponing or putting off?	*I have stopped seeing friends as much as before. I spend a lot more time sitting and worrying about problems and I don't go out much. I hardly do any enjoyable activities at the moment.*
Make a list of different types of activity	We can think about three different types of activity: • **Enjoyable activities:** things that you do (or used to do) for enjoyment, or new activities you would like to try, such as seeing friends, playing games, hobbies and interests. • **Routine activities:** important activities in your daily routine such as cooking, cleaning, shopping for food, laundry, having a bath or shower, walking the dog, going to the gym. • **Necessary activities:** these are essential activities which will have negative consequences if avoided, such as paying bills, claiming benefits or having a health check. Make a list of as many different activities in each category that you can think of.	**Enjoyable activities:** • Meeting a friend for lunch • Going for a walk in the park • Playing a game with my grandson • Crafts such as knitting • Reading a book • Having my nails done or a haircut **Routine activities:** • Having a shower every day • Putting on make-up • Preparing meals • Washing up • Going to the gym • Walking the dog **Necessary activities:** • Paying bills • Doing my tax return • Going to the dentist • Picking up my prescription • Remembering to take my medication

Box 4.16 – contd			
	Choose an activity to try	Choose one activity to try. Start with easier activities! Remember, social activities and physical exercise are often helpful to improve low mood and anxiety.	*Playing with my grandson*
	What am I going to do?	Be specific about what you plan to do: what, when, where, who with and how long for? Choose a specific date and time to carry out the activity. You might find it helpful to write this on your activity diary.	*I am babysitting for him at the weekend so I can play a game of cards with him instead of just watching TV*
	How achievable is this activity?	On a scale of 1–10 how achievable is this activity? 1 – 2 – 3 – 4 – 5 – 6 – 7 – 8 – 9 – 10 Aim for a score of at least 8. For anything less, can you make it easier to carry out?	*8/10*
	Do it! Carry out the activity!	Keep a record of whether you carried out the activity.	*I did it!*
	What happened?	Notice what happened. What was the outcome? What was helpful? What obstacles got in the way? How could I make it easier next time?	*I enjoyed playing cards with him and I felt pleased with myself as he enjoyed it too*
	What next?	Go back to the list of activities and choose a new one to try. Try to include a balance of enjoyable, routine and necessary activities in your day. Keep adding new activities to the list that are important.	*Next I would like to get back to regularly walking my dog with my husband*

Values-based activity setting

Values represent what matters most to people. They involve the person asking themselves some 'big' questions such as:

- What do I care about? What kind of person do I want to be?
- What qualities do I want to encourage?
- What do I want out of life?

Values are like a compass, which provide direction, meaning and purpose to life, rather than focusing on a specific outcome (see *Box 4.17*). For example, a value might involve education rather than passing an exam, or connecting with my friends, rather than going out on any particular occasion.

Understanding people's values can help to motivate change. Values depend on behavioural actions to be brought to life. We can take 'towards actions' that are in the direction of our values (e.g. going for a walk if our value is physical exercise) or 'away actions' which move us away from the things we care about (e.g. avoiding seeing people we care about because of anxiety).

Box 4.17 | **Examples of values**

ACTIVE – to live a physically active life

APPEARANCE – to take care of my own appearance

AUTONOMY – to be able to choose my own path

BALANCE – to avoid extremes and find balanced perspectives or life choices

CARING – to be supportive and nurturing to myself and others

CHALLENGE – to solve problems, stretch my own limits and test my abilities

COMPETENCE – to develop knowledge, skills and ability to carry out particular tasks or roles

CONNECTION – to feel connected and close to the important people in my life

CONTRIBUTION – to make a lasting or meaningful contribution to the world

COURAGE – to be brave and make positive choices in the face of fear, uncertainty, difficulties and setbacks

CREATIVITY – to express my own new and original ideas

FAMILY – to be part of a close and loving family

FINANCIAL – to have financial security and stability

FITNESS – to build physical fitness

FLEXIBILITY – to adapt to new circumstances and changes

FRIENDSHIP – to spend time with important friends

FUN – to play and to find pleasure and joy in life

FUTURE – to plan where I would like my life to take me

GLOBAL – to care about important world or environmental issues

GROWTH – to change, grow and adapt

HEALTH – to look after my physical health

HONESTY – truthfulness, sincerity and clarity

HOPE – to believe in future possibilities and that it is possible keep going through current difficulties

HUMOUR – to laugh and find humour in the world

INDEPENDENCE – to make my own decisions and care for myself

INTIMACY – to safely share my innermost experiences and thoughts with other

KINDNESS – to relate to myself and others with kindness and compassion

LEARNING/EDUCATION – to learn new things and develop and stimulate my mind

LEISURE – to participate in activities that I find enjoyable, relaxing or fun

LOVE – to find and express love and affection

OUTDOORS – to spend time in the outdoor environment

Box 4.17 – contd		

PEACE – to find a sense of tranquillity, harmony, calmness or stillness

PERSISTENCE – to keep going with tasks or challenges, despite difficulties or setbacks

PRESENCE – to be mindful and aware of the present moment

PURPOSE – to have meaning and direction in my life

RECOGNITION – to acknowledge the existence and validity of my own contribution and actions

RELAXATION – to find ways of calming and relaxing

RESILIENCE – to cope with life's difficulties without losing self-esteem or confidence

RESPECT – to treat myself and others with consideration, respect and fairness

RESPONSIBILITY – to take ownership and responsibility for important duties, decisions or roles

RISK – to be willing to take risks and chances in life

SAFETY – to feel physical and emotional safety and security and a sense of trust in self and others

SPACE – to find physical space and time for myself

SPIRITUALITY and RELIGION – to develop spiritual or religious beliefs and practices

SELF-ESTEEM – to feel pride and care for myself

TRADITION – to value and uphold respected patterns from the past or a particular culture

UNDERSTANDING – to build understanding and knowledge about myself and others

OTHER – anything else that is important to me

Choose 4–6 of the listed values which are most important for you at the moment. You can add any other values that are important if they are not mentioned on the list. For each value, ask:

Why have you chosen this value?

What does it mean to you? How is it important for you?

What actions or activities are linked to this value?

Asking patients about values:

- *"Who and what is important in your life?"*
- *"Which are your most important values at the moment?"*
- *"Is anxiety interfering with any of your important values?"*
- *"How might overcoming your anxiety help you to connect more fully with these values?"*
- *"How can reducing anxiety help you to achieve or continue to enjoy the things that are important in your life?"*
- *"How important might it be to learn new ways to manage your anxiety and get back in touch with your values?"*

Values can be used to support setting relevant goals in behavioural activation or graded exposure. People can be encouraged to take small behavioural steps towards their values, even if this may mean a transient increase in anxiety.

- *"What tiny or micro-steps might take you in the direction of your most important values...?"*
- *"Are you able to take this step, even if you experience some anxiety...?"*

> **Case example 4.1: Emma**
>
> **Discussing values**
>
> Emma is a 25-year-old woman with anxiety and frequent attendances at the surgery with headaches. Dr Patel recognises the huge impact that Emma's anxiety is having on her life, including marked behavioural restriction and reduced quality of life. He decides to take some time to explore her values, with the aim of using brief values-based behavioural activation to increase positive and meaningful activities, and to help move consultations away from repeatedly discussing her physical symptoms and her anxiety about her health.
>
> Dr Patel asks Emma to choose 4–6 of her most important values from the list in *Box 4.17*. Emma is initially surprised, but is willing to carry out the activity. She chooses the following values:
>
> - FRIENDSHIP: my friends are very important to me but I'm not seeing much of them because I'm so worried about my health that I haven't felt like going out.
> - FAMILY: my mum and my sister are very important to me, but I seem to spend a lot of time talking about my health worries with them.
> - RELAXATION: I constantly feel on edge and anxious and I would love to feel more relaxed and calm.
> - FITNESS: I used to be proud of being very fit and active but I have cut down physical activity because of worry about my headaches.
> - BALANCE: I would like to get more balance in my life, so that I am spending time on things that are important and not getting so caught up in worrying about my headaches that I ignore other parts of my life.
>
> This discussion was extremely useful in helping Dr Patel understand more about Emma and how he might be able to support her. It also identified several possible behavioural changes that might improve Emma's quality of life, such as increasing physical exercise and spending time with friends and family.

Micro-goals

Micro-goals are tiny targets which are easily achieved and which can help with developing positive habits (see *Box 4.18*). Micro-goals are extremely brief, ideally taking no longer than 2–5 minutes. Although such changes are small, they offer an achievable strategy for changing long-standing, habitual negative behavioural patterns and for increasing the individual's belief in their own ability to make changes in their lives (self-efficacy). The focus should be on the process of learning to make life changes through taking tiny steps, rather than on achieving a specific outcome. The aim is to help people recognise that they do not have to remain stuck in repetitive patterns of unhelpful behaviour. Ideally, micro-goals are actions that move people towards an important value in some way, although the step may be very small.

Box 4.18	**Examples of micro-goals**

- Finding my trainers in the garage and putting them by the front door (ready for increased exercise)
- Short walk to the postbox to post a letter
- Making eye contact and smiling at the shop assistant when I buy my paper
- Buying myself a magazine at the same time as the weekly shopping
- Sending a text to an old friend
- Driving a new route home from work
- Practising attention training while brushing my teeth each morning and evening
- Asking my wife how her day was
- Thinking about one thing that went well during the day as I drop off to sleep

4.5 Other strategies

Mindfulness and relaxation

Self-care strategies for anxiety may include mindfulness or relaxation activities. There are many available mindfulness resources (see *Section 4.7*). Breathing exercises to reduce hyperventilation such as 'square breathing' and prolonged exhalation are discussed in *Chapter 6* (panic disorder).

Attention training

Attention training involves learning to move the mind away from catastrophic and frightening thoughts about problems and difficulties that might happen in the future, by learning to focus on the present moment and pay attention to what is happening in the 'here and now' (see *Box 4.19*). This is a useful skill that can help reduce the impact of anxiety, enabling people to concentrate more fully on important activities in daily life.

Attention training does not involve trying to control worry thoughts or make them go away. These thoughts can be acknowledged and observed in the mind, but do not have to be engaged with. Rather than continually running through thoughts and worries, the person can shift their attention back to whatever they are doing in the present moment.

Improving sleep

Many anxiety disorders are associated with problems sleeping, which may include difficulty falling asleep or staying asleep at night. Anxiety and worry can interfere with sleep by preventing the mind from settling at night. Experiencing loss of sleep is also likely to contribute to increasing anxiety, tension and feeling on edge, with a lowering of mood.

Giving advice about managing sleep can help to improve mood and quality of life. Strategies for improving sleep are summarised in *Box 4.20*.

Box 4.19

Attention training: focus on your daily activities

Choose an activity to focus on. This might be an everyday routine task such as eating, brushing your teeth, walking or taking a shower. Try to choose something that is important or relevant to your current daily routine.

Whilst carrying out the task, try to give it your complete and full attention. Focus on the sensory aspects of carrying out the activity and use these to anchor your attention to the task at hand.

Each time you find your mind has wandered away, try to bring it back to the task by thinking about:
- **touch**: what does the activity feel like? Where on your body are you touching an object? What is the texture like – is it rough, smooth, soft or hard? Is the temperature warm or cold?
- **sight**: what can you see? What shapes or patterns are there? What colours and shades can you notice? How about noticing light or shadows?
- **hearing**: what can you hear? What sounds can you become aware of? What sounds are far away or close at hand? What are the loudest and quietest sounds?
- **smell**: what smells or aromas can you notice? How do these affect you?
- **taste**: can you notice any particular taste or flavours? How many different tastes can you become aware of? Do the tastes change?

Box 4.20

Sleep hygiene tips

- Keep a regular sleep pattern: stick to fixed times for going to bed and waking up and avoid sleeping in after a poor night's sleep.
- Avoid daytime naps.
- Regular exercise during the daytime helps sleep at night but try to avoid strenuous exercise in the 4 hours before bedtime.
- Create a comfortable sleeping environment: ensure your bedroom is dark, quiet, not too cluttered, that your bed is comfortable, and the room is a good temperature for sleeping.
- Avoid caffeine, nicotine, and alcohol within 6 hours of going to bed. Consider complete elimination of caffeine from the diet.
- Avoid eating a heavy meal late at night.
- Plan a relaxing activity before going to bed.
- Avoid watching or checking the clock throughout the night.
- Avoid late-night technology: looking at bright screens late at night disrupts the sleep–wake cycle.

Stimulus control: retrain your sleep habits
- This involves retraining the body and mind to associate bed with sleep, rather than with lying awake being unable to sleep, so that you fall asleep quickly when you go to bed (within 15 minutes).

Box 4.20 – contd

- Only try to sleep when you feel tired or sleepy, rather than spending a lot of time lying awake in bed.
- Get up and try again later: if you haven't been able to get to sleep after about 20 minutes, get out of bed and do something calming or boring, such as sitting in another room in a dim light, until you feel sleepy. Don't do anything overly simulating or interesting. Then return to bed and try to sleep again. Repeat the process if you still can't sleep.
- Only use the bedroom for sleep and sexual activity. Keep electronic gadgets such as phones, computers, TVs and other devices out of the bedroom.

Sleep restriction
- This is one of the most effective methods of improving 'sleep efficiency' (the proportion of time in bed that you are asleep).
- Use a sleep diary (see *Box 4.21*) to work out your average amount of actual sleep per night. Don't include time spent lying in bed awake. Then plan to stay in bed for only the length of your calculated average sleep time.
- Choose a regular wake-up time that suits you and stick to this every day.
- Set your bedtime by subtracting the number of hours of sleep needed from your wake-up time.
- Follow the planned bedtime and wake-up time for at least one week.
- After a week, assess how well you are sleeping. If you are feeling sleepy before your bedtime, falling asleep more quickly and sleeping more soundly through the night, you can increase your time in bed by 30 minutes, by going to bed 30 minutes earlier.
- Do not extend your time in bed if you are awake during the night for longer than 30 minutes. Continue the initial routine for another week and then review again.
- Extend your sleep by another 30 minutes at the end of each week until you feel you are getting sufficient sleep that is good quality, with less than 30 minutes of wake time during the night.
- Decrease your time in bed if your excessive wakefulness or poor sleep returns.
- Once you find your ideal bedtime and sleep schedule, try to stick with it regularly.
- Sleep restriction will often make you more tired at first, so avoid it if you are driving or operating heavy machinery. Wait until you have a holiday to try it out.

Manage your expectations about sleep
- Be realistic with your sleep expectations: many people do not need as long as 7–8 hours' sleep.
- Remind yourself that even a small amount of sleep is valuable. Try not to focus so much on getting a specific amount of sleep each night.
- It can be completely normal to have interrupted sleep, waking after around 4 hours and dropping back to sleep again. Try not to worry or panic if this happens. Simply accept that you've woken and lie quietly. Often, you will drop back to sleep again.
- Use a sleep diary for at least 2 weeks to get the accurate facts about your own sleep patterns, rather than making assumptions. You can repeat this a few months later to see how you are progressing.

Box 4.20 – contd

Tips for putting anxiety and worry aside
- Use 'worry time' to write down any problems or worries that might keep you awake at night. Do this well before bedtime. Try to include ideas for how you could cope with any difficulties.
- Keep a notebook next to your bed and write down any new worries that pop up at night. Then put it aside and tell yourself that you will deal with this in the morning.
- Problem-solving can help reduce anxiety, stress and worry which may keep you awake at night.
- Try not to sleep: trying to force ourselves to sleep only increases anxiety and tension. Trying not to sleep may make it easier to drop off.
- You can cope better than you think! Rather than thinking about all the problems from lack of sleep, remind yourself that you have coped without sleep before, and that a night without sleep is not a disaster.

Box 4.21

Sleep diary

What time did you go to bed last night?	
How long did it take for you to drop off to sleep?	
After falling asleep, how many times did you wake up in the night?	
How long did you sleep in total last night? (e.g. 5 hours 30 minutes)	
If you found it difficult to sleep, what did you do whilst you were awake?	
What time did you wake up in the morning?	
What time did you get up?	
How long did you spend in bed in total last night (including time spent awake)?	
How long did you spend asleep last night?	
How would you rate the quality of your sleep last night?	1 2 3 4 5 6 7 8 9 10 Poor Excellent
How many drinks containing caffeine did you drink yesterday (e.g. tea, coffee, fizzy drinks)?	
How many after 6pm?	

Box 4.21 – contd	How much alcohol did you drink yesterday?	
	Did you have any naps during the day yesterday? How many, and for how long were you asleep?	
	How much moderate to vigorous exercise did you carry out yesterday? (e.g. swimming, brisk walking, dancing, aerobics, gardening)	
	Did you take any sleeping tablets last night?	
	Did you take any other drugs? If yes, which ones?	
	Did you have any particular stresses or other problems yesterday?	
	Anything else important?	

4.6 Summary and key points

- 10 minute CBT involves the use of CBT principles and communication skills in 'bite-sized' chunks within routine brief primary care consultations.
- The **Re-FRESHER** model offers one approach to using CBT-based communication skills within GP consultations:
  - **Re**cognise anxiety and **R**aise the issue
  - **F**rame the session: manage time effectively
  - **R**ecent **E**xample: explore a specific recent example using a CBT framework
  - **S**ummarise: reflect back the discussion and highlight any vicious cycles that are present
  - **H**andover and **H**omework: strategies to hand over responsibility and encourage self-efficacy and self-management by the patient include setting relevant brief homework tasks
  - **E**xplanation: provide an empowering explanation of the problem
  - **R**eview and check understanding of the discussion.
- Cognitive 10 minute CBT strategies include:
  - highlighting and labelling of thoughts – learning to recognise and view thoughts as simply mental processes rather than facts (cognitive defusion)
  - distraction – to reduce focus on anxiety and enable re-engagement with daily activities
  - building coping strategies and problem-solving to overcome difficulties

- learning to cope with uncertainty and reduce worry
- expanding perspective to support restructuring of negative thoughts
- 'two-tracks' approach to managing both physical and emotional aspects of health in primary care.
- Behavioural strategies:
  - brief graded exposure to reduce anxiety through habituation
  - reduction of unhelpful anxiety behaviours such as reassurance-seeking and body-checking
  - behavioural activation and activity scheduling to increase participation in important and meaningful daily activities
  - values-based activity setting – planning 'towards actions' in the direction of core values may help with motivation to carry out behavioural changes
  - setting 'micro-goals' to build self-efficacy and strengthen self-belief in the person's own capacity to make changes in their life.
- Other useful strategies include mindfulness and relaxation, attention training and strategies to improve sleep.

4.7 Useful self-help online resources

Centre for Clinical Interventions	Australian website offering downloadable comprehensive workbooks on a number of mental health topics, including insomnia, health anxiety, perfectionism, procrastination, worry and rumination	www.cci.health.wa.gov.au/Resources/Looking-After-Yourself
E-couch	Australian self-help interactive programme with modules for depression, generalised anxiety and worry, social anxiety, relationship breakdown, and loss and grief	www.ecouch.anu.edu.au/welcome
Get Self-Help	Online leaflets and information based on CBT	www.getselfhelp.co.uk
Living Life to the Full	Free online life skills course based on CBT on how to tackle and respond to issues/demands which we all meet in our everyday lives	www.llttf.com
Mind	Wide range of downloadable leaflets on mental health topics	www.mind.org.uk/information-support/a-z-mental-health
MoodGym	Australian interactive, online self-help programme based on CBT, which teaches skills to prevent and manage symptoms of depression and anxiety	www.moodgym.com.au
Northumberland, Tyne & Wear NHS Trust leaflets	Comprehensive range of downloadable self-help leaflets about common mental health conditions	https://web.ntw.nhs.uk/selfhelp/
Royal College of Psychiatrists	Downloadable mental health leaflets covering a wide range of mental health conditions and problems	www.rcpsych.ac.uk/mental-health/treatments-and-wellbeing

Chapter 5
Generalised anxiety disorder

GAD quick reference guide

What is generalised anxiety disorder (GAD)?	Persistent, uncontrollable anxiety and worry about multiple everyday situations and problems usually associated with multiple physical symptoms such as fatigue, headache, muscle tension, irritability or insomnia.
How common is it?	Prevalence of around 4.4% in the UK. One of the commonest anxiety disorders in primary care, affecting around 7–8% of patients.
Risk factors	These include psychosocial stressors and socioeconomic deprivation, a family history of psychiatric disorders, experiencing childhood abuse or bullying, and being female. People suffering from chronic physical health conditions are also more likely to develop GAD.
Co-morbid conditions	As many as 90% of people with GAD will develop a co-morbid psychiatric disorder including depression, other anxiety disorders, substance misuse and suicide.
Usual course	Usually starts in adolescence/young adulthood and is often chronic, waxing and waning in the course of the person's life, with a high risk of relapse in response to life stresses.
Common presentations	People with GAD typically present frequently with concerns about their health or other persistent worries, including concerns about coexisting physical health conditions. They may also present with recurrent physical or somatic symptoms.
How to make the diagnosis	Screening can be carried out with GAD-2. Also ask: *Do you worry about a lot of things? Is it hard to stop worrying? Is worry stopping you from participating in any important activities?* GAD-7 and HADS are both useful for diagnosis and monitoring.
What else could it be?	Differential diagnosis and possible co-morbid conditions include other anxiety disorders, depression, substance misuse, somatoform or bodily distress disorders, and underlying physical causes of somatic symptoms.
Self-management strategies	General self-care including physical exercise and sleep hygiene are often helpful. Help patients to understand their condition by giving clear explanations of GAD and the person's specific symptoms. Self-management strategies using 10 minute CBT include activity scheduling, postponing worry, mindfulness and problem-solving skills.

Treatment of GAD	Low intensity CBT is offered for mild to moderate cases. For moderate to severe, or persistent symptoms, high intensity psychological therapy (CBT or applied relaxation) is equally effective as medication. First-line drug treatment is with an SSRI and should continue for at least one year. Mindfulness group sessions may also be beneficial.
When to refer	Severe or complex GAD with marked functional impairment or when there are concerns about risk such as self-neglect or self-harm, or a lack of response to primary care treatment strategies.
Follow-up	Due to the chronic nature of the disorder, GAD is likely to benefit from long-term follow-up in primary care.

CBT framework for GAD

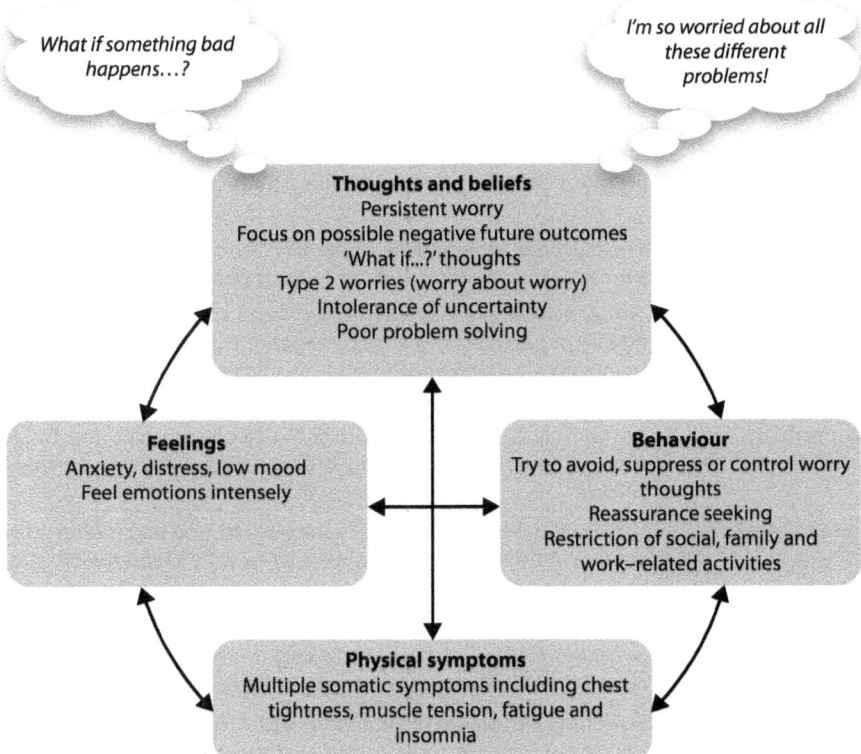

5.1 Introduction

Generalised anxiety disorder (GAD) is associated with persistent and widespread worry. Despite being one of the commonest anxiety disorders in primary care, affecting around 7–8% of patients, GAD often goes unrecognised and consequently untreated. People with GAD tend to be frequent attenders in both primary and secondary care settings, presenting with persistent anxiety and numerous somatic symptoms, and represent the most resource-intensive patient group of all the anxiety disorders. GAD is associated with significant disability and an impaired quality of life which is equivalent to that of chronic physical conditions such as arthritis and diabetes.

5.2 What is GAD?

GAD is characterised by persistent, uncontrollable anxiety and worry about multiple everyday situations and problems, including family, health, work, finances and relationships. The worry is out of proportion to the actual threat or risk of the situation and often feels difficult to control. In some cases, the anxiety may be 'free-floating' and associated with a general sense of apprehension without any particular focus. People with GAD often describe themselves as sensitive or 'a worrier'.

The disorder is also commonly associated with a range of physical symptoms including restlessness, fatigue, disturbed sleep, muscle tension and difficulty concentrating (see *Box 5.1*). Some of the physical symptoms are physiological responses to anxiety, whilst others may be medically unexplained or be associated with coexisting physical health problems. These somatic symptoms typically wax and wane over time.

These anxiety and somatic symptoms lead to significant distress and interfere with the individual's ability to function in daily life.

Box 5.1	**Diagnostic criteria for GAD**

- Marked anxiety, tension and worry persisting for several months, which may involve:
  - o 'free-floating anxiety' or general apprehension
  - o excessive worry about multiple everyday events and problems including family, health, finances, school, work, etc.
- Multiple physical symptoms associated with autonomic arousal including:
  - o palpitations and chest pain
  - o sensation of a lump in the throat, difficulty with breathing or swallowing, or feeling of choking
  - o sweating, trembling or shaking; dry mouth
  - o nausea, churning stomach and other gastrointestinal symptoms
  - o feeling light-headed, dizzy or unsteady; numbness and tingling
  - o muscle tension, aches and pains; being restless, on edge and unable to relax
  - o difficulty concentrating, irritability and poor sleep
- The symptoms result in significant distress or impairment in important areas of functioning (e.g. family, relationships, social interaction, education and work)

5.3 Epidemiology

GAD affects around 4.4% of adults in England. In the USA, GAD has an estimated lifetime prevalence of 5% and a 12-month prevalence of 3%. About two-thirds of people diagnosed with GAD are female, and prevalence is highest in those between 35 and 55 years of age. GAD is one of the commonest disorders in primary care, affecting between 7 and 8% of patients.

5.4 Aetiology

The aetiology of GAD is usually multifactorial, involving psychological, social and biological factors. Risk factors for GAD are summarised in *Box 5.2*.

Box 5.2

Risk factors associated with GAD (NICE, 2017)

- Female sex
- Family history of psychiatric disorders
- Childhood adversity including:
  - maltreatment (e.g. sexual or physical abuse)
  - parental problems such as witnessing domestic violence, alcoholism, drug use and mental illness
  - exposure to an overprotective or overly harsh parenting style
  - bullying or peer victimisation among young people
- Environmental stressors including:
  - physical or emotional trauma
  - domestic violence
  - unemployment
  - low socioeconomic status
  - lack of social support, e.g. being divorced or separated; living alone or as a lone parent
- Substance dependence or exposure to organic solvents
- Chronic and/or painful physical health conditions such as arthritis

---

5.5 CBT model of GAD

The CBT model explains the development of GAD as arising from persistent worry. Worry involves a chain of repetitive thoughts, which are predominantly verbal, about a wide range of potential bad things that may happen in the future. Worry thoughts often include 'What if...?' fears about the future such as: *What if I lose my job? How would I cope? What if I become ill and cannot provide for my family? What if my son has an accident?*

The purpose of worry is an attempt by the mind to be vigilant for possible threat and to try to mentally solve problems that have not yet happened. This is a normal process and in the absence of an anxiety disorder, worry thoughts are usually short-lived and lead either to some form of positive action to resolve the problem or are 'let go' as the mind moves on to a different train of thought. However, in GAD, worry becomes a problem because people spend disproportionate and unhelpful amounts of time worrying, have difficulty disengaging from their negative thoughts and are left stuck in an endless repeating loop of persistent negative self-talk about the future, which worsens anxiety and low mood over time. This process is associated with underlying beliefs such as:

> The world is dangerous, and I may not be able to cope with any problems that arise in the future, so I must anticipate all bad things that might happen, so that I can avoid them or prepare for them.

A summary of the CBT model of GAD is shown in *Figure 5.1*.

Type 1 and type 2 worries in GAD

There are two main types of worry in GAD:
- Type 1 worries relate to feared future events; these may be current real problems or relate to hypothetical or potential situations which have not yet occurred.

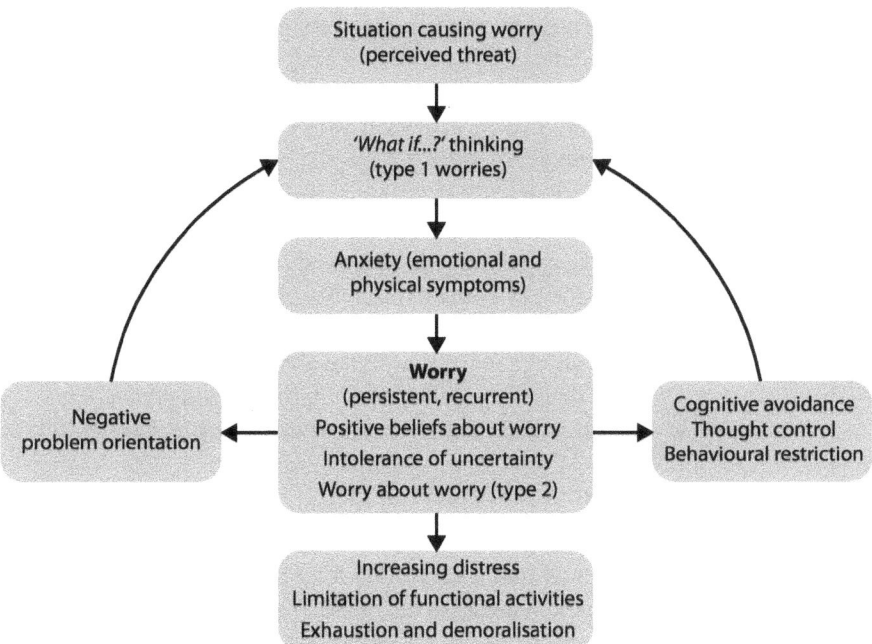

Figure 5.1 CBT model of GAD.

- Type 2 worries involve negative beliefs or 'worry about worry'. These are often beliefs that worrying is dangerous and uncontrollable, and will cause either physical or mental harm, e.g. *"If I keep worrying I will go crazy or become ill"*.

Some individuals with GAD may also hold positive beliefs about the benefits of worry, which encourages them to give increased time and attention to worry thoughts, such as:
- *"If I keep worrying, I can stop something bad happening to me"*
- *"Worrying helps me solve problems and motivates me to do things"*
- *"Worrying helps me to prepare for the worst and shows that I care"*.

Excessive attention on worries

Individuals with GAD often find it hard to draw their attention away from their worries and to pay attention to their daily activities. This negative focus fuels the belief that they are unable to control their worries and leads to a worsening of anxiety and mood.

Thought control strategies

GAD typically involves a range of cognitive and behavioural strategies which are attempts to try to avoid, suppress or control worry thoughts. Unfortunately, thought control strategies are ultimately ineffective because attempts to suppress thoughts typically have the paradoxical effect of making that thought occur even more often and lead to increased worry over time. These strategies often include:
- telling themselves to 'stop worrying' or 'don't think about it'
- trying to reason with their worry thoughts: *"The likelihood of that bad thing happening is so small"*
- distraction: trying hard to focus on something else
- thinking positively: *"Everything will be fine!"*
- seeking excessive reassurance from others to ease their concerns (e.g. constantly phoning a relative to check if they are OK)
- excessive information seeking, e.g. repeatedly searching the internet to check things they are worried about
- using drugs or alcohol to numb their feelings of worry
- avoiding situations that trigger worry, e.g. not watching the news.

Intolerance of uncertainty

Individuals with GAD tend have a pervasive fear of the unknown, and consequently find it very difficult to tolerate uncertain or ambiguous situations. They may hold negative beliefs such as:
- *"Uncertainty makes life intolerable and stops me from functioning"*
- *"I need to be completely certain or I cannot feel safe or at ease"*.

This leads to increased levels of stress and further worry behaviour as a vicious cycle.

Emotional dysregulation

Emotional regulation relates to how an individual manages, expresses and responds to emotion. People with GAD tend to experience emotions more intensely and quickly than others. They also often have a limited understanding of their emotional experiences, including having difficulty in identifying, labelling and describing emotions. Negative cognitive reactivity involves holding unhelpful beliefs about the negative consequences of experiencing emotions and leads to unhelpful strategies to try to manage difficult feelings, such as the use of worry or other cognitive control strategies.

Negative problem orientation

Negative problem orientation involves taking a negative or unhelpful approach towards coping with life problems. Individuals with GAD get stuck in worry thoughts and fail to engage in effective problem-solving or coping behaviour. This can arise due to beliefs about their own lack of ability to cope with the problem as well as pessimism about possible outcomes. Being constantly fixated on future problems also prevents the individual from engaging and interacting with the real world that is around them.

Physical symptoms in GAD

Physical and somatic symptoms are often a presenting feature of GAD in primary care. These symptoms may be associated with the fight or flight response, such as palpitations, breathlessness, restlessness, irritability and poor concentration. Because of the chronic nature of GAD, it is also common to have symptoms associated with long-term anxiety and low mood, including fatigue, muscle aches and sleep difficulties. Functional disorders such as irritable bowel syndrome, chronic pain and chronic fatigue syndrome may also be associated with GAD.

5.6 Co-morbidity

As many as 90% of people with GAD will develop another psychiatric disorder during their lifetime. There is a significantly increased risk of major depression, social anxiety disorder, alcohol and drug misuse, and suicidal ideation and attempts.

People suffering from physical health conditions are also more likely to develop GAD, including those with chronic pain syndromes, asthma or COPD, and inflammatory bowel disease.

5.7 Course and prognosis of GAD

GAD often develops in early childhood or adolescence and typically has a chronic, fluctuating course throughout life, with symptoms that wax and wane in response to life stressors and relatively low rates of complete spontaneous remission. It is often controlled rather than cured. Only around 40% of those diagnosed with GAD are likely to have recovered after 12 years and the duration of illness in GAD may be as long as 20 years. After a remission from GAD, the risk of relapse over the next year has been found to lie between 15 and 30%. Because of this, long-term support and education are frequently required in primary care.

5.8 Presentation of GAD

I've been having headaches, palpitations, muscle pains and I get tired so quickly these days. I'm worried there's something serious wrong...

I feel really fed up and exhausted. I worry about everything and I can't seem to stop myself. It's really hard to make decisions...

I'm worried about my son; he's having problems at school. I'm having some issues at work too. Plus, my mum was very ill last year. I just keep wondering what's going to go wrong next...

People with GAD typically attend primary care frequently, with persistent anxiety or worry about a wide range of different issues. They may often also present with physical or somatic symptoms, or worry about their health, including persistent anxiety about a coexisting chronic physical health problem. This can make it harder to make the diagnosis initially, because health professionals may focus on physical rather than emotional symptoms. It is therefore important to remain alert to the possibility of the diagnosis. Over time, and after a succession of consultations, it may become more apparent that an individual has multiple worries and that reassurance only has a temporary impact, which can then highlight the need for an assessment for an anxiety disorder such as GAD (*Box 5.3*).

Box 5.3

Tips for spotting GAD

- Consider the possibility of GAD in people who present frequently with anxiety or concerns about their health or other worries/multiple life problems
- Remember that GAD is also more common in patients with chronic physical health conditions, who may attend regularly with concerns about their condition
- Notice how you feel after seeing a particular patient – if you are experiencing feelings of anxiety yourself, this can be a clue that the patient is also highly anxious
- GAD may also be present in a patient with long-standing or recurrent depression, and anxiety may persist following treatment for low mood

---

Case example 5.1: Sebastian

How might GAD present?

Sebastian, a 28-year-old IT support technician, attends the surgery asking for a sleeping tablet to help his persistent poor sleep. His GP, Dr Long, asks for more details about what is stopping him from sleeping. He explains that he finds it very hard to get to sleep and is wakeful through the night with a racing mind. He often lies awake at night feeling agitated and tense, and "worrying about everything in my life".

Dr Long asks, "What kinds of things do you worry about?" Sebastian replies by saying: "I worry about virtually everything. I worry about money and whether I might lose my job. I keep wondering if I've made a mistake at work or upset one of my colleagues and that I will get into trouble. I also worry about my girlfriend and whether she might leave me."

Dr Long asks about physical symptoms and Sebastian describes tension in his shoulders and back, and general muscle aches. He has fatigue and exhaustion most days and is finding it hard to concentrate at work.

Dr Long asks how Sebastian reacts to the worries, and what he does to try to feel better. Sebastian says: "I try to stop myself from worrying and try to think about other things, but I can't control all these worry thoughts, they keep coming back into my mind over and over and keep me awake." He checks his work repeatedly and this is making it difficult to meet deadlines for his latest projects. Sebastian also frequently texts his girlfriend to check that everything is OK. He has been drinking more alcohol to try to help himself sleep.

Case example 5.1: *contd*

His GP uses the information given during the consultation to complete a brief CBT framework for when Sebastian is lying awake at night worrying:

Thoughts
Repeated worry thoughts such as:
- Have I made a mistake at work?
- I might get into trouble with my boss.
- What if I lose my job?
- Will I be able to pay for everything this month?
- What if my girlfriend leaves me?

Feelings
Anxious
Agitated and tense at night

Behaviour
Tries not to worry
Seeks reassurance by texting his girlfriend
Repeatedly checks his work or asks colleagues for advice
Drinks more alcohol

Physical symptoms
Poor sleep
Tension in shoulders and back
Muscle aches
Fatigue and exhaustion
Difficulty concentrating

With this history, Dr Long has identified that Sebastian's difficulty sleeping is one symptom of a more widespread anxiety disorder which involves persistent worry about a wide range of different problems. She suspects that the problem may be due to generalised anxiety disorder and goes on to carry out a more thorough assessment with this condition in mind.

5.9 Management of GAD

GAD is largely managed in the primary care setting, and GPs are likely to take a central role in coordinating care. The main goals of treatment in GAD are to improve symptoms of anxiety, restore daily functioning and prevent relapse. Treatment should follow a stepped care approach.

Making the diagnosis

As described above, it can be challenging to make a diagnosis of GAD, often because patients may present with concerns and worries about physical health problems. Some strategies for raising the subject of anxiety are shown in *Box 5.4*.

Diagnostic and screening tools
GAD-2 is a useful screening tool which involves asking two questions about anxiety symptoms over the past two weeks (see *Section 2.3*) and has high sensitivity and specificity for identifying people with GAD.

Box 5.4 | **Starting to talk about anxiety**

- Reflect back when you notice that a patient seems anxious and identify their main concerns: *"This condition seems to be worrying you a lot... What are you most concerned about?"*
- Express empathy for the distress associated with experiencing continual anxiety and worry: *"It must be difficult and exhausting to be constantly worrying about different problems..."*
- Broaden the conversation to explore whether worry is a problem in other aspects of their life: *"Do you worry about a lot of things? Do you find it hard to stop worrying? Would you describe yourself as 'a worrier'?"*
- Ask for a specific example: *"Can you give me an example of a time that you were worrying about this? What was going through your mind...?"*
- Look for the functional impact of worry: *"Is anxiety or worry about your health or other problems having a major impact on your life?"*

GAD-7 is a self-administered patient questionnaire which is highly sensitive and specific as a screening tool and severity measure for GAD (see *Section 2.3*). A score of 10 or more is suggestive of significant anxiety, and further assessment and evaluation would be recommended. The anxiety questions of the HADS can also be used to identify GAD.

What else to consider

The differential diagnosis should include physical and mental health conditions that can cause widespread anxiety and worry (see *Box 5.5*).

Box 5.5 | **Differential diagnosis for GAD**

- Health anxiety: anxiety about health features in both GAD and health anxiety; however, sufferers of GAD will also worry about a wide range of other issues, whereas in health anxiety the worry and preoccupation are localised to concerns about health and illness
- Other anxiety disorders including social phobia, panic disorder, OCD and PTSD
- Depression
- Substance misuse disorder
- Somatoform or bodily distress disorders: pervasive anxiety caused by the presence of a variety of distressing physical symptoms including chronic fatigue syndrome (CFS), chronic pain or medically unexplained symptoms (MUS)
- Underlying physical health condition mimicking anxiety or causing symptoms which lead to excessive worry (note that GAD may also coexist with a physical health condition)

Initial assessment of GAD

Initial assessment of GAD may involve ruling out physical causes of symptoms if you (the clinician) are worried, but watchful waiting may also be appropriate. If you do decide to carry out any tests, it is helpful to anticipate a negative result: *"I am checking your thyroid as occasionally this can cause similar symptoms, but I am expecting the result to be normal."*

GAD may also be present in the context of a co-morbid physical health anxiety, so try not to over-focus on physical symptoms and broaden the discussion to include emotional and psychological aspects of the problem. *"How are the symptoms affecting your life? Is worry about your health problem becoming a problem for you?"*

Initial assessment of GAD should cover the following key areas:
- The number, severity and duration of symptoms.
- The degree of distress and functional impairment.
- The presence of other mental health conditions, including anxiety disorders, depression and substance misuse.
- Ensure that any co-morbid medical conditions are optimally managed, as this is likely to improve overall functioning.
- Review any important environmental stressors which may be contributing to GAD, such as physical or emotional trauma, employment or financial worries, poor living conditions, or problems with interpersonal relationships.
- Assess the level of functional impairment – how much are symptoms interfering with the person's life and ability to carry out important activities and roles?
- Assess for suicidal intent in people with marked low mood or depression.

Exploring GAD using a CBT framework
It is often helpful to explore anxiety symptoms using a CBT framework. Some useful questions to aid in assessment of GAD are shown in *Box 5.6*.

Initial management in primary care

Explain the diagnosis
One of the most important goals for management of GAD is to explain the disorder in a way that helps the person to cope more effectively with the problem. It is often helpful to use a CBT framework to make the explanation as clear as possible.

Psychoeducation about the role of worry in GAD. Giving psychoeducation about anxiety and worry and how they affect people with GAD is also important. A key message is that having worry thoughts is not a problem per se, but it is how we respond to these negative thoughts that can cause difficulties. Conversely, offering repeated reassurance about health concerns without addressing underlying worry is unlikely to reduce anxiety and may lead to excessive and repeated presentations for further reassurance.

| Box 5.6 | **A CBT framework for assessment of GAD in primary care** |

Thoughts
- Do you have a lot of 'what if...' thoughts about future possible problems?
- Do you worry about a lot of different things?
- Is this new for you or have you always been someone who worries?
- Do you find it hard to stop worrying or to control your worries?
- Are you able to cope well when the future is uncertain?

Feelings
- How are you feeling generally?
- You seem quite anxious about this? Is it worrying you a lot?
- Do you tend to experience intense emotions?
- How is your mood? Has persistent worry led to you becoming low or demoralised about the future?

Behaviour
- Do you spend much of your time worrying?
- What do you do to try to stop yourself worrying?
- Do you often seek reassurance from others?
- Are you avoiding anything to try to stop yourself from worrying?
- Do you use alcohol or drugs to try to numb your feelings?

Physical symptoms
- Do you have any physical symptoms related to anxiety or worry (e.g. feeling exhausted, problems sleeping, headaches or muscle tension)?
- Are there any other physical health problems you are concerned about?

Environmental factors and triggers
- What's happening in your life? Are there any particular stresses at the moment? Are you well supported at home?
- How is the worry affecting your life? Does it get in the way of your day-to-day life at home or work?
- In the past, did anyone in your family tend to worry a lot?

General self-care

Regular exercise is beneficial for physical health and is associated with reduced anxiety; it is usually best initiated in small steps to avoid excessive fatigue and problems with 'boom–bust' patterns of activity which are less likely to lead to improved fitness and exercise tolerance. Reducing caffeine intake, smoking cessation, and improving sleep habits may also be beneficial.

Box 5.7	**Explaining GAD**

Negative thoughts such as worries are completely normal and happen to everyone but can become a problem if they arise too frequently, get stuck inside our head or prevent us from living a full and enjoyable life.

In GAD, people get stuck in loops of persistent worries that are out of proportion to the actual risk of the problem. The worries feel hard to control and lead to a lot of emotional distress. People with GAD often spend so much time worrying that it gets in the way of other important life activities, which can lead to low mood and reduced quality of life. Many people with GAD even worry about the fact that they worry so much!

Worry causes physical symptoms by the release of adrenaline, a chemical that prepares us for fight or flight. This makes us feel on edge, causes chest tightness, palpitations and headaches. These symptoms often trigger more worries, such as thinking: 'Could there be something serious going on?'.

Worry also affects people's behaviour. We may try to block out our worries but find we can't. We may forget to plan ways to cope with possible problems. We might seek reassurance from friends, family members and doctors, but it doesn't last, and the worries are soon back. We might avoid certain activities, restrict our lives or use alcohol and drugs to ease our distress.

Constant worrying does not make us safer! But it will make us feel on edge and exhausted, and lower our mood. There are things you can do to help you look at your worries differently and help you find better ways to deal with them. I would be happy to discuss how you might start to go about this...

Self-help books and websites

Self-help strategies can be particularly helpful for people with mild to moderate GAD. These include:

- providing written information about GAD and how it affects people
- highlighting relevant self-help books and websites based on CBT principles
- providing information about local and national support groups for anxiety
- self-help materials based on principles of CBT.

10 minute CBT strategies for primary care

10 minute CBT strategies involve brief interventions that can be used by GPs and other primary care health professionals to encourage positive self-management and reduce unhelpful ways of coping with anxiety symptoms in GAD.

Behavioural strategies. Some of the most practical and useful 10 minute CBT strategies involve making small changes in behaviour that are aimed at breaking vicious cycles of anxiety, as well as increasing the time spent carrying out valued and meaningful activities, which is likely to lead to an improvement in mood and wellbeing. Useful behavioural strategies are covered in detail in *Chapter 3*, and include:

- activity scheduling and behavioural activation, particularly in long-standing GAD associated with low mood and marked restriction of daily activities
- reduction of unhelpful anxiety behaviours such as excessive checking, reassurance seeking or searching for information about health concerns on the internet
- brief graded exposure to situations that are being avoided due to anxiety.

Managing worries – the 'worry tree'. The 'worry tree' provides a series of simple steps for coping when worries arise (*Figure 5.2*). Changing the focus of attention involves choosing an engaging activity to carry out instead of worrying. When anxiety levels are high, a distraction activity (see *Chapter 3*) may be helpful. Choosing activities that are valued and meaningful to the individual is also important.

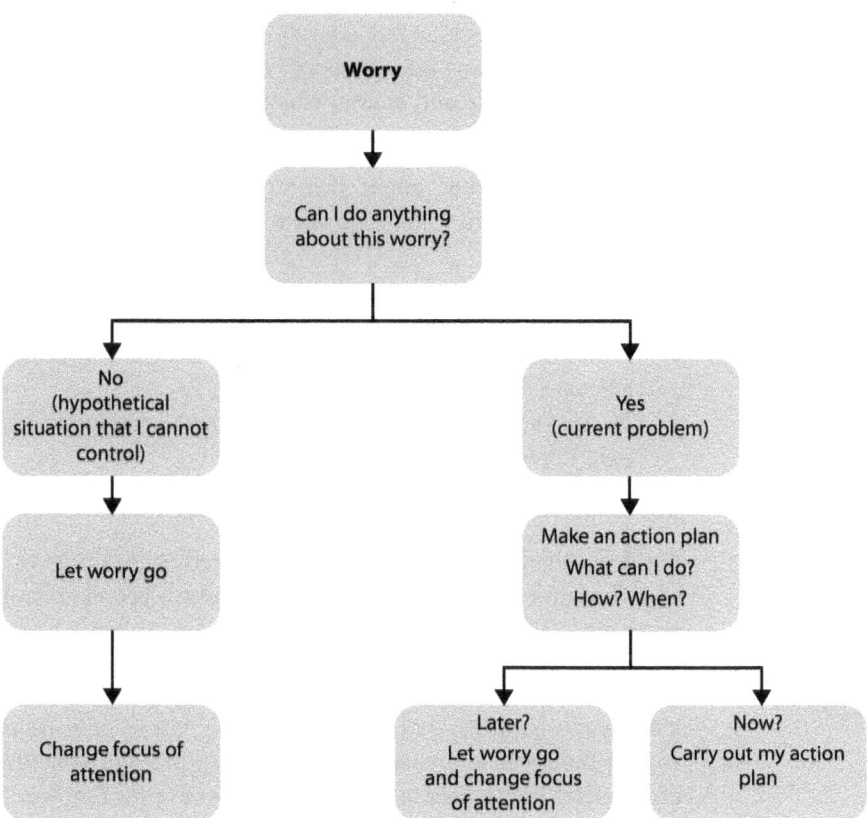

Figure 5.2 The worry tree.

Postpone worry – 'worry time'. Encourage patients with GAD to confine their worrying to a set daily 'worry time' (*Box 5.8*). Postponing worry is different from trying to suppress worry thoughts, and involves recognising that it is normal and natural for negative or 'what if...?' worry thoughts to pop into the mind, but that it is not necessary to 'chase' or engage with the thought when it arises.

Reframing the role of worry

Reframing the role of worry involves discussing alternative beliefs about worry such as: *"Worry does not help protect me but simply uses a lot of my time and generates negative emotion."* This process could include:

- re-evaluation: *"what is the real risk of bad events?"*
- reframing: *"will this matter to me in a month or a year's time?"*
- taking a wider perspective: *"I do not have control over most events but can still live a meaningful life."*

Coping with uncertainty. In GAD, patients use worrying as a strategy to prepare for the worst and to predict and plan for problems. This leads to a reduction in the sense of uncertainty or unpredictability about the world and can temporarily make the anxious person feel safer. However, the reality is that worrying does not actually make life any safer or reduce the risk that something bad might happen. It simply uses time and energy which could be better used on meaningful or valued life activities.

Some questions that might help to prompt a discussion that encourages individuals to begin to develop their ability to cope with uncertainty (see also *Box 4.10*) include:

- *"Is it possible to be certain of everything in life?"*
- *"What are the pros and cons of trying to be certain about everything?"*
- *"Is the amount of time you spend trying to be certain about things the best use of your time?"*
- *"Do you know anyone who is able to cope with uncertainty about things? What might you learn from them?"*

Use of the 'ABLE' method of managing uncertainty is covered in *Chapter 4*.

Problem-solving. Patients with GAD often lack skills in problem-solving, and consequently get stuck worrying about a problem rather than planning strategies for overcoming it. Feeling more able to understand and cope with problems will lead to an increased sense of control over the world, and reduced anxiety. This may involve simply switching focus from *"What if the worst happens...?"* thoughts towards *"Then what would I do to cope...?"* coping thoughts. A structured approach to problem-solving involves a series of practical steps (*Box 5.9*). See also *Chapter 4* for further information about problem-solving.

Box 5.8

Postponing worries – setting a daily 'worry time'

Choose a dedicated 15–30 minutes for worrying each day, ideally at the same time and in the same place. Try to avoid doing this just before bedtime. When a worry arises outside of the planned worry time, simply tell yourself: *"It's OK to have this worry, but I'm going to put off thinking about it until my worry time."*

It may be helpful to carry a notebook to quickly write down the worry thought and then close the book until worry time. Don't be concerned if the same thought pops back again very quickly – this is common and to be expected in GAD. Simply repeat the same process: accept the thought, write it down and then park it for later.

During worry time, you can review your list of worries. It is not necessary to think about particular worries if they are no longer an issue – simply cross them off the list. Try to include some problem-solving ideas. Ask yourself: *"Is there anything I can do to help this situation?"*

At the end of worry time, try to move quickly on to another activity that is likely to lift your mood, such as exercise, listening to music or calling a friend.

Box 5.9

Steps in structured problem-solving

1. Identify the problem
2. Brainstorm a list of possible solutions and their pros and cons
3. Choose one solution to try first and break it down into smaller steps
4. Plan how to cope with any difficulties that might arise when carrying out this solution
5. Try out the solution and review the outcome
6. Decide what the next step should be and repeat the process

Treatment in primary care

If an individual with GAD has marked functional impairment or does not improve with self-management, the next step is to offer psychological therapy or drug treatment. In GAD, both approaches appear to be equally effective. The choice of first-line treatment should consider a number of factors including:

- patient preference
- local availability and waiting lists for psychological therapy
- previous response to treatment
- co-morbid physical and mental health conditions.

Drug treatment

First-line drug treatment for GAD is with an SSRI. NICE recommends sertraline first-line but acknowledges that this is an unlicensed use. SSRIs which are licensed for the treatment of GAD in the UK are escitalopram and paroxetine. If the first choice of SSRI is ineffective, then it is recommended to offer an alternative SSRI or an SNRI such as venlafaxine. Duloxetine, although not mentioned by NICE, is licensed for the treatment of GAD.

Pregabalin is also an option for treatment of GAD, and it may have an earlier onset effect than antidepressants. Side-effects include dizziness and drowsiness, and discontinuation symptoms may arise. There are some reports of pregabalin abuse, and it should be avoided in people with a history of drug misuse or addiction.

If the condition does not respond to the first-line drug treatment, the individual can be offered either a psychological intervention or an alternative medication as recommended above. If the condition partially responds to a drug treatment, it may be beneficial to combine drug and psychological approaches.

Initiation and monitoring of drug therapy should follow recommended guidelines, which are summarised in *Chapter 3*.

Drug treatments to avoid in GAD. Avoid use of benzodiazepines except as a short-term measure (maximum 10–14 days) during crises. Similarly, beta blockers and MAOIs are not usually considered appropriate options for GAD. Antipsychotics should also be avoided.

Psychological therapy

Low intensity psychological therapy. This may be offered to people with mild to moderate GAD. It typically involves either:

- individual guided self-help supported by a trained practitioner, using written or electronic materials; this usually consists of five to seven weekly or fortnightly face-to-face or telephone sessions, each lasting 20–30 minutes
- CBT-based psycho-educational groups facilitated by trained practitioners. These usually have a group size of no larger than 12 participants per practitioner and involve around six weekly 2-hour sessions.

Intensive psychological therapy. The most effective psychological treatment for moderate to severe GAD involves individual, high intensity CBT or applied relaxation (see *Box 5.10*). CBT is as effective as medication, but with a reduced risk of relapse after treatment is discontinued. The optimum duration of CBT in GAD is 16–20 sessions lasting around 1 hour, which reflects the long-standing nature of the condition.

CBT enables individuals to reduce the behaviour of worrying and find new strategies to manage their anxiety, cope with life stressors, and manage any distressing anxiety-related physical symptoms. As individuals undergo CBT therapy, they begin to recognise that:

- they cannot control their fears, but can control how they respond to their fears

Box 5.10	**Psychological approaches used in GAD**

Psychoeducation	Understanding the CBT model for GAD; learning to recognise worry thinking and the vicious cycle of anxiety associated with attempts at thought control or avoidance.
Worry exposure	Patients mentally expose themselves to worry by thinking about the feared events; for example, by bringing to mind a thought or image relating to the most feared expectation and focusing on this for a prolonged period of around 25 minutes. This leads to both habituation to the feared image, with a reduction in associated anxiety, and contributes to changing the perceived meaning of the feared situation. This may be one of the most important and effective aspects of CBT.
Reducing avoidance and other behavioural interventions	Strategies aimed at reducing unhelpful anxiety-related behaviours which act to maintain and worsen anxiety as a vicious cycle, including situational avoidance, checking, reassurance-seeking and excessive planning.
Behavioural activation	Structured approach to progressively increase time spent each day in carrying out valued, meaningful and important life activities, including increasing social interaction, physical activity and participation in enjoyable activities such as hobbies.
Applied relaxation	Developing skills in self-monitoring and early recognition of anxiety symptoms, along with skills in cue-controlled muscle relaxion that are carried out during 'real life' anxiety-provoking situations.
Structured problem-solving	Developing skills in coping with life problems can reduce anxiety and increase a sense of self-efficacy and control over life.
Cognitive restructuring	Looking for balanced alternative perspectives for worry thoughts and beliefs about worry.
Meta-cognitive therapy and learning to manage uncertainty	Identifying and challenging positive and negative beliefs about worry (type 2 worries) and learning new and more effective ways of relating to negative thoughts, including coping with uncertainty.
Mindfulness and acceptance strategies	Using mindfulness practices and meditation to adopt a more accepting relationship with cognitions and experience, allowing disengagement from worry thoughts without directly trying to challenge or change them.

- persistent worrying offers no protective value and does not help to manage potentially negative future problems
- worry reinforces negative thinking and leads to an increase in anxiety over time
- they are able to cope with whatever future challenges come their way.

Applied relaxation teaches the patient how to relax rapidly during anxiety-provoking situations and should be differentiated from general relaxation. It typically involves 12–15 weekly sessions. It appears to be as effective as CBT although the evidence base is currently less robust than for CBT.

Mindfulness-based interventions may also be effective and are associated with a reduction in symptoms of anxiety and co-morbid depressive symptoms. These are typically offered in a group format with eight weekly sessions lasting around 2.5 hours and often an additional extended practice session lasting up to a full day.

When to refer

Refer to specialist mental health services if there is severe, complex or treatment-refractory GAD associated with marked functional impairment, or when there are concerns about risk such as self-neglect or a high risk of self-harm. It may also be important to refer if there is significant co-morbidity such as substance misuse, personality disorder or complex physical health problems.

Treatments that may be offered at this stage include:
- involvement of multi-agency teams, including crisis intervention, outpatient and inpatient care when appropriate
- optimisation of drug therapy
- high intensity psychological treatment.

Combining treatment approaches, including psychological and drug treatments, may be considered, although evidence for the effectiveness of this approach is lacking. Combination treatments should be undertaken only by practitioners with expertise in the psychological and drug treatment of complex anxiety disorders that are refractory to treatment.

Summary of primary care management of GAD

Stepped care approach	What to offer	What does this involve?
Initial presentations of mild to moderate anxiety	General self-care	Offer advice about general self-care including regular, graded exercise and sleep hygiene
	10 minute CBT advice about managing anxiety	• Explain the diagnosis of GAD using a CBT framework, including how thoughts, feelings and behaviour can cause vicious cycles in anxiety • Give explanations for the patient's specific distressing physical and somatic symptoms • Use activity scheduling and brief behavioural activation to increase participation in meaningful and important life activities • Encourage a reduction in unhelpful anxiety behaviours such as excessive checking, reassurance seeking or internet health-checking behaviour • Use a 'worry tree', 'worry time', distraction and problem-solving to help cope with worry symptoms
	Signpost to self-help resources	Provide information about CBT-based books and websites for understanding and managing anxiety
Moderate anxiety or lack of response to initial measures	The choice between psychological intervention or drug treatment should be guided by the person's preference (no evidence that either approach is more effective for GAD)	
	Refer for primary care psychological therapy	• Less severe cases: low intensity CBT involving guided self-help or group-based CBT • More severe cases (marked functional impairment or lack of response to other treatments): individual, high intensity longer-term (16–20 sessions) CBT or applied relaxation
	Pharmacological treatment	• First-line drug treatment for GAD is with an SSRI. NICE recommends that sertraline is most cost-effective (although unlicensed for GAD); continue drug treatments for at least 1 year due to high risk of relapse • If an SSRI is ineffective, consider trying an alternative SSRI or switch to an SNRI • Consider pregabalin third-line • Avoid use of benzodiazepines (except short-term during a crisis)
Severe or complex problem or lack of response to primary care treatment	Refer to specialist services	• Refer to specialist services if severe or complex GAD with marked functional impairment or if there are concerns about risk such as self-neglect or self-harm • Also refer if there is significant co-morbidity such as substance misuse, personality disorder or complex physical health problem • Also refer patients with persistent and marked symptoms who have not responded to primary care treatment strategies

5.10 Monitoring and follow-up

Because of the high risk of relapse and chronicity of GAD, long-term support and education are frequently required in primary care. It is sometimes helpful to use a questionnaire such as GAD-7 to monitor outcomes and pick up relapses at an early stage. This can be printed out in advance, enabling the patient to complete the form at home prior to the GP appointment.

When commencing medication for GAD, patients should be reviewed every 2–4 weeks for the first 3 months and around 3-monthly thereafter. Drug treatments should be continued for at least 1 year due to the high risk of relapse following treatment.

Case example 5.2: Anita

Diagnosis and management of GAD

Anita is 42 years old and is married with two children. She attends her GP surgery frequently for a variety of symptoms including abdominal pain and bloating, headaches, muscle pains and poor sleep. She has been seen for these problems by many different GPs and has been given diagnoses of irritable bowel syndrome and tension-type headaches. She takes occasional paracetamol for headaches, but no other medications. She attends the surgery again sounding agitated and distressed, saying, "I can't cope with all these symptoms. I'm so worried about everything. I've been coming to the surgery for such a long time, and no one seems to take me seriously."

Anita tells her GP, Dr Tan, that she is currently very anxious about her physical health. She worries that the symptoms haven't gone away and sometimes wonders if they are due to a more serious problem such as cancer. She also discloses that she worries about a wide range of other problems. Her job as a school secretary is busy and stressful, and she has an unsupportive line manager. She says that she has always been 'a bit of a worrier' but things have got a lot worse over the past year since her husband was made redundant. He has now found another job, but Anita has found it difficult to recover from the extra financial stress. Her sleep is poor. She finds it hard to drop off at night due to a 'racing mind' and is very restless and wakeful throughout the night. Over the past few months, she has found it increasingly difficult to stop worrying, and sometimes fears that the worries "will make me even more ill". Lately, it has become harder to concentrate at work because she gets preoccupied and finds it hard to "switch my mind off once it gets going". Because of her concerns about her physical symptoms and her fatigue, she has stopped going to her regular exercise class and has cut back on seeing friends.

Case example 5.2: *contd*

Dr Tan uses a CBT framework to help provide some structure when exploring Anita's experiences:

Thoughts
I can't cope with the symptoms
No-one is taking me seriously
Maybe the symptoms are due to
    something serious like cancer
The worries might make me even
    more ill
Racing mind and constant worry

Feelings
Anxious
Distressed

Behaviour
Stopped going to exercise class
Not seeing friends

Physical symptoms
Tummy pain and bloating
Headaches
Muscle pains
Poor sleep, restless
Hard to concentrate

Environmental factors
Work as a school secretary is stressful and line manager is unsupportive
Husband was made redundant – causing financial stress

Dr Tan asks Anita to complete a GAD-7 questionnaire to assess her anxiety symptoms, which reveals a score of 13, and is consistent with moderate anxiety. She shares the result with Anita and asks for her perspective on whether anxiety could be part of the problem. She reassures Anita that discussing anxiety does not mean that she will now ignore Anita's physical health, but that anxiety may be having a major impact on Anita's quality of life. They discuss the features of generalised anxiety disorder and Anita is surprised to discover that she does recognise many of the common features of GAD. "I thought I was going mad," she says. "It helps to understand what's happening to me."

They discuss the treatment options. Anita prefers to avoid medication at this stage and decides to self-refer to the local psychological therapies service. Whilst on the waiting list for therapy, Dr Tan recommends several websites and leaflets to help her understand more about GAD and how to cope with anxiety. In particular, the GP uses brief behavioural activation to encourage Anita to restart important activities such as her exercise class and seeing her friends, which has a marked impact on improving her low mood.

Case example 5.3: Joseph

Diagnosis and management of GAD

Joseph is 35 years old and works in a bank. He attends his GP surgery regularly with multiple symptoms including headache, 'shooting pains' in his chest and low back pain. He also experiences epigastric discomfort, fatigue and irritability. Investigation of his physical symptoms has revealed nothing of concern, but the symptoms have persisted. Joseph has tried over-the-counter remedies for his symptoms including herbal tablets for sleep and vitamins to boost his energy levels, but nothing has helped. His symptoms are starting to affect his work and family life.

During the consultation, Joseph admits that he has been increasingly worried over the past few years. In particular, he spends a lot of time worrying about work, finding it hard to stop thinking about the possibility of losing his job. He often lies awake at night thinking about this. This started a few years ago after several of his colleagues were made redundant. Things have been even worse over the past 9 months after his wife developed a breast lump. This was found to be benign, but since then he has become increasingly preoccupied about the health of his family. At the time of his wife's health problems, Joseph's own physical symptoms of headaches, chest pain, back pain and fatigue became a lot worse, and he now finds it difficult to engage in normal family activities with his wife and children, due to both physical discomfort and worrying.

During the consultation, Joseph remains quite preoccupied with his health and the possibility of having a serious illness, and returns to this question on a number of occasions. His GP agrees to carry out a thorough physical and mental health assessment and takes time to listen to his concerns, taking a thorough history for each physical symptom, with appropriate examination. She also assesses his mood and asks about suicidal thoughts. They agree to carry out some initial blood tests, although the GP tells Joseph that she is expecting the results are likely to be negative, and that she believes many of his symptoms may also relate to anxiety. She gives him a GAD-7 questionnaire to complete and asks him to fill it in and return to see her with the results of the investigations.

When Joseph returns to see his GP, the initial test results are all normal. His GAD-7 score is 16, which indicates severe anxiety. His GP explains that she believes his symptoms are arising from a condition known as GAD and discusses it with him, giving him a leaflet to look at after the consultation is finished. He acknowledges that he has a lot of anxiety and worry but also remains concerned about his health. The GP agrees to continue to monitor his physical health, but suggests that they could also treat his anxiety at the same time. They discuss options and he is keen to start treatment straight away, rather than waiting for referral for psychological therapy. They talk through the option of medication in detail and the GP agrees to start a prescription of an SSRI medication and review Joseph the following week. She also recommends several self-help resources to understand and manage anxiety and worry using CBT, and strongly encourages Joseph to re-engage in important family activities as much as possible. She also gives him information about sleep hygiene and mindfulness to try to improve his sleep patterns.

At the first review appointment, Joseph reports that his anxiety appears to have worsened slightly with SSRI treatment, which had been explained might happen, so he was willing to continue taking it for another week. Over the next 6 weeks, his anxiety gradually started to improve. A repeat GAD-7 after 3 months of therapy had reduced to 9, which is in the normal range. He continued medication for a further 18 months before reducing the dose gradually with a view to weaning off.

5.11 Summary and key points

- GAD is the most common anxiety disorder in primary care but it can be difficult to recognise in practice.
- Frequent attendance at GP surgeries and experiencing multiple physical symptoms may both be a sign of underlying GAD.
- GAD is also more common in people with coexisting chronic physical health conditions.
- Characteristic features of GAD include persistent and uncontrollable worry about a wide range of everyday situations.
- Somatic symptoms such as muscle tension, restlessness and poor sleep and difficulty concentrating are common.
- Features of the CBT model of GAD:
  - repetitive chains of negative thoughts about possible future problems and often also about the dangers of worry itself
  - lack of positive action or attempts to resolve the difficulty
  - intolerance of uncertainty and fear of the unknown
  - experiencing emotions more intensely than others
  - behavioural reactions are designed to avoid, suppress or control worry thoughts, but typically act to reinforce and worsen anxiety over time.
- Appropriate screening tools for GAD include GAD-7 and HADS questionnaires.
- Giving psychoeducation, which explains what worry is and how it affects people with GAD, is a very important role for GPs in primary care.
- Self-help strategies for GAD include behavioural activation, postponing worries using a daily 'worry time', using a 'worry tree' to deal with worries, problem-solving strategies and mindfulness.
- Psychological treatment for GAD is with CBT or applied relaxation; mindfulness may also be helpful for some individuals.
- Drug treatment involves an SSRI first-line; alternatively an SNRI or pregabalin may be considered, and should be continued for at least a year due to the high risk of relapse.

5.12 GAD resources

- Centre for Clinical Interventions information on generalised anxiety and worry: www.cci.health.wa.gov.au/Resources/For-Clinicians/Generalised-Anxiety-and-Worry
- Northumberland, Tyne & Wear NHS Foundation Trust self-help leaflet on anxiety: https://web.ntw.nhs.uk/selfhelp/leaflets/Anxiety%20A4%20 2016%20FINAL.pdf
- Kennerley, H. (2014) *Overcoming Anxiety*, 2nd edition. Robinson.
- Meares, K. and Freeston, M. (2015) *Overcoming Worry and Generalised Anxiety Disorder*, 2nd edition. Robinson.

Chapter 6
Panic disorder

Panic disorder quick reference guide

What is panic disorder?	Recurrent, short-lived episodes of intense fear or anxiety which arise unexpectedly and are associated with intense physical symptoms including palpitations, breathlessness and chest pain or tightness. Catastrophic misinterpretations of bodily symptoms, such as thoughts about having a heart attack or suffocation, lead to rapidly escalating anxiety symptoms as a vicious cycle.
How common is it?	Prevalence is 1.7% in the UK. Panic disorder affects around 7% of patients attending primary care.
Risk factors	More common in women, in people with a family history of panic disorder and with coexisting physical health conditions causing cardiac and gastrointestinal symptoms. Panic attacks may also be triggered by stressful life events.
Co-morbid conditions	Panic disorder commonly occurs in association with other anxiety disorders, depression, suicidal behaviour and substance use disorders, including nicotine dependence. Around one-third of people with panic disorder also have agoraphobia. It is also associated with chronic physical health conditions including mitral valve prolapse, migraine and hypertension.
Usual course	Typically begins with occasional panic attacks which gradually increase in frequency and eventually lead to a pattern of recurrent anxiety and widespread avoidance. It is particularly likely to become a chronic and relapsing condition when associated with agoraphobia.
Common presentations	Patients with panic disorder may be high users of health services and may present in primary care and emergency settings with severe somatic symptoms such as chest pain, which mimic those of serious physical illness and may lead to the disorder being unrecognised.
How to make the diagnosis	Diagnosis in primary care is largely clinical. Screening with GAD-2 questions does not specifically ask about symptoms of panic but may also identify people with panic disorder.
What else could it be?	Where appropriate, rule out underlying physical causes for symptoms of panic, including side-effects of prescribed medication. Routine physical investigation is not required if there is a typical history of panic disorder. The differential diagnosis also includes other anxiety disorders such as social anxiety and PTSD, or substance misuse.

Self-management strategies	Provide clear and accurate explanations of an individual's feared symptoms that arise during a panic attack. Use graded exposure, breathing techniques to reduce hyperventilation and distraction to manage panic symptoms.
Treatment of panic disorder	First-line treatment is with 7–14 sessions of individual CBT, which is more effective than drug therapy. Guided self-help may be offered in mild–moderate cases. SSRIs are first-line choice of medication.
When to refer	Refer to specialist mental health services if the person continues to experience significant symptoms after treatment with two interventions (any combination of psychological intervention, medication or bibliotherapy).
Risk of relapse	Relapse rates after stopping medication are between 55% and 77% but may be reduced in patients with chronic or relapsing symptoms using maintenance therapy. Relapse rates are lower after CBT.
Follow-up	Chronic relapsing cases will require long-term follow-up and monitoring. Drug therapy should be continued for 6–12 months, after which the dose can be tapered.

CBT framework for panic disorder

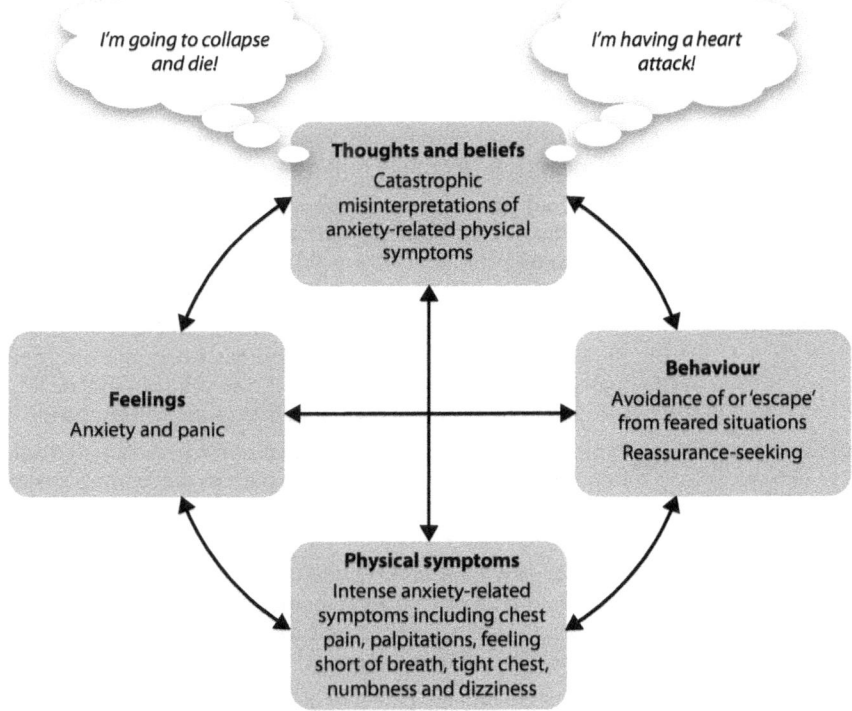

6.1 Introduction

Panic disorder is common and can be a severe and disabling illness which involves repeated, short-lived and sudden bursts of intense fear and anxiety, which are highly distressing. Patients with panic disorder have a high use of medical services, an impaired social and work life, and a reduced quality of life overall.

They may present to primary care or emergency services with somatic symptoms that can be extremely severe and mimic those of serious physical illness.

6.2 What is panic disorder?

Panic disorder is characterised by recurring, unpredictable panic attacks, usually associated with worry about having another attack, and a significant change in behaviour related to the episodes. The first panic attack may be associated with a stressful situation or experience, but gradually the attacks become dissociated and occur 'out of the blue'.

A panic attack is defined as a discrete episode of intense subjective fear. The symptoms arise rapidly and usually peak within 10 minutes and can last for 20–40 minutes but will rarely persist beyond one hour. Patients often develop a fear of experiencing further panic attacks. During a panic attack, sufferers experience intense anxiety-related physical symptoms such as chest pain and tightness, rapid heart rate, hyperventilation, sweating, shaking and gastrointestinal symptoms.

Around two-thirds of patients with panic disorder also experience agoraphobia, defined as fear in places or situations from which escape might be difficult, such as in crowded shops or trains (see *Chapter 7*). Experiencing panic attacks without meeting the ICD-10 criteria for panic disorder (*Box 6.1*) is also common, but these attacks can still have a significant effect on quality of life and ability to function in daily life.

Box 6.1

Diagnostic criteria for panic disorder

Panic attacks:
- Discrete episodes of intense fear
- Episodes arise rapidly and peak within 10 minutes, usually lasing for around 20–40 minutes
- Accompanied by intense anxiety-related physical symptoms such as palpitations, chest pain, sweating, trembling, shortness of breath, dry mouth, numbness, dizziness or light-headedness
- Associated with catastrophic fears, such as choking, having a heart attack or imminent death

Panic disorder:
- Recurrent panic attacks which arise unpredictably or 'out of the blue' without a specific trigger
- Persistent fear of having another panic attack leads to marked avoidance behaviour
- Significant impairment in important areas of functioning
- Symptoms are not caused by substance misuse, medical conditions or other psychiatric disorders

6.3 Epidemiology

Panic disorder has a prevalence of approximately 1.7% in the UK and affects about 7% of patients attending primary care. Panic attacks are even more common, and as many as 13% of the population are likely to experience a panic attack at some stage in their life.

The prevalence of panic disorder is also affected by the presence or absence of agoraphobic symptoms (see *Box 6.2*).

Panic disorder most commonly develops in the third decade, although it may develop at any time of life. It is 2–3 times more common in women than in men. It is also more common in patients presenting with cardiac and gastrointestinal symptoms. In the USA, up to 25% of patients presenting to emergency departments with chest pain may meet criteria for panic disorder.

Box 6.2	Prevalence of panic disorder with and without agoraphobia		
		12-month prevalence	Lifetime prevalence
	Panic disorder without agoraphobia	1.5%	4%
	Panic disorder with agoraphobia	0.5%	1%

6.4 Aetiology

Panic disorder is 2–3 times more common in women. Factors that may be associated with its development include:
- genetic factors: the risk of panic disorder increases around 5-fold among first-degree relatives, and twin studies suggest a strong familial component
- biochemical theories: these involve a possible abnormality of neurotransmitter function leading to increased sensitivity of the autonomic nervous system in response to stress
- environment: major life events or life stresses increase background anxiety and may trigger the onset of panic attacks
- physical health conditions: panic disorder is more common in patients presenting with cardiac and gastrointestinal symptoms.

6.5 CBT model of panic disorder

In a CBT model, panic attacks are viewed as spiralling levels of anxiety associated with catastrophic misinterpretations of harmless, often anxiety-related, bodily symptoms (*Box 6.3*). The patient incorrectly interprets these

Box 6.3

Catastrophic misinterpretations in panic disorder

Physiological change	Physical symptom experienced by patient	Examples of catastrophic thoughts and fears	Examples of associated 'safety behaviour'
Rapid heart rate Muscle tension in chest wall	Palpitations and muscular chest pain	*Maybe I'm having a heart attack* *I'm going to collapse and die!*	Resting to avoid heart rate getting faster Calling an ambulance or presenting to A&E
Hyperventilation	Feeling short of breath, chest feels tight Tingling around mouth and in hands Light-headed and dizzy	*I can't get enough air. I'm going to suffocate!* *I'm going to collapse or faint!* *Maybe I'm having a stroke!*	Trying to take deeper breaths, leading to worsened tightness and discomfort
Reduced saliva production	Dry mouth and tightness in throat; globus	*I've got a lump in my throat* *I'm choking!*	Repeated swallowing as a checking behaviour (makes it even harder to swallow)
Reduced concentration	Racing thoughts, forgetfulness	*I'm losing control* *Maybe I'm going crazy*	Attempts to control thoughts Avoiding challenging tasks Escape from a situation whenever anxiety arises (leads to reduced confidence and limits daily function)
Anticipation and fear of panic attacks	Increased background anxiety levels General sense of apprehension and fear	*I'm terrified of having another panic attack* *I must try not to get anxious!* *I might make a fool of myself in public*	Trying to mentally suppress fears (leads to paradoxical increase in worry thoughts) Avoidance of public places or only going with someone with whom we feel safe

physical experiences as indicating imminent disaster such as a heart attack, suffocation or going mad. The anxiety that develops in response to these fears results in further symptoms, such as an increasingly rapid heartbeat, dizziness or difficulty concentrating, which are further misinterpreted, rapidly increasing anxiety as a vicious cycle.

Behavioural reactions to feelings of anxiety and panic act to further reinforce fears and compound the problem over time (*Figure 6.1*). Typical behaviour associated with panic disorder includes avoidance of or 'escape' from feared situations and reassurance-seeking. 'Safety behaviours' designed to protect the person from their most feared outcome include sitting near exits in public places, avoiding exercise, staying near other people or opening the window to 'get more air'.

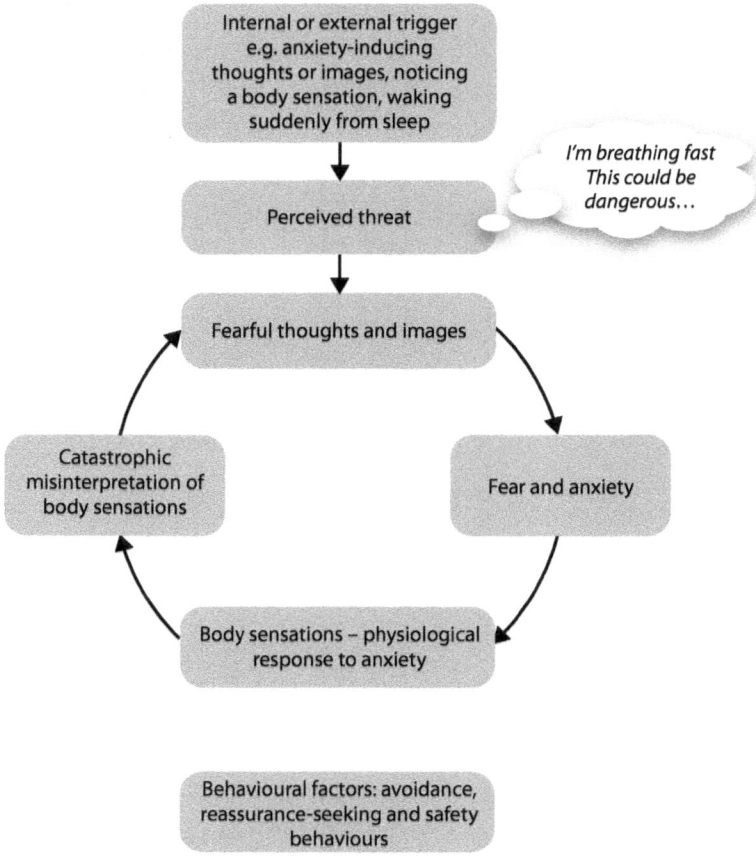

Figure 6.1 CBT model of panic disorder.

6.6 Co-morbidity

Mental health conditions

Panic disorder is highly co-morbid with other anxiety, mood and substance use disorders, including nicotine dependence. There is a significant association with depression, with lifetime prevalence rates as high as 50–60%. There also appears to be a higher risk of suicide attempts than in the general population.

Around one-third of people with panic disorder have coexistent agoraphobia. This is more common in women and is associated with greater severity and a chronic relapsing course with poorer outcomes from therapy. Social anxiety disorder may also coexist and is diagnosed where the situations avoided are predominantly social and interactive in nature (see *Chapter 9*).

Physical health conditions

Panic disorder is also associated with chronic medical conditions including mitral valve prolapse, migraine and hypertension, although the cause of the association is not yet clear. It can also coexist with independent physical disorders, which may complicate the clinical picture, especially where these disorders affect cardiac or respiratory function.

6.7 Course and prognosis of panic disorder

Panic disorder typically begins with occasional panic attacks which gradually increase in frequency and eventually lead to a pattern of recurrent anxiety and widespread avoidance. In the longer term, panic disorder can become a chronic and relapsing condition, particularly when associated with agoraphobia.

CBT and antidepressant medication are both effective for panic disorder, although some individuals with good initial treatment responses may develop recurrent symptoms following remission. This may be higher amongst people with marked agoraphobic avoidance. Rates of relapse of panic disorder after stopping medication are estimated to be between 55% and 77%. Relapse may be lower after successful completion of CBT, particularly if people are offered maintenance therapy.

6.8 Presentation of panic disorder

Patients with panic disorder may present with anxiety or with physical symptoms that arise as part of a panic attack. They may be high users of health services with frequent attendances in primary care and emergency settings with severe somatic symptoms, such as chest pain, which mimic those of serious physical illness, and this may lead to the disorder being unrecognised.

> *I've got this terrible chest pain and a tight chest – I think I'm having a heart attack!*

> *I've got a difficult boss and now I'm struggling to go to work. I keep feeling dizzy as if I'm about to pass out in meetings…*

> *I keep getting a tight chest. It's really scary and comes on out of the blue. Could it be my asthma?*

Panic attacks which arise unexpectedly and without any obvious triggering situation or event are characteristic of panic disorder without agoraphobia. Those that arise in a predictable way as a follow-on to a given anxiety-provoking situation or event usually reflect a phobia, such as agoraphobia or social phobia.

Case example 6.1: Nisha

How might panic disorder present?

Nisha, a 22-year-old first-year university student, attends the surgery. She describes waking in the middle of the night with a pounding heart, hot flushes and difficulty breathing. The episode came on suddenly and unexpectedly, and the symptoms subsided after a few minutes. Over the last few months, she has been feeling more anxious and has experienced similar episodes in the daytime, at varying levels of intensity. As she approaches her end of year exams, the episodes have become more common and more severe. She is now worried that she might be on the verge of a "nervous breakdown" and describes being overly aware of her "fast breathing and pounding heart".

Her greatest fear during the episode was that she was about to suffocate and collapse, because her chest felt so tight. She has been avoiding going to lectures and has been staying with her boyfriend due to increasing fears about sleeping alone. Her university studies have been suffering and it has been harder than usual to concentrate on her work. She also admits to sometimes drinking excessive alcohol to try to prevent the episodes at night.

Her GP uses the information that Nisha gives during the consultation to complete a brief CBT framework for Nisha's experience during a recent panic attack:

Case example 6.1: *contd*

Thoughts
Am I having a nervous breakdown?
I'm going to suffocate or collapse

Feelings
Anxious and panicky

Behaviour
Avoiding going to lectures
Staying with boyfriend to avoid
being alone
Drinking excess alcohol

Physical symptoms
Difficulty breathing
Tight chest
Pounding heart
Hot flushes
Difficulty concentrating

With this history, Nisha's GP strongly suspects that the episodes are due to panic disorder and goes on to carry out a more thorough assessment with this condition in mind.

6.9 Management of panic disorder

GP management of panic disorder begins with recognition and an initial assessment of the condition. The role also includes the provision of support and information, and in collaboratively making initial decisions about management. This may include providing advice about lifestyle changes, making decisions about prescribing medication, and making referrals for psychological interventions or specialist services. A stepped care approach to management is often recommended.

Making the diagnosis

Screening and diagnostic tools

NICE guidelines suggest that there is insufficient evidence to recommend any screening tool for the diagnosis of panic disorder and recommend that clinicians rely largely on consultation skills to elicit the key information.

For screening, use of the two GAD-2 questions may help to identify patients with panic disorder (see *Chapter 2*). GAD-7 was designed for assessment of generalised anxiety disorder but there is evidence that it is also sensitive in detecting panic-related symptoms and could be used as part of a broader assessment of anxiety. However, it does not specifically ask about panic symptoms.

The Panic Disorder Severity Scale (PDSS) is a 7-item measure assessing the frequency, avoidance, degree of distress, and functional impairment of panic attacks but is relatively long to complete in the primary care setting.

Discussing panic symptoms

Some patients with panic disorder will be aware that their symptoms are likely to be due to anxiety. Others will present with somatic symptoms that they fear are due to an underlying physical health condition and may be more resistant to accepting the diagnosis of panic disorder. Some useful questions for asking about anxiety in patients presenting with somatic symptoms are shown in *Box 6.4*.

Ruling out underlying physical causes

An important role of primary care is to look for underlying physical causes for symptoms of panic. This might include ruling out hyperthyroidism and investigation of physical symptoms such as chest pain, palpitations, dizziness or shortness of breath.

Many drugs can also trigger panic attacks, including prescribed medication such as SSRIs, or withdrawal from medication such as benzodiazepines or zopiclone, or withdrawal from alcohol, or even just caffeine and nicotine. Illegal substances, particularly stimulants, can also be associated with panic symptoms.

Whilst it is important not to miss likely physical causes, it is not necessary to routinely investigate or refer a patient presenting with typical symptoms of panic

---

Box 6.4 **Starting to talk about panic attacks**

- Reflect back when you notice that a patient seems anxious or panicky about their symptoms: *"This symptom seems to be worrying you a lot…"*
- Identify which symptom(s) are giving rise to high levels of anxiety: *"Which is the most severe symptom or the one that worries you the most…?"*
- Ask for a specific example: *"Can you give me an example of a time that you started to feel tight in your chest? Where were you and what were you doing?"*
- Identify the person's fears and health beliefs at the time of a panic attack: *"What went through your mind when you were experiencing the chest pain? What was the worst thing that it might be?"*
- Tentatively explore whether they had considered the possibility of anxiety: *"Do you think that anxiety or panic might be a cause of your symptoms? How do you feel about this possibility?"*
- Ask about avoidance and the functional impact of panic attacks: *"How much are the symptoms affecting your life? Are you avoiding any situations to stop yourself getting them?"*

disorder. Over-investigation or unnecessary referrals can make it difficult for patients with panic disorder to accept an emotional disorder as an explanation for their symptoms.

What else to consider

The differential diagnosis should include physical and mental health conditions that can cause acute episodes of anxiety or symptoms which mimic anxiety (*Box 6.5*).

Initial assessment

The initial assessment should explore the nature and frequency of the panic attacks, whether they are spontaneous or associated with specific triggers and whether agoraphobia has developed. Asking questions using a CBT framework can be very helpful when later explaining the condition to patients, as it is easy to highlight the vicious cycles of panic using this model (*Box 6.6*).

It is helpful to explore the specific fears held by each patient about the meaning of their physical symptoms, particularly what they fear most when the panic attack is at its height. This can help to identify the most relevant explanations about the nature of anxiety and how it may be affecting this individual. Remember that the process of recalling thoughts and feelings during a panicky episode can trigger further anxiety in some people. The discussion should therefore be carried out sensitively, whilst remaining vigilant to possible increased anxiety or distress in the patient during the discussion.

It is also important to assess for the presence of co-morbid conditions such as depression or substance misuse.

Box 6.5 **Differential diagnosis for panic disorder**

- Physical health conditions mimicking or triggering panic attacks: e.g. cardiac or respiratory conditions, hyperthyroidism
- Substance misuse: symptoms caused by the effects of substance use or as a result of withdrawal
- Agoraphobia: panic attacks are predictable and associated with specific situations from which escape may be difficult
- Social anxiety: symptoms are provoked specifically by anticipated and actual exposure to social and performance situations and are associated with a fear of embarrassment or negative evaluation by others
- PTSD: episodes of acute anxiety or panic triggered by trauma-related cues following a traumatic experience

| Box 6.6 | A CBT framework for assessment of panic disorder in primary care |

Thoughts
- At the time of the panic attack, what did you fear happening most?
- What might be the most serious explanation of the symptoms?
- Do you fear having another attack or worry about the consequences of the attack?

Feelings
- How do you feel during the episode?
- Do you have sudden episodes of intense fear or discomfort that are unexpected or out of the blue?
- Do they arise rapidly, usually within minutes?
- How long do the intense feelings last for?

Behaviour
- What do you do when you start to feel panicky?
- Do you do anything to try to prevent a panic attack coming on?
- Are you avoiding any places, situations or activities for fear of having a panic attack?

Physical symptoms
- What are the typical physical or bodily sensations that you experience?
- Which ones concern you the most?

Environmental factors and triggers
- Does the panic attack occur spontaneously or in reaction to a particular place, person or event?
- How often do the episodes occur?
- Are there any particular life stresses or difficulties at the moment?

Initial management in primary care

The next step is to offer treatment in primary care. The choice of treatment should be made through a process of shared decision-making with the patient. Psychological therapy, medication and self-help have all been shown to be effective for panic disorder. Self-help strategies can also be used as an adjunct to other treatments.

Explaining panic disorder

One of the most important goals for management of panic disorder in primary care is to provide explanations which help people to better understand the nature of anxiety and the 'fight or flight response' (*Chapter 1*), ideally using a CBT framework to make the explanation clearer. In panic disorder, fear leads to a vicious cycle of rapidly spiralling anxiety. This can be markedly reduced by giving clear and credible explanations about the cause of the person's most feared physical symptoms during a panic attack.

Explanations should be tailored to address the person's specific concerns. For example, someone fearing fainting or collapse may benefit from learning that blood pressure typically rises during a panic attack, so they are highly unlikely to faint, and that the feeling of dizziness actually stems from a combination of hyperventilation and feeling disorientated. Someone fearing choking may benefit from an explanation of what choking is, and a practical experiment of how the throat can feel very tight after repeated swallowing (ask the patient to swallow five times rapidly to demonstrate this).

Self-help strategies

Self-help strategies can be particularly helpful for people with mild to moderate panic disorder. These include:

- providing written information about panic disorder and how it affects people
- highlighting relevant self-help books and websites based on CBT principles
- providing information about local and national support groups for anxiety
- lifestyle modification: physical exercise, reducing caffeine intake, smoking cessation and improving sleep habits may all be beneficial.

Box 6.7 **Explanation of a panic attack**

In panic attacks, people experience very intense bouts of anxiety that come on extremely quickly, when they feel under threat. It involves a physical reaction known as the fight or flight response, where the body starts preparing to cope with potential danger. This creates powerful physical sensations. You might notice that you are breathing more quickly and deeply to get more oxygen into the system and that your heart is racing as it pumps more blood around your body to help your muscles prepare to fight or run. The muscles of your chest wall tense up and are working harder, which leads to pain in your chest.

In panic attacks, people usually find these symptoms very frightening, which leads to further anxiety and more physical symptoms as a vicious cycle.

However, although it can feel very unpleasant, remember that symptoms of anxiety are not harmful or dangerous. Try to accept what is happening and do not run away from the situation. If you wait, the fear will pass. Concentrate on exhaling slowly or using 'square breathing' to reduce hyperventilation. Distraction can also be helpful. Focus on your surroundings or carry out a mental exercise, check your phone or count backwards from 100 until your symptoms begin to improve.

10 *minute CBT strategies for panic disorder*

These brief interventions can be used to encourage positive self-management and reduce unhelpful ways of coping during a panic attack.

Cognitive defusion. Cognitive 'defusion' involves learning to disconnect or distance ourselves from negative or unhelpful thoughts, and to recognise them as simply words and ideas, rather than absolute facts. It involves a process of pausing, stepping back and observing what is happening in our mind and body. This can be a helpful way to 'unhook' from fearful or catastrophic thoughts about the meaning of physical symptoms in panic attacks. The process of becoming less 'fused' with thoughts leads to a thought becoming less believable and allows the person to consider alternative perspectives.

Using defusion is often more helpful in a time-pressured GP consultation than attempts to persuade or convince the person that a thought is unhelpful or inaccurate. Strategies to encourage cognitive defusion include:

- labelling thoughts: *"That sounds like a really scary thought..."*
- reflecting back: *"It sounds like you were thinking that the pain might be due to a heart attack, and that was a very scary idea..."*
- writing it down: seeing our thoughts as written words on paper allows us the opportunity to step back and view them from a different perspective
- using the sky and the clouds metaphor: *"Look up at the sky and watch the clouds moving slowly across it. Your mind is the sky, the clouds are your thoughts. Clouds come and go, and the weather may change, but the sky is constant and still. If we wait, a cloud, or a difficult thought can pass, allowing the sun to shine through again."*

Graded exposure. It is often helpful to encourage patients with panic disorder to gradually reduce avoidance of feared situations, using a brief form of graded exposure. This should be carried out in very small steps, setting 'micro-goals' for making change. The patient can be encouraged to carry this out whilst also

---

Box 6.8 | **Steps for graded exposure**

1. Make a list of a variety of situations that are being avoided due to anxiety or panic
2. Choose one of the easiest or least anxiety-provoking situations to try first, breaking it down into much smaller steps if needed
3. Aim to complete the task and remain in the situation despite feeling anxious; it can be helpful to plan strategies for coping with any anxiety that arises, e.g. breathing exercises or distraction
4. Try out the task and repeat it until it is more easily achievable without the use of any safety behaviours
5. Repeat with a slightly more challenging experience

using some form of CBT-based self-help material, such as a book or website, which will enable the patient to take the lead in this process.

Behavioural activation. Using brief behavioural activation strategies to increase participation in any meaningful or enjoyable activities, with a goal of improving general wellbeing and mood, can also be extremely important.

Reducing hyperventilation. Using breathing techniques can help to reduce hyperventilation during a panic attack. These should be practised several times each day when the individual is not feeling anxious, so that they will be more easily recalled and used in a panicky situation. Techniques include:

- square breathing (*Figure 6.2*): breathe in for a slow count of 4, hold for 4, breathe out slowly for 4 and hold again for 4; repeat this process for 4 minutes
- slow exhale (*Figure 6.3*): breathe out as slowly as possible, creating a gentle audible sighing sound, while counting upwards in your head to as high a number as possible, inhale and then repeat the slow exhale
- vigorous exercise such as a brisk walk or jog, or running up and down the stairs, provides distraction and will reduce symptoms arising from hyperventilation.

Distraction. Distraction can be a useful strategy to help reduce anxiety at the peak of a panic attack, enabling the individual to remain in the situation and leading to a reduced anxiety over time. It involves shifting attention away from

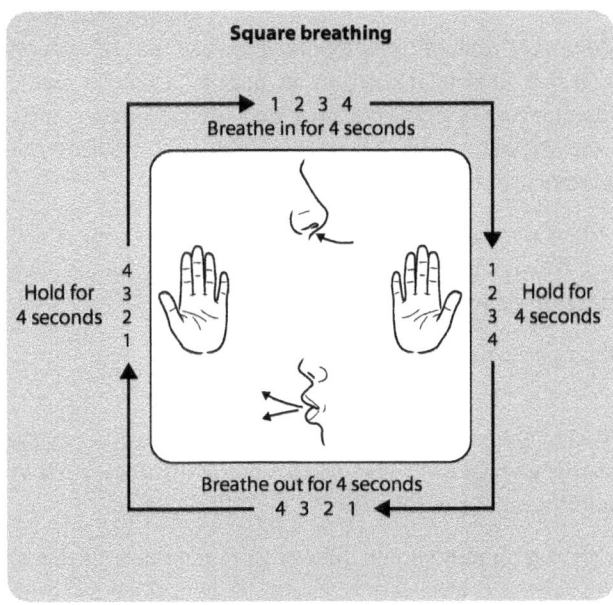

Figure 6.2 'Square breathing'.

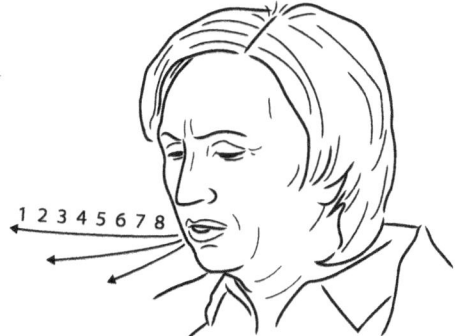

Figure 6.3 Prolonged exhalation.

catastrophic thoughts and fears, by paying attention to something else. To be effective in a panic attack, the activity needs to engage the mind when anxiety levels are very high, and therefore should not be overly complex or difficult. However, distraction techniques should not be overused as they can become counterproductive if used as a method of avoiding feared situations.

Examples of distraction activities include:
- counting backwards or in sevens or simple mental arithmetic
- focusing on the immediate environment: mentally describe the sights, sounds, smells around you or count the objects that can be seen
- simple puzzles, crosswords, word searches or sudoku; drawing a diagram or picture
- raising activity levels – going for a short walk or running up and down the stairs
- electronic distraction: sending an email or a text message, or using an app or game on the phone (note – this should be used with caution as it has a particularly high risk of leading to avoidance).

Treatment of panic disorder in primary care

Psychological therapy
CBT is the first-line treatment for panic disorder and is more effective than medication. It usually involves between 7 and 14 weekly one-to-one sessions, with the process of therapy rarely lasting longer than 4 months. Briefer CBT (i.e. less than 7 sessions) may also be used in combination with structured self-help materials in mild–moderate cases.

Importantly, research does not currently support the use of relaxation techniques such as progressive muscle relaxation as part of CBT for panic disorder. Relaxation strategies are ineffective and may even inadvertently increase anxiety as they may detract from the patient's ability to tolerate the anxiety and some patients may use them as safety behaviours.

Factors which may lead to poorer outcomes from CBT include a younger age of onset, longer duration of the disorder, poor motivation and individuals with high levels of social dysfunction or avoidance.

Core components of CBT for panic disorder are shown in *Box 6.9*.

Drug treatment
Drug therapy is less effective than CBT but may be helpful in some cases. First-line treatment is usually with an SSRI licensed for panic disorder, such as sertraline, citalopram, escitalopram or paroxetine.

Initiation and monitoring of drug therapy should follow recommended guidelines, which are summarised in *Chapter 3*. Medication should be continued for 6–12 months after the optimal dose is reached, after which the dose can be tapered.

Box 6.9 | **Core components of CBT for panic disorder**

Psychoeducation	• Understanding the panic model and the CBT approach to panic disorder • Education that panic symptoms are not dangerous but reflect the body's automatic response to danger • The role of avoidance in maintaining the problem

Cognitive restructuring (CR)	• Discussion and verbal processing to help the patient identify and restructure the thoughts that arise during a panic attack
	• CR can be used to address unhelpful thinking styles such as over-estimation of danger or catastrophising about anxiety-related physical symptoms through:
	  o learning to treat the thought as a hypothesis or theory
	  o looking at evidence for and against the thought being accurate
	  o identifying a balanced, alternative conclusion based on the evidence
	• CR may also involve looking for alternative thoughts that promote coping behaviour and reduce avoidance of feared situations

Graded exposure	• Repeated graded exposure to situations that are being avoided due to anxiety or panic, building up through a gradually increasing hierarchy of difficulty • The patient remains in the situation until anxiety symptoms have subsided (habituation), leading to tolerance and eventual resolution of the anxiety • Patient must not carry out any safety behaviours, avoidance or distraction from the source of the anxiety • Interoceptive exposure involves doing physical exercises to provoke panic symptoms (e.g. deliberately hyperventilating, or spinning a chair to recreate dizziness) • *In vivo* exposure involves facing the real-life situations that provoke panic attacks • Imaginal exposure involves imagining being in a panic-provoking situation and visualising coping with it
Core beliefs	Some patients may need to address underlying core beliefs that lead to increased anxiety and tendency to panic (e.g. "*I must be in control all the time*")
Relapse prevention	Review what has been learned, identify potentially difficult situations that may trigger an attack and identify strategies to prevent future attacks or to manage their anxiety should a panic attack occur

At the end of treatment, withdraw the SSRI gradually, as dictated by patient preference, and monitor for relapse for as long as is appropriate to the individual.

If there is no improvement after a 12-week course of SSRI medication, or an SSRI is not suitable, consider trial of an alternative SSRI or a TCA such as imipramine or clomipramine. Alternatives include an SNRI such as venlafaxine, or an anticonvulsant such as gabapentin or sodium valproate.

Benzodiazepines, sedative antihistamines and antipsychotics are not recommended for panic disorder and should be avoided. Propranolol has also been shown to lack efficacy in panic disorder and may even contribute to its maintenance as a safety behaviour and should therefore be avoided in most cases. Where possible, 'as required' medication should also be avoided, which can worsen anxiety by reinforcing fears about the dangers of panic attacks.

If there is insufficient response to medication, then consider psychological treatment, if this has not previously been tried.

When to change treatments
After around 12 weeks of first-line therapy, an assessment of the effectiveness of the initial treatment should be made, and a decision made whether to continue or consider an alternative intervention if there is insufficient improvement. This might involve changing to an alternative SSRI, trying a different class of antidepressant medication or offering psychological therapy if it has not so far been tried. Conversely, medication may be offered to patients who have not improved after undergoing psychological therapy.

When to refer

Offer referral to specialist mental health services if the person continues to experience significant symptoms after treatment with two interventions (any combination of psychological intervention, medication, or bibliotherapy), or in severe cases where there are concerns about a risk of self-harm or neglect, or significant functional impairment.

Specialist mental health services should conduct a thorough, holistic reassessment of the individual, their environment and social circumstances. Care should be based on the individual's circumstances and shared decisions made. Management options at this stage include:
- CBT with an experienced therapist, if not offered already, including home-based CBT if attendance at clinic is difficult, e.g. due to agoraphobic symptoms
- structured problem-solving
- alternative options for medication
- assessment for and treatment of co-morbid mental health conditions
- day support to relieve carers and family members
- referral to tertiary centres for advice, assessment or management in severe cases.

Summary of primary care management of panic disorder

Stepped care approach	What to offer	What does this involve?
Initial presentations of mild to moderate panic disorder	Explain the diagnosis and the person's feared symptoms	• Give clear and accurate explanations of the patient's feared symptoms and how these symptoms can arise as a consequence of a panic attack • Use the CBT framework and the fight or flight response to increase understanding of the nature of anxiety and its effect on the body
	10 minute CBT advice about managing anxiety	• Discuss the role of graded exposure to reduce avoidance to feared situations • Use brief behavioural activation to increase participation in any meaningful or enjoyable activities • Reduce hyperventilation using strategies such as 'square breathing' and slow exhalation • Use distraction to help reduce anxiety during a panic attack, enabling the individual to remain in the situation and leading to reduced anxiety over time
	Signpost to self-help resources	Provide information about CBT-based books and websites for understanding and managing anxiety
Moderate panic disorder or lack of response to initial measures	CBT is the most effective treatment for panic disorder and should be first-line choice of treatment	
	First-line: refer for primary care psychological therapy	• Less severe cases: low intensity CBT involving guided self-help or group-based CBT • More severe cases: 7–14 sessions of individual CBT over a maximum of 4 months
	Second-line: pharmacological treatment	• Initial choice of drug treatment for panic disorder is an SSRI licensed for panic disorder such as sertraline, citalopram, escitalopram or paroxetine; therapy should be continued for 6–12 months and can then be tapered • Maintenance therapy may reduce the risk of relapse • Second-line therapy could involve a TCA (imipramine or clomipramine), SNRI or anticonvulsants (gabapentin or sodium valproate) • Benzodiazepines, sedative antihistamines and antipsychotics should be avoided • Where possible, avoid 'as required' medication as this may act as a safety behaviour and worsen panic
Severe or complex problem or lack of response to primary care treatment	Refer to specialist services	• Refer if the person continues to experience significant symptoms after treatment with two interventions (any combination of psychological intervention, medication or bibliotherapy), or in severe cases of significant functional impairment or a risk of self-harm or neglect

6.10 Monitoring and follow-up

Patients with panic disorder should undergo regular review in primary care, particularly in the early stages of starting medication. Individuals receiving self-help interventions should be offered regular review every 4–8 weeks so that progress can be monitored, and alternative interventions considered if appropriate.

Follow standard guidelines for monitoring during initiation and maintenance of antidepressant medication (see *Chapter 3*). There is a risk of relapse after discontinuation of drug therapy, which may be reduced using maintenance therapy in patients with recurrent or relapsing symptoms.

Case example 6.2: Richard

Diagnosis of panic disorder

Richard is 38 years old and presents to the surgery for the second time in 4 weeks with sudden-onset chest pain, rapid heart rate, sweating, dizziness and shortness of breath. He works in a high-pressured job in a large bank and the attacks have worsened recently when his new boss has been putting him under pressure to achieve higher targets.

He worries about having these episodes in public and other places where getting help would be difficult. He has stopped driving his car and is avoiding crowded areas for fear of bringing on further attacks. He never goes anywhere without his mobile phone, in case he needs to call his wife for help. Past medical history is unremarkable and cardiac investigations have always been completely normal.

Dr Khan has never met the patient previously, so he starts by taking a full history, carrying out a physical examination and reviewing the medical record including all letters from emergency services and hospital letters. The GP is aware that Richard seems very anxious and agitated, and reflects this back with empathy during their conversation, whilst exploring Richards fears and health beliefs: *"You seem very anxious… This must be very frightening… What is the most frightening part for you? What is the worst thing that might happen?"*

Richard explains that when he experiences these episodes, he believes that he is going to faint, which he describes as both embarrassing and dangerous, saying, *"I could never return to work if I fainted in front of my boss. And what if it gets so bad that I stop breathing? I could suffocate!"*

Dr Khan uses labelling to highlight Richard's catastrophic fearful thoughts: *"It sounds like you were having a lot of very frightening thoughts. You were thinking that you might faint or even stop breathing or suffocate…? That sounds very scary…"*

He also asks Richard to describe the physical sensations that are making him anxious, using non-judgemental language, by asking: *"Can you tell me the physical sensations that you are having that make you feel like you might faint or stop breathing…?"*

Case example 6.2: *contd*

Dr Khan uses a CBT framework to write down Richard's experiences:

Thoughts
I'm going to faint
I could never return to work if I
    fainted in front of my boss
I might stop breathing or
    suffocate

Feelings
Anxious and agitated
Panicky
Embarrassed

Behaviour
Stopped driving
Avoids crowded areas
Takes mobile phone for
    reassurance

Physical symptoms
Chest pain, rapid heart rate
Sweating, dizziness and
    shortness of breath
Tight chest and light-headedness

Environment
High pressured job in a bank; new boss and higher targets

Dr Khan notices that Richard seems to be getting anxious when talking about his feared physical symptoms. So, he shows Richard how to carry out a brief 'square breathing' exercise. By concentrating on this, Richard is able to reduce his anxiety levels and engage more fully in the discussion again.

The GP explains that he believes Richard is experiencing panic attacks, saying: *"You have described experiencing a very severe tightness in your chest and a feeling of light-headedness. That physical sensation led to thoughts that you might faint or suffocate."*

Dr Khan then gives a credible physiological explanation for Richard's symptoms: *"An alternative explanation for your symptoms is that they are due to severe anxiety. It's possible that this was a panic attack. When you have high levels of anxiety, your body releases the chemical adrenaline, which triggers the fight or flight response as it prepares for possible danger. So you start to breathe faster and deeper, and can 'hyperventilate' causing tightness and discomfort in the muscles of your chest wall. This over-breathing can also make you feel light-headed, although you are actually far less likely to faint because your blood pressure rises during periods of anxiety..."*

Dr Khan explains that the most effective treatment for panic disorder is CBT but that medication may also be an option in some cases. He gives Richard a leaflet about panic disorder and invites him to return for a follow-up consultation to discuss the treatment options.

6.11 Summary and key points

- Panic disorder is characterised by recurrent episodes of intense fear and highly distressing somatic symptoms.
- Individuals with panic disorder make catastrophic misinterpretations about the risks of harmless, anxiety-related physical symptoms, leading to rapidly escalating anxiety as a vicious cycle.
- Avoidance or safety behaviours maintain the disorder over time and lead to significant functional impairment.
- Assessment of panic disorder involves clinical interview and there is no recommended specific screening tool, although HADS or GAD-7 may be helpful to monitor background levels of anxiety.
- Underlying physical causes should be ruled out when clinically indicated, including physical health conditions, prescribed or over-the-counter medications, and illicit substances.
- Psychoeducation involves providing a credible alternative medical explanation for an individual's specific feared physical symptoms that arise during a panic attack.
- CBT is the most effective treatment for panic disorder, and is associated with a lower risk of relapse after successful treatment than antidepressants.
- Relaxation training is not recommended in panic disorder and may even worsen long-term anxiety by reinforcing fears about the dangers of panic attacks and acting as a form of safety behaviour.
- SSRI antidepressants are first-line medication for panic disorder; other drug treatments include SNRI antidepressants and tricyclics. Benzodiazepines and beta blockers are not recommended.

6.12 Panic disorder resources

- Centre for Clinical Interventions: www.cci.health.wa.gov.au/Resources/For-Clinicians/Panic
- Northumberland, Tyne & Wear NHS Foundation Trust Self Help leaflets: https://web.ntw.nhs.uk/selfhelp/leaflets/Panic%20A4%202016%20FINAL.pdf
- Manicavasagar, V. and Silove, D. (2017) *Overcoming Panic: A self-help guide using cognitive behavioural techniques*, 2nd edition. Robinson.

Chapter 7
Agoraphobia

Agoraphobia quick reference guide

What is agoraphobia?	Anxiety and fear of places or situations from which escape might be difficult or help might not be available in the event of having a panic attack. Avoidance of anxiety-provoking situations results in a significant limitation of daily activities.
How common is it?	It is one of the least common anxiety disorders. The 12-month prevalence of agoraphobia without panic disorder at 0.8% is lower than that of panic disorder with agoraphobia at 1%.
Risk factors	Agoraphobia usually develops as a complication of panic disorder, affecting up to one-third of sufferers.
Co-morbid conditions	Most cases of agoraphobia occur in association with panic disorder. Other co-morbidities include other anxiety disorders, depression and somatoform disorders. Substance misuse may sometimes develop as an attempt to manage chronic anxiety symptoms.
Usual course	Tends to have a chronic, persistent course and complete remissions are rare.
Common presentations	Patients with agoraphobia may present with behavioural manifestations of their anxiety such as a restricted lifestyle and reduced functioning in important life areas or with panic attacks associated with specific feared situations. Agoraphobic symptoms may also be present in patients with medically unexplained symptoms or a chronic physical health disorder.
How to make the diagnosis	Screening can be carried out with GAD-2. Also ask: *"Do you worry about a lot of things?" "Is it hard to stop worrying?" "Is worry stopping you participating in any important activities?"* GAD-7 and HADS are both useful for diagnosis and monitoring but do not ask specifically about agoraphobic symptoms.
What else could it be?	Differential diagnosis includes panic disorder without agoraphobia, other anxiety disorders and depression. It can also arise in patients with physical health conditions.
Self-management strategies	Help patients to understand their condition by giving clear explanations of agoraphobia and how behavioural avoidance leads to a worsening of anxiety over time. Self-management strategies using 10 minute CBT include graded exposure to feared situations, use of coping statements, behavioural activation, and strategies to cope with anxiety such as distraction, reducing hyperventilation and mindfulness.

Treatment of agoraphobia	CBT involving graded exposure is the most effective treatment for agoraphobia but may need a longer duration of therapy than in panic disorder (12–20 sessions). First-line medication involves SSRIs, although this is less effective than CBT. Alternative drugs include TCAs (clomipramine and imipramine), venlafaxine, gabapentin and sodium valproate. Long-term drug therapy may be required due to the high risk of relapse.
When to refer	Refer if the person continues to experience significant symptoms after treatment with two interventions (any combination of psychological intervention, medication or bibliotherapy), or in severe cases of significant functional impairment or a risk of self-harm or neglect.
Follow-up	Due to the chronic nature of the disorder, agoraphobia is likely to benefit from long-term follow-up in primary care. Severe agoraphobia is associated with difficulties attending appointments in health settings, and some patients may benefit from telephone support or even home visits on some occasions.

CBT framework for agoraphobia

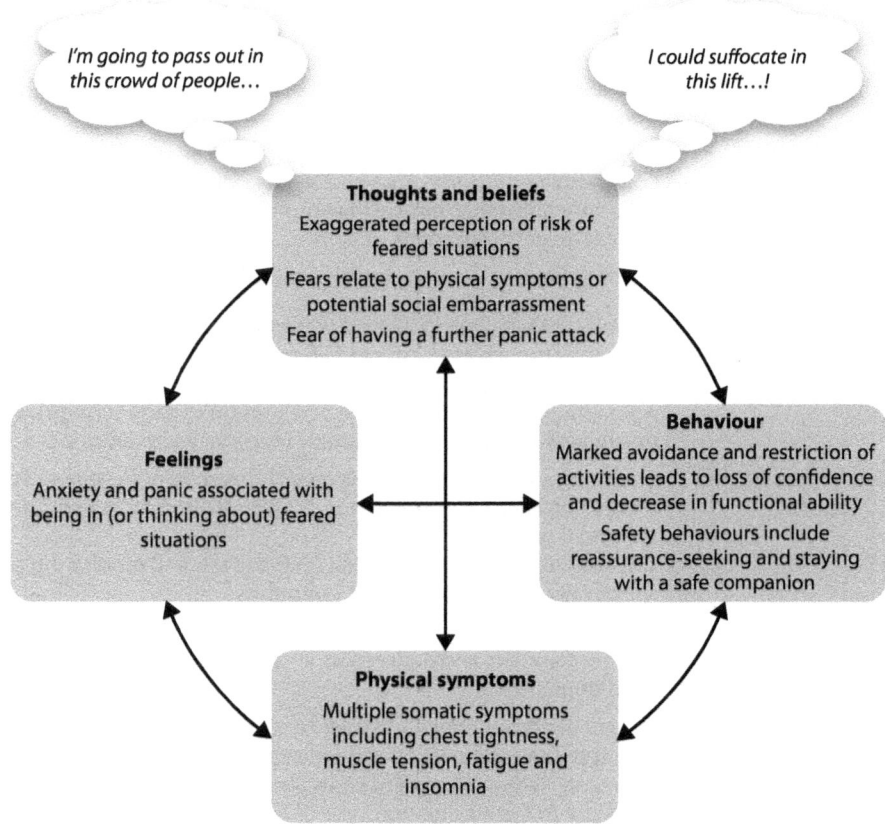

7.1 Introduction

Agoraphobia involves a fear of being in situations in which the person perceives that escape may be difficult or embarrassing. The condition usually develops as a complication of panic disorder. It is one of the least common anxiety disorders but can be very debilitating for sufferers when present.

7.2 What is agoraphobia?

Agoraphobia is an anxiety disorder characterised by an intense fear of being in places or situations from which there is no easy escape, or where help cannot be obtained in the event of developing panic-like symptoms or some other incapacitating reaction such as fainting, vomiting or a seizure.

Common situations associated with anxiety in agoraphobia include:
- crowded shops, theatres or cinemas
- travelling on public transport – e.g. buses, trains or planes
- open spaces – e.g. car parks or bridges
- being in queues or crowds of people
- being outside of the home alone in other situations or alone at home.

The fear or anxiety that arises is severe and out of proportion to actual danger posed by the situation and may lead to the development of a panic attack. In an attempt to minimise or control anxiety, people with agoraphobia typically avoid feared situations, endure them with dread, or are only able to enter them in the presence of a secure companion.

Box 7.1

Diagnostic criteria for agoraphobia

- An intense fear of being in situations from which escape might be difficult or help might not be available
- Fear is out of proportion to actual danger posed by the situation and may lead to a panic attack
- Typical situations causing anxiety include: shops, theatres, crowds, public places, travelling away from home or travelling alone
- The individual is consistently anxious about these situations due to a fear of specific negative outcomes such as panic attacks or other incapacitating or embarrassing physical symptoms
- The situations are avoided or only entered in the presence of a trusted companion, or endured with intense fear or anxiety
- Physical symptoms of anxiety include palpitations, chest pain, shaking, sweating and dry mouth
- Symptoms persist for at least several months and cause significant distress or impairment in important areas of functioning

Agoraphobia is also associated with a range of anxiety-related physical symptoms including sweating, shaking, difficulty breathing, feeling dizzy and gastrointestinal symptoms.

A broad spectrum of severity of symptoms of agoraphobia is possible. Some people are able to continue to manage their daily lives with difficulty, whilst others are severely affected, and the progressive restriction of anxiety may even lead to some individuals becoming completely housebound. Impairment of social roles, such as being able to work, is also common in agoraphobia.

Diagnostic criteria for agoraphobia disorder are shown in *Box 7.1*.

7.3 Epidemiology

Epidemiological data for agoraphobia is limited but it is thought to be one of the least prevalent of all anxiety disorders. The 12-month prevalence of pure agoraphobia (without panic disorder) at 0.8% is lower than that of panic disorder with agoraphobia at 1%. Agoraphobia is about twice as common in women as in men and has an average age of onset between 25 and 30 years.

7.4 Aetiology

Agoraphobia usually develops as a complication of panic disorder, affecting up to one-third of sufferers. Factors that increase the likelihood of developing agoraphobia in people suffering from panic disorder include female gender, more severe dizziness during panic attacks, cognitive factors, dependent personality traits and social anxiety disorder.

7.5 CBT model of agoraphobia

The CBT model of agoraphobia has many similarities with that of panic disorder (*Chapter 6*), but includes a very marked behavioural component with avoidance of anxiety-provoking situations. This behaviour reinforces anxiety and is associated with poorer outcomes than panic disorder without agoraphobia.

A CBT framework for agoraphobia is shown in *Box 7.2*.

7.6 Co-morbidity

Agoraphobia is rarely seen alone and is most commonly seen in association with panic disorder. Other co-morbidities include other anxiety disorders, including social phobia, specific phobias and generalised anxiety disorder, as well as depression and somatoform disorders. Agoraphobia may also be associated with substance misuse disorders, including inappropriate use of prescribed medications, which may develop as a result of attempts to manage symptoms of anxiety.

Box 7.2 **CBT framework for agoraphobia**

Thoughts

Recurrent worries and exaggerated perception of risk of feared situations

Thoughts about danger associated with feared situations (*"I'm not safe when I travel alone"*)

Fears may relate to physical symptoms (*"The chest pain means I might be having a heart attack!"*)

Other fears relate to potential social embarrassment (*"I would be publicly humiliated if I fainted in public"*)

It is common to fear having a further panic attack (*"Having another panic attack would be unbearable!"*)

Feelings

Anxiety and panic symptoms associated with being in (or thinking about being in) feared situations

Behaviour

Avoidance of feared situations – leads to a reduction in confidence and gradual decrease in functional ability over time

Escape from feared situations – e.g. going home if starting to feel anxious

Safety behaviours include:
- reassurance-seeking, including staying with a safe companion when out
- sitting near exits to enable easy escape if anxiety arises
- carrying objects to increase perceived sense of safety (e.g. a lucky charm, a phone or a benzodiazepine tablet)

Physical symptoms

Anxiety-related physical symptoms including:
- palpitations (heart racing)
- chest tightness and discomfort
- hyperventilation (feeling as though breathing is difficult)
- gastrointestinal symptoms including butterflies in the stomach and nausea
- sweating
- shaking and trembling

7.7 Course and prognosis of agoraphobia

Agoraphobia tends to have a chronic, persistent course, in which complete remissions are rare. The presence of severe agoraphobia is associated with a reduced chance of complete remission and greater risk of relapse of panic disorder. The prognosis for untreated agoraphobia is likely to be poor and may persist for years with patients becoming increasingly impaired.

Treatment with a combination of medication and/or CBT is effective for agoraphobia and many people are able to gradually reduce their feelings of fear and anxiety to the point where they can function normally and enjoy life again. Nevertheless, many patients continue to experience some level of agoraphobic symptoms in the long term. Despite treatment 40–50% will have residual symptoms after 3–6 years. Relapse is also common, with 25–50% experiencing a relapse within 6 months of discontinuation of medication.

7.8 Presentation of agoraphobia

I get chest pains and dizziness whenever I try to go out alone or travel on public transport…

I need a home visit… I'm too anxious to leave the house… No, I can't possibly come to the surgery or attend hospital appointments…

Patients with agoraphobia often present with the behavioural manifestations of their anxiety – a highly restricted lifestyle and reduced functional capacity. This may be in the context of medically unexplained symptoms or a chronic physical health disorder. It is helpful to ask about agoraphobia symptoms in frequently attending patients with complex or repeated somatic or physical symptoms.

Other people may present with panic attacks which are associated with specific feared situations. The symptoms of agoraphobia and avoidance can make it difficult for patients to seek help, due to fears about leaving the home and attending healthcare settings. Some patients may request home visits due to anxiety about attending the GP surgery, and others may avoid health professionals altogether.

7.9 Management of agoraphobia

There are few specific guidelines about the management of patients with pure agoraphobia. In general, patients with agoraphobia can be treated following the same guidelines as panic disorder (see *Section 6.9*).

Case example 7.1: Sarah

How might agoraphobia present?

Sarah is a 25-year-old receptionist who presents to her GP surgery with symptoms of anxiety which have been worsening over the past year. It developed three months previously after she had a flu-like illness and had continued to commute to work on the train when feeling unwell. At this time, she felt light-headed and thought she might faint in public. She found this extremely distressing and experienced a panic attack on the train. She was later sent home from work with a friend, as she felt unable to travel alone, and had two weeks off work.

She attends her GP asking whether there might be some underlying medical reason why she still has not fully recovered from her flu-like illness. She still feels exhausted, lethargic and "fuzzy-headed".

On further questioning, Dr Andrews takes a full medical history and examines Sarah. She also asks how the symptoms are affecting Sarah's life at the present time. This question helps to identify the significant behavioural and functional impact of Sarah's symptoms.

Since the initial episode, Sarah describes becoming increasingly fearful of travelling on public transport for fear of fainting again. She notices that she often feels anxious, tight-chested, experiencing palpitations, and that she can start to feel faint at even the thought of travelling on the train. She has had several panic attacks before going to work, which have led to her taking a significant amount of time off work. Her boss is starting to make negative comments about her attendance, which she is distressed about as she enjoys the job.

Dr Andrews asks Sarah which symptom causes her most distress and what she most fears might happen during a panic attack. Sarah has severe anxiety at the idea of fainting. "Maybe I would stop breathing or else completely lose control in front of everyone and have to be taken to hospital."

Sarah says that she feels safer if she can travel with a friend and tries to work from home whenever possible. She has also started to develop similar anxiety when driving and in crowded public places such as busy shopping centres and has started to avoid going out with her friends to bars and restaurants.

This information can be summarised in a CBT framework, as follows:

Thoughts
I might faint in public
I could stop breathing
I might lose control in front of others

Feelings
Anxious
Panicky

Behaviour
Takes time off work or works from home
Travels with a friend if possible
Avoids crowded public places
Avoids going to bars and restaurants with friends

Physical symptoms
Exhausted, lethargic
"Fuzzy-headed"
Faint
Tight chest and palpitations

Triggers for anxiety
Driving, public places such as shopping centres, bars and restaurants

This history demonstrates many features of agoraphobia, enabling Dr Andrews to carry out a further assessment of Sarah's mental health, and enabling her to reach a diagnosis of panic disorder with agoraphobia.

Making the diagnosis

Screening and diagnostic tools

As with panic disorder, there is no specific recommended screening tool for the diagnosis of agoraphobia, and the diagnosis is largely clinical. GAD-2 can be used to screen for anxiety, and GAD-7 or the anxiety questions of the HADS can be used to assess background levels of anxiety. However, these tools do not specifically ask about agoraphobic symptoms.

Discussing symptoms of agoraphobia

Agoraphobia should be suspected in patients with anxiety or panic attacks which arise consistently in specific situations such as in crowds, public places or public transport. Some useful questions for asking about symptoms of agoraphobia are shown in *Box 7.3*.

What else to consider

As in panic disorder, the differential diagnosis should include physical and mental health conditions that can cause anxiety or symptoms which mimic anxiety.

Box 7.3 | **Starting to talk about agoraphobia**

- Does anxiety frequently arise in any specific situations?
- Can you give me an example of a time that you started to feel anxious? Where were you and what were you doing?
- How did you cope with the situation or try to reduce your anxiety?
- Are you avoiding any situations in order to stop yourself becoming anxious?
- Is this having an impact on how you are able to live your life? Are you missing or avoiding any important activities because of anxiety?

Box 7.4 | **Differential diagnosis for agoraphobia**

- Panic disorder (without agoraphobia) or other anxiety disorders such as PTSD, GAD or social anxiety
- Physical health conditions mimicking or triggering anxiety or panic symptoms: e.g. cardiac or respiratory conditions, hyperthyroidism
- Depression leading to marked avoidance behaviour associated with low mood and withdrawal
- Substance misuse: leading to reduced participation in important roles and causing anxiety-like symptoms due to the effects of substance use or as a result of withdrawal

Initial assessment of agoraphobia

Initial assessment should explore anxiety and identify the specific situations that tend to trigger anxiety, or which are being avoided. Try to establish what the particular fears are that are leading to the avoidance behaviour. It is also important to assess for symptoms of panic disorder as it is highly likely to be a co-morbid disorder.

Agoraphobia can be a chronic and debilitating disorder. Over time, it may also become associated with low mood and depression. In this case, it is also important to assess for suicidal thoughts and intent.

A CBT framework can be very helpful in making a structured assessment of the condition and may identify a number of vicious cycles that may be maintaining the problem (*Box 7.5*).

Initial management in primary care

The next step is to offer treatment in primary care. Management of agoraphobia may be complicated by the fact that the patient's condition prevents them from leaving the house to access treatment. In some cases, it may be helpful to seek domiciliary psychological therapy in the home, if this service is available locally. If this service is not available, then telephone treatment or medication combined with self-help approaches may be alternative options.

The choice of treatment should be made through a process of shared decision-making with the patient. Psychological therapy, medication and self-help have all been shown to be effective for panic disorder. Self-help strategies can also be used as an adjunct to other treatments.

Explaining agoraphobia
The first step is to explain agoraphobia to the patient (*Box 7.6*). When giving the explanation, it is helpful to have a clear understanding of the individual's particular thoughts and fears, and to tailor the explanation to fit the person's own experiences and behaviour.

As in panic disorder, it is often helpful for health professionals to provide clear and accurate physiological explanations for any feared physical or somatic symptoms that are contributing to the patient's avoidance behaviour, such as chest tightness or dizziness when in a public place.

Self-help strategies
Self-help strategies can be helpful for people with mild to moderate agoraphobia, although there is not a strong evidence base for their effectiveness. These include:
- providing written information about agoraphobia and how it affects people
- highlighting relevant self-help books and websites based on CBT principles
- providing information about local and national support groups for anxiety

| Box 7.5 | A CBT framework for assessment of agoraphobia in primary care |

Thoughts
- What went through your mind when you started to feel anxious?
- What is the worst thing that might happen if you went into this situation?
- What might happen if you stayed in the situation rather than leaving when you start to feel anxious?

Feelings
- How do you feel emotionally?
- Is the anxiety out of proportion to the actual danger or threat in the situation?
- Do you ever experience panic attacks?
- How is your mood? Do you ever feel low, despondent or demoralised?

Behaviour
- Are you avoiding any situations due to your anxiety?
- Do you ever need to take someone with you to help you face a feared situation?
- What do you do to try to stop yourself worrying?
- Do you often seek reassurance from others?
- Do you do anything else to help combat your anxiety (e.g. drinking alcohol or taking drugs)?

Physical symptoms
- Do you have any distressing or disabling physical symptoms which affect you?
- What physical reactions are you aware of when you are in a difficult situation?

Environmental factors and triggers
- Do you feel particularly anxious or uneasy in situations that you might find it difficult to leave or escape, or if there is no one around to help you?
- In which situations are you most likely to feel anxious?
- Do you have a family history of anxiety or panic attacks?

- lifestyle modification: physical exercise, reducing caffeine intake and smoking cessation may all be beneficial.

10 *minute CBT strategies for agoraphobia*

The main focus for supporting self-management of agoraphobia is to encourage people to gradually expand their life activities and reduce unhelpful coping behaviours such as avoidance, that are common in agoraphobia.

| Box 7.6 | **Explaining agoraphobia to patients** |

In agoraphobia, people develop **feelings** of anxiety and fear about being in certain situations, especially when escape might be difficult or embarrassing. This fear arises from **thoughts or worries** that something bad might happen, such as having a panic attack in public. You might also worry about the **physical symptoms** that arise when you start getting anxious, such as palpitations, dry mouth or breathing quickly. These physical reactions can be very unpleasant and quite scary but are not really dangerous.

People with agoraphobia often react by avoiding many situations that might make them anxious, such as public transport, supermarkets or standing in queues. This is a type of **behaviour**. Many people also carry out 'safety behaviours' to make them feel less anxious, such as only going out with someone that they trust, or carrying a specific book, phone or medication. These behaviours reduce anxiety in the short term but cause major problems in the longer term by reducing confidence in your ability to cope in these situations and markedly restricting your life. Some people are unable to work or even leave their home for fear of getting anxious – life has become about continually trying to avoid feeling anxious, rather than doing the things that matter to you.

Graded exposure. People with agoraphobia tend to avoid or escape from situations that make them anxious. This rapidly relieves anxiety in the short term but leads to long-term problems and maintains the cycle of anxiety over time. Graded exposure involves facing up to fears and staying in a feared situation until the anxiety falls. This process is known as habituation (see *Figure 7.1*). By repeating this process, the anxiety will gradually reduce, enabling the individual to carry out previously feared activities without becoming anxious. The three key features of exposure are that it should be:

- **graded**: facing fears in gradual steps, starting with easier situations and building up to more challenging scenarios.
- **repeated**: the process must be repeated until the person feels comfortable in the situation before progressing to the next step.
- **prolonged**: the person must remain in the situation long enough for their anxiety to fall by at least half. This process usually takes between 30 and 60 minutes. It can be helpful to plan strategies for coping with any anxiety that arises, such as using breathing exercises or distraction techniques.

Gradually reducing the use of safety behaviours may also be included within the exposure ladder.

As with panic disorder, graded exposure for agoraphobia involves creating a hierarchy of feared situations and gradually working upwards through increasingly more challenging scenarios (*Box 7.7*).

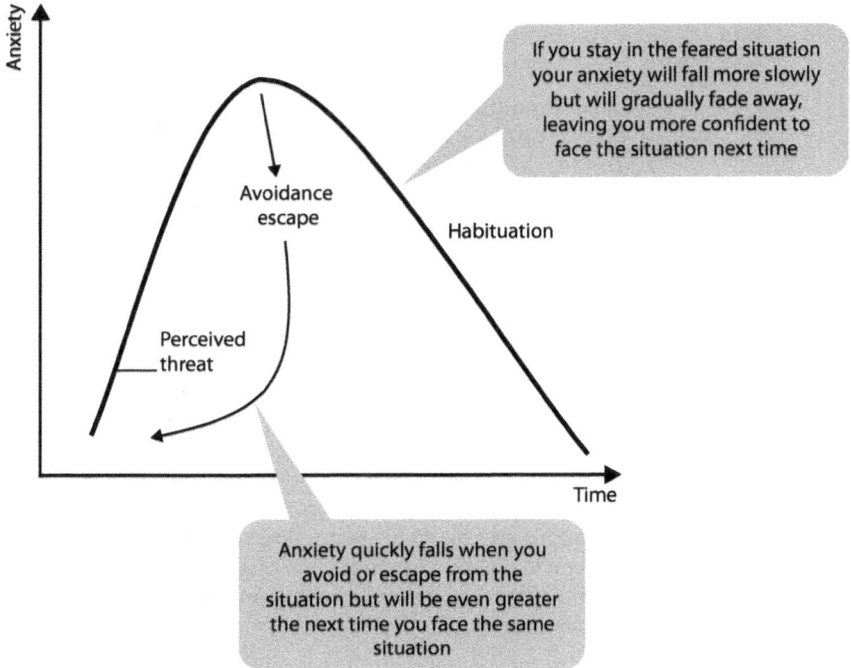

Figure 7.1 Reducing anxiety through habituation.

Example ladder of situations for graded exposure

- Walking around the block with a family member
- Walking around the block alone
- Going to the local shop with a friend
- Going to the local shop alone
- Going to the supermarket at a quiet time (accompanied)
- Going to the supermarket at increasingly busy times
- Going to the supermarket alone
- Travelling on a train (accompanied and then alone)

Coping statements. It may be helpful for the individual to plan out some written coping statements that will help them to successfully carry out behavioural tasks such as exposure, e.g.:

- Anxiety will not harm me.
- I don't want to let anxiety rule my life.
- If I stay in this situation, the anxiety will soon pass.
- Although this is very unpleasant right now, it will help me to reduce anxiety in the long term and will improve my life in the future if I stay here and don't leave the situation.

- The physical symptoms of anxiety are quite unpleasant but are a normal part of the body's fight or flight reaction.

Behavioural activation in agoraphobia. Behavioural change in agoraphobia does not solely need to focus on exposure and reducing avoidance. Particularly in severe agoraphobia, the process of exposure can be very challenging and may require one-to-one formal CBT to carry out successfully.

Behavioural activation is particularly important for patients with chronic agoraphobia, who may have developed low mood as a consequence of the prolonged avoidance and restriction of life activities. It involves increasing any activity that is meaningful, enjoyable or valued by the individual in tiny steps. Examples include spending time with friends and family, self-care activities, relaxation, hobbies and physical exercise.

Other strategies. Other useful strategies are similar to those used in panic disorder and include reducing hyperventilation during a feared situation, which may be triggering distressing symptoms. It may also be helpful to use distraction to help the person to cope with any anxiety that arises and to remain in a feared situation. Mindfulness may also be helpful.

Treatment of agoraphobia in primary care

Psychological therapy

CBT is the most effective treatment for agoraphobia and largely involves graded exposure. The duration of therapy may need to be longer than in panic disorder, often lasting 12–20 sessions, due to the chronic nature of the problem. Outcomes of CBT tend to be poorer if there is severe avoidance or high levels of social dysfunction. The therapy process may include a focus on strategies to reduce the risk of future relapse, such as writing a 'relapse prevention plan' which is a review of what has been learned through therapy, and planning specific strategies for coping with potentially difficult future situations that may trigger anxiety.

Drug treatment

Medication is an option in agoraphobia, although it is less effective than CBT. Treatment should follow guidelines for panic disorder (see *Chapter 6*). First-line treatment for agoraphobia is usually with an SSRI such as sertraline, citalopram, escitalopram or paroxetine. Second-line medications that may be considered include TCAs (clomipramine and imipramine), venlafaxine, gabapentin and sodium valproate. Initiation and monitoring of drug therapy should follow recommended guidelines which are summarised in *Chapter 3*. Long-term drug therapy may be required for many patients due to the high risk of relapse after discontinuing medication.

As with panic disorder, benzodiazepines, sedative antihistamines, antipsychotics and propranolol are not usually recommended. Where possible, 'as required' medication should also be avoided, as it can worsen anxiety by reinforcing fears about the dangers of panic attacks.

Combined treatment

Patients with severe agoraphobia may benefit from combined treatment with medication and CBT, which may be more effective than either treatment alone.

When to refer

As with panic disorder, offer referral to specialist mental health services if the person continues to experience significant symptoms after treatment with two interventions (any combination of psychological intervention, medication or bibliotherapy), or in severe cases where there is significant functional impairment or concerns about a risk of self-harm or neglect.

Specialist mental health services should conduct a thorough, holistic reassessment of the individual, their environment and social circumstances. Care should be based on the individual's circumstances and shared decisions made. Management options at this stage include:

- CBT with an experienced therapist, if not offered already, including home-based CBT if attendance at clinic is difficult, e.g. due to agoraphobic symptoms
- structured problem-solving
- alternative options for medication
- assessment for and treatment of co-morbid mental health conditions
- day support to relieve carers and family members
- referral to tertiary centres for advice, assessment or management in severe cases.

Summary of primary care management of agoraphobia

Stepped care approach	What to offer	What does this involve?
Initial presentations of mild to moderate agoraphobia	Explain the diagnosis and the person's feared symptoms	• Give clear and accurate explanations of vicious cycle of avoidance and anxiety associated with agoraphobia • Identify the thoughts and beliefs associated with specific feared situations • Provide physiological explanations of any important symptoms that are causing distress
	10 minute CBT advice about managing anxiety	• Discuss the role of graded exposure to reduce avoidance to feared situations • Use 'coping statements' to help the patient engage in important activities that may cause anxiety • Use brief behavioural activation to increase participation in any meaningful or enjoyable activities • Reduce hyperventilation using 'square breathing' and slow exhalation • Use distraction to help the individual to remain in an anxiety-provoking situation
	Signpost to self-help resources	Provide information about CBT-based books and websites for understanding and managing anxiety

Stepped care approach	What to offer	What does this involve?
Moderate agoraphobia or lack of response to initial measures	CBT is the most effective treatment for agoraphobia and should be first-line choice of treatment	
	Refer for primary care psychological therapy	• Less severe cases: low intensity CBT involving guided self-help or group-based CBT • More severe cases: up to 12–20 sessions of individual CBT
	Pharmacological treatment	• First-line drug treatment for panic disorder is with an SSRI, such as sertraline, citalopram, escitalopram or paroxetine • Therapy should be continued for at least 6–12 months and can then be tapered but may need to be continued longer-term due to the high risk of relapse • Second-line therapy could involve a TCA (imipramine or clomipramine), SNRI or anticonvulsants (gabapentin or sodium valproate) • Benzodiazepines, sedative antihistamines and antipsychotics should be avoided • Where possible, avoid 'as required' medication as this may act as a safety behaviour and worsen anxiety symptoms
Severe or complex problem or lack of response to primary care treatment	Refer to specialist services	• Refer if the person continues to experience significant symptoms after treatment with two interventions (any combination of psychological intervention, medication or bibliotherapy), or in severe cases of significant functional impairment or a risk of self-harm or neglect

7.10 Monitoring and follow-up

Patients with agoraphobia should undergo regular review in primary care, particularly in the early stages of starting medication. This can be challenging for health services if patients are severely agoraphobic and find it difficult to attend appointments in health settings. A combination of telephone and face-to-face review, and even occasional home visits in extreme cases, may help to overcome this problem. Patients can also be encouraged to set goals to attend health service appointments as part of psychological therapy treatment plans. Due to the chronic nature of the disorder, the follow-up in primary care may be a long-term process.

Case example 7.2: Diane

Diagnosis and management of agoraphobia

Diane is a 56-year-old woman with a long history of anxiety. Over the last 10 years she has found it increasingly difficult to leave the home and has not been out at all for over a year. She registers with a new GP and requests a home visit to assess her chest tightness and palpitations as she says she is unable to attend the surgery.

In view of the physical symptoms, her GP, Dr Baird, agrees to visit her to make an assessment. He discovers that Diane has high levels of anxiety at the thought of leaving the house, which have led to her becoming completely housebound. Her husband is her main carer who does all her shopping and physical care at home. Her chest symptoms and palpitations are always associated with anxiety.

The anxiety first developed about 10 years ago after she experienced an episode of chest pain when out shopping and lifting some heavy bags out of her trolley. An ambulance was called and she was sent to hospital. The medical records state that she was not found to have any cardiac cause for the pain, but Diane remains convinced that she experienced a kind of "heart attack", which might recur if she over-exerts herself, and she therefore avoids going anywhere for fear that medical help may not be available quickly. She describes experiencing further "heart attacks" around three times per week, usually when her husband is out of the house.

Dr Baird asks Diane the GAD-2 screening questions, which are suggestive of anxiety; she responds positively to the third question ("Do you find yourself avoiding places or activities and does this cause you problems?"), which confirms marked behavioural avoidance.

Dr Baird carries out a physical examination, which is normal. However, Diane refuses to leave the house to attend any appointments for any further medical investigations or psychological treatment. Her previous GP has been treating Diane with diazepam to manage the anxiety and she has been taking 10–15 mg daily for the past 3 years without any reduction in her anxiety symptoms or chest pain. She is keen to continue this prescription.

Dr Baird recognises that this is a complex and long-standing problem having a marked functional impact on Diane's life, which is likely to require a long-term approach to support and management. He suspects that the likely underlying diagnosis is agoraphobia, because of Diane's high levels of anxiety and behavioural avoidance. He documents clearly that he has recommended further physical investigation and assessment and that the patient has declined, but also recognises that her decisions are stemming from severe anxiety and is able to remain empathetic and begin to develop a supportive relationship that avoids blame or negativity.

Dr Baird agrees to continue to prescribe diazepam for another 2 weeks and plans to return to assess Diane further with a HADS questionnaire to look for low mood and anxiety symptoms. He explains the problems associated

Case example 7.2: *contd*

with long-term benzodiazepine use including dependence, tolerance and lack of long-term efficacy. He suggests that an alternative approach to treatment might be more helpful and they agree to discuss this further at the next appointment.

What should be the approach to treatment in the longer term?

CBT is likely to be the most effective treatment for Diane but options for therapy may be limited if domiciliary or telephone therapy is not available in the region. Alternative treatment options could involve initiating treatment with SSRI medication such as sertraline. It is likely to be helpful to commence at extremely low doses and build the dose up gradually to minimise the risk of discontinuing medication due to side-effects. Any improvement in her anxiety symptoms may also facilitate attendance for face-to-face psychological therapy in future.

It may also be helpful to encourage a very slow and gradual reduction in diazepam, at a rate which avoids withdrawal effects, over a period of 3–12 months. This may be more achievable after the patient has been established on SSRI therapy or after psychological therapy. If a patient is unwilling or highly resistant to reducing benzodiazepines, NICE recommends that they are advised of the benefits of stopping, and any concerns about stopping should be explored and addressed, but they should not be pressurised or forced to stop. The decision can be reviewed and further discussed at a later stage.

Any treatment options can be combined with brief self-management advice, particularly encouraging Diane to re-engage with important and meaningful daily activities in small steps using brief behavioural activation.

7.11 Summary and key points

- Patients with agoraphobia have a marked fear of situations in which they perceive that escape may be difficult, or help may be difficult to obtain in the event of a panic attack or other incapacitating or embarrassing symptoms.
- Agoraphobia usually occurs with panic disorder and its presence is associated with a worse prognosis.
- For a diagnosis of agoraphobia to be made, the patient must experience anxiety in at least two different situations.
- Agoraphobia is characterised by marked behavioural avoidance and restriction of life activities, and can have a very significant impact on social and occupational functioning.
- Management is very similar to that of panic disorder and first-line treatment typically involves CBT or SSRI antidepressants.

- Progressive graded exposure is effective for agoraphobia and involves repeatedly remaining in feared situations until anxiety gradually reduces (habituation), leading to reduced anxiety and increased self-confidence.
- Agoraphobia is a chronic condition with high rates of relapse after stopping medication and many patients may benefit from long-term or maintenance drug therapy.

7.12 Agoraphobia resources

There are relatively few specific resources for agoraphobia alone, but resources addressing panic disorder also include symptoms of agoraphobia:

- Centre for Clinical Interventions: www.cci.health.wa.gov.au/Resources/For-Clinicians/Panic
- Lovell, K. (1999) *Overcoming Agoraphobia* leaflet. Available at: www.anxietyuk.org.uk/wp-content/uploads/2010/05/overcoming-agoraphobia-lovell-1999.pdf
- Northumberland, Tyne & Wear NHS Foundation Trust Self Help leaflets: https://web.ntw.nhs.uk/selfhelp/leaflets/Panic%20A4%202016%20FINAL.pdf
- Manicavasagar, V. and Silove, D. (2017) *Overcoming Panic: a self-help guide using cognitive behavioural techniques*, 2nd edition. Robinson.

Chapter 8
Specific phobias

Specific phobia quick reference guide

What is a specific phobia?	An extreme and unreasonable fear of a specific single object or situation, such as dentists, spiders, lifts, flying or seeing blood, which is out of proportion to the actual danger or threat. Symptoms of anxiety such as nausea, sweating, increased heart rate and shaking occur when the person encounters or thinks about the object or situation. Anxiety leads to avoidance of the source of the phobia.
How common is it?	Specific phobia is the commonest anxiety disorder, with a lifetime prevalence of around 12%. Onset is usually in children aged 5–13 years.
Risk factors	Phobias are more common in women than in men. Some phobias develop as a conditioned response to a threatening or distressing experience, or as a learned response from the observation of others, such as parents or siblings. However, there is often no precipitating factor to the development of a phobia. Genetic factors may also play a role, but there is currently very limited research in this area.
Co-morbid conditions	Co-morbidity rates between specific phobia and other mental health disorders are very high, including depression, anxiety, eating disorders and substance misuse. Around 70% of people with specific phobia also report more than one clinically relevant fear and this is associated with increased risk of co-morbid conditions. The development of specific phobia often precedes the onset of other disorders and may represent an early life indicator of vulnerability to psychopathology.
Usual course	Specific phobias usually arise in childhood and can persist for decades if untreated. However, many children also experience transient specific fears which do not persist or develop into a lasting phobia. The fear and avoidance in specific phobias frequently result in a restricted lifestyle with considerable impact on sufferers' daily lives, and impairment of role is comparable with other anxiety and substance use disorders.
Common presentations	Patients may attend requesting treatment such as benzodiazepines to cope with feared situations such as flying. Phobias about medical interventions such as fears about blood, needles or injections may lead to lack of compliance with testing or treatment for conditions such as diabetes. Some individuals with specific phobia will present with secondary or co-morbid conditions such as depression. Patients with specific phobia can be high users of healthcare services.

How to make the diagnosis	There is no specific screening tool for the diagnosis of specific phobia, but if suspected it is helpful to ask directly about phobic symptoms. Useful questions include: • *"Do you have an intense fear of a particular object, situation or animal?"* • *"Do you feel anxious, nervous or panicky when confronted by it?"* • *"Do you try hard to avoid coming into contact with it?"* When screening with GAD-2, consider adding a third question, *"Do you find yourself avoiding places or activities and does this cause you problems?"* to help identify individuals with phobic avoidance.
What else could it be?	The differential diagnosis includes other disorders with distress or avoidance related to anxiety including panic disorder with agoraphobia, social phobia, OCD, PTSD and health anxiety.
Self-management strategies	Provide clear and accurate explanations of an individual's feared symptoms that arise during a panic attack. Use graded exposure, breathing techniques to reduce hyperventilation and distraction to manage panic symptoms.
Treatment of specific phobia	First-line treatment is with 7–14 sessions of individual CBT which is more effective than drug therapy. Guided self-help may be offered in mild–moderate cases. SSRIs are first-line choice of medication.
When to refer	Refer to specialist mental health services if the person continues to experience significant symptoms after treatment with two interventions (any combination of psychological intervention, medication or bibliotherapy).
Risk of relapse	Relapse rates after stopping medication are between 55% and 77% but may be reduced in patients with chronic or relapsing symptoms using maintenance therapy. Relapse rates are lower after CBT.
Follow-up	Chronic relapsing cases will require long-term follow-up and monitoring. Drug therapy should be continued for 6–12 months, after which the dose can be tapered.

8.1 Introduction

A specific or simple phobia is an extreme form of fear or anxiety triggered by a particular situation or object, even when there is no danger. Phobias are important to recognise, as they represent one of the most common and treatable psychiatric conditions.

Complex phobias such as agoraphobia or social phobia tend to have a more disruptive or disabling impact on people's lives and are covered separately in *Chapters 7* and *9*, respectively.

8.2 What are phobias?

A specific phobia is an intense, extreme and persistent fear of a specific and discrete object or situation, which is out of proportion to the actual danger or threat. *Box 8.1* lists the commonest types of phobia.

CBT framework for specific phobias

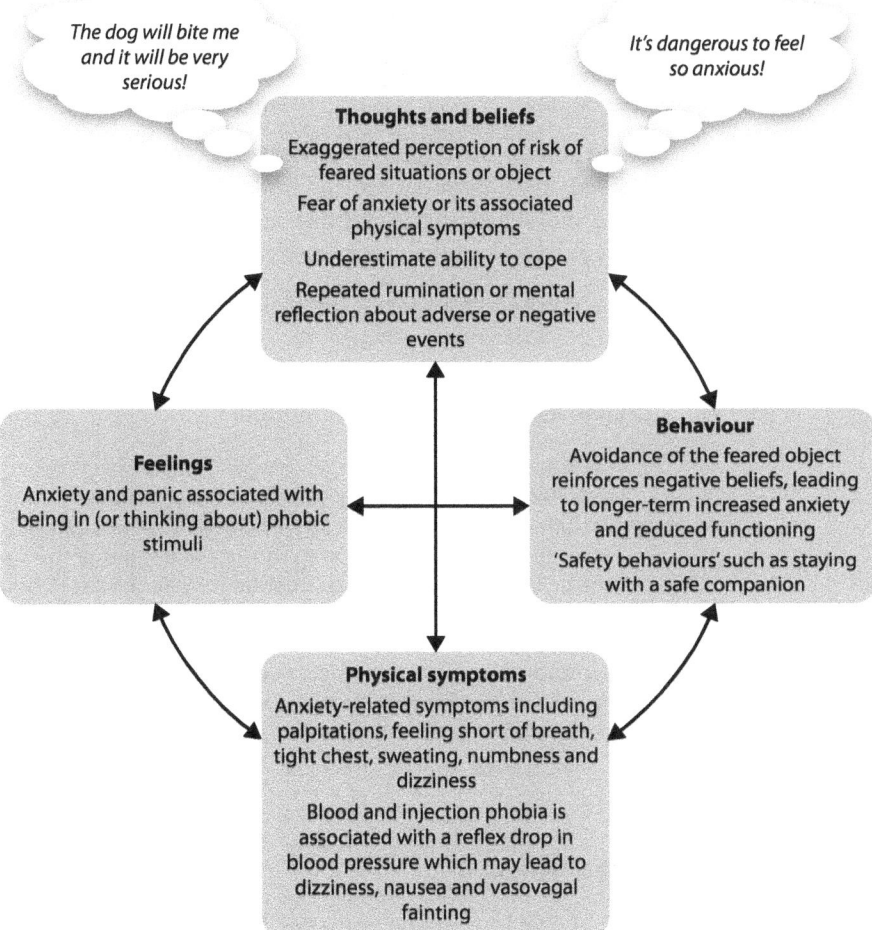

Box 8.1   **Common types of phobia**

- Animal: including snakes, insects, spiders and dogs
- Situational: such as driving, flying or enclosed spaces
- Natural environment: such as heights and the dark
- Blood, injuries, medical experiences: including blood tests, injections and other medical procedures such as visiting the dentist
- Other: including fear of choking, vomiting, loud noises and clowns

Specific fears of objects, animals, people or situations are widespread in children, adolescents and adults, but only a minority of affected individuals reach the full diagnostic criteria for specific phobia.

A fear becomes a phobia if it lasts for at least several months and has a significant impact on how the person is able to live their day-to-day life.

Fear and anxiety are triggered immediately on actual or anticipated exposure to the feared object or situation, and lead to avoidance or extreme distress. Many affected individuals have multiple fears, and this is associated with greater severity and impairment and more frequent psychiatric co-morbidity.

Diagnostic criteria for specific phobias are shown in *Box 8.2*.

Box 8.2   **Diagnostic criteria for specific phobia**

- Marked and excessive fear or anxiety that consistently occurs when exposed to one or more specific objects or situations (e.g. proximity to certain animals, flying, heights, enclosed spaces, sight of blood or injury)
- Anxiety is out of proportion to the actual danger of the situation and contact with the triggering situation may evoke panic symptoms
- Phobic objects or situations are avoided or endured with intense fear or anxiety
- Symptoms persist for at least several months and result in significant distress or impairment in personal, family, social, educational, occupational or other important areas of functioning

---

8.3 Epidemiology

Specific phobia is the commonest of all anxiety disorders. Lifetime prevalence is around 12% and 12-month prevalence is around 9%.

The commonest phobias are:
- animals (3.8%)
- blood, injuries and medical experiences (3%)
- high places (2.8%)
- natural phenomena, including water or weather events (2.3%)
- fear of flying; this has the lowest prevalence (1.3%) and is understandably more common in high income countries.

Phobias are 2–3 times more common in women than in men. The onset of specific phobia is usually in children aged between 5 and 13 years.

8.4 Aetiology

A phobia may sometimes develop as a conditioned response to a threatening or distressing experience. Onset can also occur as a learned response from the observation of others, such as parents or siblings, reacting fearfully to a particular stimulus. However, there is often no precipitating factor to the development of a phobia.

Certain stimuli, such as snakes, may be more likely to induce phobias due to their evolutionary threat relevance. There is some suggestion that genetic factors may also play a role in the development of phobias, but there is currently very limited research in this area.

8.5 CBT model of phobias

Behaviour in phobias

Behaviour is one of the most important factors acting to maintain phobias and is the focus of the first-line treatment in exposure therapy.

Avoidance and escape
Avoidance and escape are common unhelpful behaviours seen in phobias. Avoidance refers to behaviours that attempt to prevent exposure to a fear-provoking stimulus. Escape means to quickly leave an anxiety-provoking situation.

Avoidance and escape both act to reduce anxiety in the short term but are responsible for maintaining the phobia in the long term as a vicious cycle, and also lead to a decrease in functioning. Avoidance prevents the extinction of anxiety that normally occurs through repeated exposures to a phobic stimulus. In addition, the relief that is felt each time the phobia is avoided encourages the person to continue avoidance in future. Avoidance also prevents the person from learning that their fears about the phobic stimulus are exaggerated and are unlikely to come true. It also prevents people from learning that anxiety symptoms are not harmful and that they are able to cope when confronted by the phobia, if given the opportunity to do so.

Safety behaviours
People may develop safety behaviours to help them feel safe or to cope with their phobia, such as staying with a trusted person, only sitting in very isolated or secluded areas of a restaurant or visiting shops during very quiet times of the day. Safety behaviours also act to maintain the vicious cycle of anxiety in phobias by preventing people from learning that they can cope with the phobia by themselves without needing any additional support.

Feelings

Feelings in phobia include anxiety and may be severe enough to lead to a panic attack when the person comes into contact with a feared situation or object.

Thoughts

People's unhelpful thoughts and predictions can often make it more difficult for them to overcome their phobia. Typical thoughts in phobias involve information processing biases with overestimation of the likelihood of a negative event occurring if they were to face their phobia ("*I will get trapped in this lift and run out of air*"). People with phobias also underestimate their ability to cope with anxiety. This makes it very difficult for them to face and overcome their fear ("*I will be unable to cope and would pass out immediately if I got into that lift*"). Cognitive rehearsal of negative outcomes through repeated rumination or mental reflection about adverse or negative events also tends to inflate the level of fear.

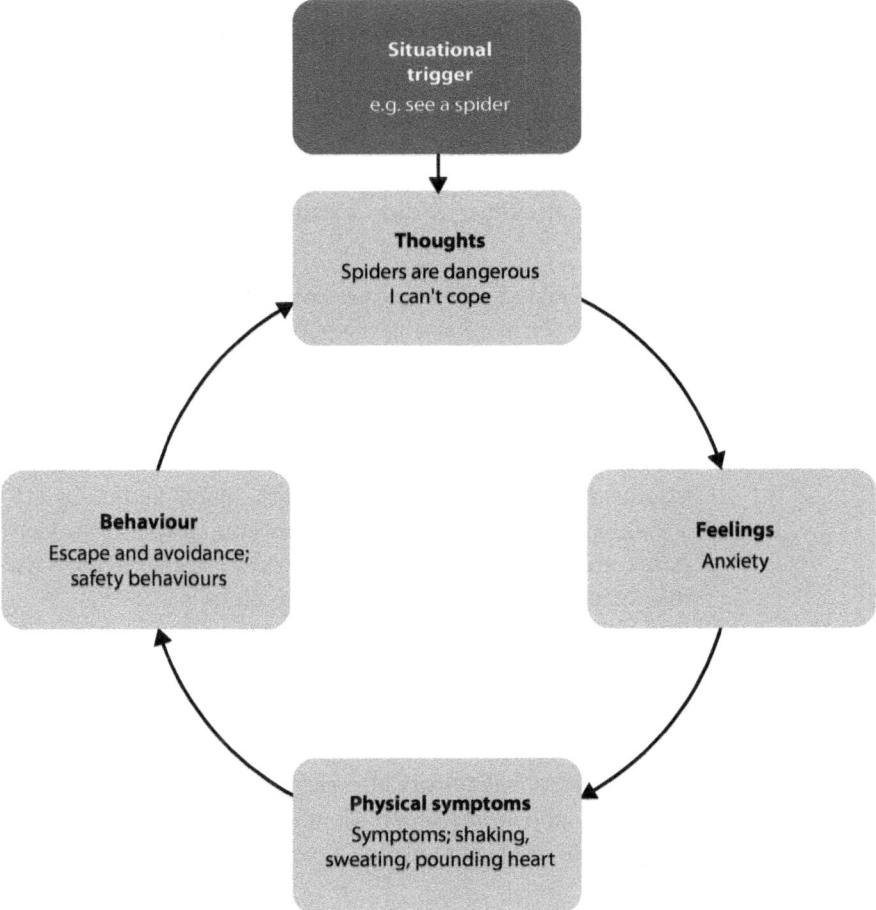

Figure 8.1 Vicious cycles of anxiety in phobias.

Physical symptoms

Physical symptoms in phobias are related to the sympathetic response to anxiety including sweating, shaking, hot flushes, feeling short of breath, choking sensations, pain or tightness in the chest, nausea and other gastrointestinal symptoms, feeling faint, a dry mouth and feeling confused or disorientated.

Blood injection injury phobias

Blood injection injury phobias differ from other phobias. Here, the increase in heart rate and blood pressure that is triggered by the anxiety-provoking trigger, such as a needle, is followed by a quick drop in blood pressure leading to dizziness, nausea and sometimes fainting. This is the only phobia where fainting may actually occur. In other phobias and anxiety disorders, the experience of dizziness is due to hyperventilation and is associated with an elevation of blood pressure, making fainting unlikely.

It is therefore important for patients who suffer from blood injection injury phobias to learn strategies to prevent fainting (see *Box 8.8*).

Fear of flying (aviophobia)

Phobias about flying may develop if an individual has persistent and excessive fear triggered by flying or the thought of flying. Typically, flying is avoided or endured with intense anxiety, which may take the form of a panic attack. There are a number of different fears which may be associated with a fear of flying:
- Fear of crashing: people typically have vivid images and replay the worst-case scenario multiple times in their heads.
- Fear of having a panic attack or becoming overwhelmed by anxiety and out of control whilst airborne.
- Other fears include enclosed spaces (claustrophobia), fear of being out of control, falling, terrorism, fires or simply having a 'bad feeling' about the flight.

The fear of flying often develops when people experience an unexpected level of anxiety when flying, and fear that these symptoms will return in a future flight.

Flight phobia may also arise as a consequence of panic disorder with agoraphobia; such individuals may fear having a panic attack whilst on an aeroplane. In this case, sufferers will experience fear and anxiety in other situations from which escape may be difficult if they have a panic attack, and not simply when flying.

8.6 Co-morbidity

Co-morbidity rates between specific phobia and other mental health disorders are very high, including depression, anxiety, eating disorders and substance misuse disorders. Importantly, the development of specific phobia often precedes the onset of other disorders.

Approximately 70% of people with specific phobia report more than one clinically relevant fear. Co-morbidity also becomes more common with increasing numbers of fear subtypes in specific phobia, suggesting that specific phobia may be an early life indicator of psychopathology vulnerability. There is also some evidence suggesting that early treatment of phobias could also alter the risk of developing other mental health disorders.

Specific phobias are associated with considerable role impairment in sufferers' daily lives, with levels that may be comparable with other anxiety and substance use disorders. They are also associated with a relatively high use of healthcare services. This functional impairment can be partly explained by high co-occurrence with other disorders but also due to the restricted lifestyle resulting from fear and avoidance.

8.7 Course and prognosis of specific phobias

Specific phobias usually arise in childhood or early adult life and can persist for decades if they remain untreated. However, parents can be reassured that many children experience transient specific fears which do not persist or develop into a lasting phobia, and this can be viewed as a normal aspect of child development.

8.8 Presentation of phobias

People rarely present directly with specific phobias, so it is often necessary to ask about them directly to make the diagnosis; for example, in children presenting

I have a phobia about snakes. I feel sick and shaky if I even hear the word...

It stops me living my life. Things that other people do without even thinking about them have become problems for me...

with anxiety. Some individuals may perceive phobias as untreatable, despite the availability of effective interventions. Others may be unwilling to face the feared object or situation in the process of exposure therapy. Some individuals may present with co-morbid anxiety or mood disorders such as panic disorder or social anxiety.

Certain phobias, such as those with fears about blood, needles or injections, may present in primary care as patients who are non-compliant with investigations and treatments such as blood tests or blood glucose monitoring in diabetes. Other medical fears include claustrophobia leading to fear of being trapped inside a scanner during imaging studies.

Patients may also present requesting medication such as benzodiazepines to cope with feared situations such as flying or dental procedures.

Case example 8.1: Douglas

How might specific phobia present?

"Can I have some diazepam to calm me down when I next take a flight…?"

Douglas, a 35-year-old business executive, attends his GP, Dr Shafi, and requests diazepam for an upcoming flight for work. He explains that he is required to fly to the USA several times a year for work, but he feels increasingly anxious at the thought of flying. His fear of flying developed two years ago following a fairly turbulent flight. At the time he had been in a very stressful job and was generally more anxious than usual. He recalls becoming highly anxious during the turbulence and is worried that this might happen again.

Since then Douglas has flown on several occasions but found each flight extremely stressful and anxiety-provoking. He now starts to feel anxious several weeks before the flight is due to take place. He was given a prescription for diazepam by another GP for the last flight and he thinks this may have helped.

At the thought of flying, Douglas describes feeling shaky and sweaty and having extreme tightness in the chest. His anxiety is triggered by the thought of being in a plane with heavy turbulence. He fears having a panic attack and getting "completely out of control" and needing to be restrained by the cabin crew.

Dr Shafi explains to Douglas that benzodiazepines are not recommended for management of phobias and that taking a sedating medication whilst flying might put him and other passengers at risk in the unlikely event of an emergency situation. Benzodiazepines do not treat anxiety but simply mask it, and there is also a risk that they might contribute to worsening anxiety in the long term by acting as a safety behaviour. They discuss how effective exposure therapy for phobias can be – in some cases as little as one session can be beneficial. Douglas agrees to look into a fear of flying course in order to permanently overcome his anxiety.

8.9 Management of phobias

Making the diagnosis

Screening and diagnostic tools

Early recognition and treatment of phobias is important as it may alter the risk of developing other anxiety disorders. There is no specific recommended screening tool for the diagnosis of specific phobia, but if suspected it is helpful to ask directly about phobic symptoms in both adults and children presenting with possible anxiety. Consider specific phobia as a differential diagnosis in other anxiety disorders if the source of anxiety is limited to one (or several) discrete triggers. Useful questions to make the diagnosis include:

- *"Do you have an intense fear of a particular object, situation or animal?"*
- *"Do you feel anxious, nervous or panicky when confronted by it?"*
- *"Do you try hard to avoid coming into contact with it?"*

GAD-2 can be used for screening for general anxiety but does not include any specific questions relating to phobias. Asking a third question, *"Do you find yourself avoiding places or activities and does this cause you problems?"*, will help to detect a number of people with phobia whose functioning is impaired but who otherwise would not be identified by the two GAD questions.

Differential diagnosis

Specific phobias must be distinguished from other disorders with significant distress or avoidance related to anxiety. Panic disorder with agoraphobia involves pervasive anxiety, which is not specifically triggered by a single stimulus, as in specific phobias. Patients with panic disorder have multiple panic attacks in a wide range of situations. In social phobia, the fear is less about the specific stimulus and more about potential negative social evaluation.

Initial assessment

Initial assessment should identify which specific objects or situations tend to trigger anxiety, or which are being avoided. Severity can be judged by assessing the number of fears, the level of anxiety, and the degree of functional impairment associated with the phobia.

Exploring the phobia CBT framework can be helpful to understand the condition, and can be used when explaining the problem, enabling the health professional to highlight any vicious cycles that are present (*Box 8.4*).

Initial management in primary care

Explaining specific phobias

The first step is to explain specific phobias to the patient, ideally using the CBT framework to illustrate the explanation. It is important to emphasise the behavioural factors that tend to maintain the cycle of anxiety in specific phobia, as this is key to successful treatment.

Self-help strategies

Self-help strategies can be particularly helpful for people with mild to moderate phobias, who may be able to self-treat the problem. These include:

- providing written information about specific phobia and how to overcome it
- highlighting self-help books and websites based on CBT principles
- providing information about local and national support groups for anxiety

Box 8.3

Differential diagnosis of specific phobias

- Panic disorder with agoraphobia
- Social phobia
- OCD
- PTSD
- Health anxiety

Box 8.4

A CBT framework for assessment of agoraphobia in primary care

Thoughts
- What would be your greatest fear(s) if you were faced by this object/situation?
- What would the worst thing that might happen if you stayed in the situation?
- Do you have any other worries or difficulties with your mood?

Feelings
- How do you feel emotionally in these situations?
- Is the anxiety out of proportion to the actual danger or threat in the situation?
- Do you ever experience panic attacks?

Behaviour
- Are you avoiding any situations due to your anxiety, or do you need to take a companion with you to help you face them?
- Do you do anything else to help combat your anxiety (e.g. drinking alcohol or taking drugs)?
- What do you do to try to stop yourself worrying?
- Do you often seek reassurance from others?

Physical symptoms
- Are you affected by any distressing or disabling physical symptoms?
- What physical reactions arise if you face (or think about) the situation/object that causes you anxiety?

Environmental factors and triggers
- Does a particular object or situation cause you extreme anxiety or even panic?
- How many different situations would cause this type of reaction?
- Is this affecting how you are able to live your life, e.g. work, relationships, family, social life, health?

Box 8.5

Explaining specific phobia

People with a specific phobia have an intense and extreme fear of a particular object, situation or animal. In phobias, people usually experience anxiety symptoms only when they are faced with the object or situation that they fear, or if they start to think about it, and are generally free from anxiety for the rest of the time.

When faced by the phobic situation or object, they will often experience fearful or catastrophic **thoughts** that they are facing serious danger. It is common to overestimate the risks posed by the situation and underestimate your ability to cope with the anxiety that arises. This leads to strong **feelings** of anxiety and sometimes panic. The fear leads to intense anxiety-related **physical symptoms**, such as shaking, sweating, nausea, palpitations and feeling breathless. These bodily sensations can also be very frightening.

Phobias become a particular problem when people begin to change their **behaviour** to avoid the feared items. Avoidance leads to a worsening of the phobia over time, by stopping people from confronting their fears and preventing them from learning that the situation is not as dangerous as they feared, and that they are able to cope with the phobia and any anxiety that arises. A restricted lifestyle also means that people with phobias miss out on many important life activities, which eventually leads to a loss of confidence and can affect mood.

It is important to discover when people are suffering from phobias, as they are one of the most treatable emotional conditions and respond extremely well to exposure therapy.

- lifestyle modification: physical exercise, reducing caffeine intake, smoking cessation and improving sleep habits may all be beneficial for improving overall wellbeing.

10 *minute CBT for specific phobia*

Graded exposure. Graded exposure is an effective treatment for phobias which can be used as a self-help strategy by people for mild to moderate phobias. This involves creating a hierarchy of feared situations which are currently being avoided due to the phobia. It is important to be as creative as possible and think of as many possible situations that might stimulate different levels of anxiety.

The next step is for the patient to begin facing some of the situations that they find difficult. This process will allow them to learn that the phobia is not as frightening as they previously thought and that they are able to cope with any anxiety that arises. As the person progresses successfully through each step of the hierarchy, their confidence is likely to grow whilst the anxiety will begin to lessen.

| Box 8.6 | **Example of hierarchy of graded exposure to a spider phobia** |

- Talking about spiders
- Looking at cartoon images of spiders
- Looking at a photograph of a small spider
- Looking at a photograph of a large spider
- Holding a toy spider
- Walking through a park or garden
- Looking at a small spider in a container from across the room
- Looking at a large spider in a container from across the room
- Looking at a small spider in a container up close
- Looking at a large spider in a container up close
- Watching a spider crawl across the table
- Watching a spider crawl on someone else's hand
- Having a spider crawling on my own hand

| Box 8.7 | **Tips for effective graded exposure** |

- Start small! Begin by choosing a situation that is only mildly threatening or anxiety-provoking and progress gradually towards situations that are more challenging.
- Repeat each exposure several times. Carry out the exposure task as often as possible, ideally on several different days, until you feel comfortable with the situation. The more often you expose yourself to items on your hierarchy, the quicker your fear will reduce.
- Stick with it when you are facing feared situations! Your anxiety will start to decrease if you stay in the situation. Stay in the situation until your anxiety has reduced by at least half. As you get higher up your hierarchy, you may find that you need more exposure time, and sometimes as long as 45 minutes, in order to feel comfortable.
- Cut out safety behaviours! Try not to use any safety behaviours during your exposure tasks. They prevent you from fully exposing yourself to your fear and learning that you can cope without them.
- Remember that anxiety is a normal physiological reaction that everyone experiences sometimes. It can be uncomfortable and unpleasant, but it is not dangerous and should not be feared or avoided.

Managing anxiety symptoms. The anxiety triggered by a phobic situation usually leads to a variety of uncomfortable physical sensations that can sometimes be frightening in themselves. Exercises such as controlled breathing and progressive muscular relaxation can be used to help people learn to tolerate and cope with anxiety-related symptoms.

However, it is important to try to avoid using relaxation exercises during exposure tasks. The purpose of exposure therapy is to enable people to habituate or get used to the anxiety that arises, until it eventually disappears. Attempts at relaxation may end up becoming safety behaviours that prevent people from fully experiencing anxiety and may actually get in the way of successful exposure therapy. For people who are very unwilling to attempt exposure without use of a relaxation strategy, it is possible to create a graded hierarchy which involves a gradual reduction in the use of safety behaviours.

Applied tension. Applied tension exercises can be used to reduce the risk of fainting when faced by blood, injection or injury, for example prior to a blood test (see *Box 8.8*).

Psychological treatments for phobias

Phobias are one of the most easily treatable anxiety disorders. Exposure therapy is the treatment of choice. Even a single session of therapy has demonstrated efficacy, although a greater number of sessions is associated with more favourable outcomes. CBT and exposure therapies have both demonstrated sustained benefits at long-term follow-up assessments.

Exposure therapy. This involves people confronting the feared situation to break the pattern of avoidance and fear. Exposure therapy leads to habituation, where the level of anxiety that arises to the feared stimulus gradually decreases over time (see *Figure 8.2*). It also challenges assumptions that feared objects, activities or situations are associated with bad outcomes and can lead to the development of new, more realistic beliefs about feared objects, activities or

---

Box 8.8

Applied tension for reducing the risk of fainting

- Sit in a chair and tense the muscles in your arms, legs and body for about 10–15 seconds.
- Hold the tension until you feel a warmth spread into your face or head. However, do not tense the muscles in your face or head, and avoid tensing your arm during a blood test procedure as this can make it more painful.
- Relax your body and release the tension for 20–30 seconds. Here, the goal is to allow your body to return to a normal state which is not overly tense nor completely relaxed.
- Repeat the exercise 5 times over a period of about 5 minutes.
- Practise several times a day for at least a week before using as part of exposure therapy to blood or needles.
- If you develop a headache when trying the applied tension technique, try to reduce the level of tension or the frequency of practice sessions.
- Try to learn to recognise the early signs of your blood pressure dropping, such as feeling light-headed, and use the applied tension technique as soon as you notice these sensations.

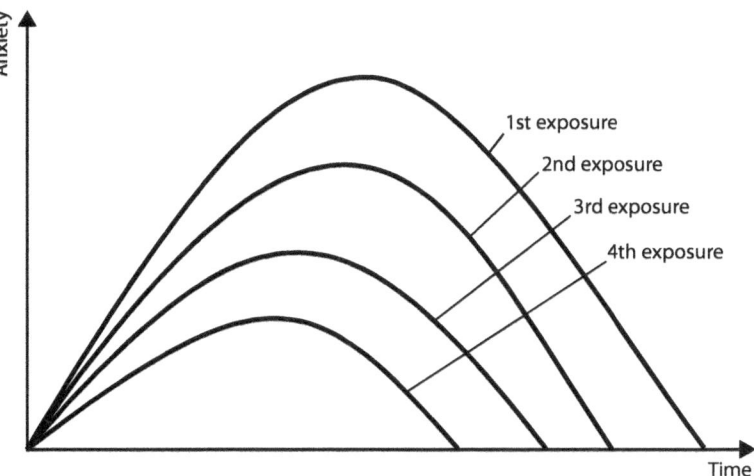

Figure 8.2 Habituation after exposure to a feared stimulus.

situations. Exposure can also build self-efficacy as the individual learns that they are capable of confronting their fears and can cope with the experience of fear and any feelings of anxiety that may arise in the previously avoided situation.

In graded exposure, the patient constructs an exposure fear hierarchy in which feared objects, activities or situations are ranked according to difficulty. The process of therapy begins with mildly or moderately difficult exposures, then progresses to harder ones.

In vivo exposure involves having patients come into direct contact with a feared object, situation or activity, such as a handling a live spider or a snake, being at heights or driving a car. This is the most rapid and effective form of treatment, particularly if exposure to the feared stimulus is provided in multiple different settings. Exposure therapy is also more effective if sessions are grouped closely together, exposure is prolonged, and involves some therapist involvement rather than being entirely self-directed. There is no evidence that either flooding or gradual exposure is more effective, but progressive exposures are generally more acceptable to patients.

Imaginal exposure involves asking the patient to imagine being exposed to the feared stimulus. Virtual reality exposure (VRE) involves use of a technology to create virtual simulation of the phobic situation, which triggers anxiety and allows the patient to emotionally process the exposure to the stimulus. Both of these approaches are less effective than *in vivo* exposure in the short term, although results are similar in the longer term and they may be more practical for treatment of certain feared situations such as fear of flying.

Applied tension. Exposure therapy combined with applied tension exercises (see *Box 8.8*) designed to prevent fainting has been shown to be effective for blood injury phobias. The patient is exposed to feared stimuli such as blood, injuries or needles, whilst being instructed to tense their muscles in order to raise blood pressure and prevent fainting in the presence of blood or injections.

Systematic desensitisation. Here, exposure is combined with relaxation exercises to make the process of exposure more manageable and to help patients learn to associate the feared objects, activities or situations with relaxation. However, this may be less effective than pure exposure theratpy.

Cognitive behavioural therapy. CBT for phobias is of similar effectiveness as pure exposure treatment, and it is not clear whether the addition of cognitive strategies is associated with enhanced treatment outcomes. CBT typically involves both behavioural exposure and cognitive approaches, such as cognitive restructuring of the faulty threat appraisals and unhelpful beliefs maintaining the phobic reaction.

Box 8.9 **Elements of CBT for phobias**

- Help the patient understand the nature of their phobic reaction(s) and identify the specific thoughts, feelings and behaviours associated with the phobia
- Explain the behavioural model of phobic anxiety and the role of avoidance and safety behaviours in maintaining symptoms
- Use of self-monitoring to improve understanding of the person's reactions to phobic situations, recognition of individual behavioural responses to the situation leading to a greater sense of mastery control
- Cognitive restructuring using guided discovery to generate alternatives to unhelpful or negative beliefs maintaining phobias, such as over-perception of risk associated with the situation
- Understanding the physiological response to anxiety and recognition of how fear of physical reactions to phobic situations may contribute to maintenance of the phobia ('fear of fear')
- Behavioural experiments involving exposure to feared situations, which also act to test the validity of negative beliefs and assumptions
- Develop a graded hierarchy of phobic objects and situations
- Exposure should be graduated, repeated and prolonged, including the use of imaginal exposure where practical problems make it hard to implement *in vivo* exposure, and interoceptive exposure for clients who are fearful of bodily sensations in the phobic situation
- Reduce avoidance or the use of safety behaviours

Drug treatment

Pharmacotherapy for the treatment of specific phobias is generally unproven and, given the effectiveness of exposure-based psychological therapies, it is not a recommended treatment in most cases. There is some limited evidence that SSRIs may be effective for specific phobias and these may be considered in patients who have marked functional impairment relating to the phobia and a lack of response to, or refusal to engage with, psychological approaches. Medication may also have a role where phobias are co-morbid with other anxiety disorders such as panic disorder or social anxiety disorder.

Benzodiazepines

Benzodiazepines are only recommended for use in clinical practice for the short-term relief of severe anxiety in acute situations. This is rarely appropriate or necessary in specific phobia, and it should be noted that benzodiazepines are contraindicated in phobic states (see *BNF*). Benzodiazepine use might rarely be considered when it is urgently necessary for a patient with a specific phobia to face a feared situation, such as a dental or imaging procedure.

There is no clear evidence as to whether concomitant use of benzodiazepines will impact upon the efficacy of psychological approaches but from a behavioural perspective, it can be argued that benzodiazepine use is likely to act as a safety behaviour which reinforces negative beliefs about the possible consequences of exposure to the feared stimulus and may therefore act to maintain anxiety over time.

Benzodiazepines are sometimes considered for management of fear of flying but again are likely to only be appropriate for emergency flight situations. Prescribers should bear in mind that benzodiazepine use may be associated with sedation, slowed thinking and longer reaction times, which may put the person and others on the flight at risk, due to being unable to act safely in the event of an emergency situation. This may be particularly marked if their use is combined with alcohol.

When to refer

Consider referral to specialist services if the person continues to experience significant symptoms after treatment with a psychological intervention. Referral may also be considered in severe cases with significant functional impairment, co-morbidity or people at high risk of self-harm or neglect.

Summary of primary care management of specific phobia

Stepped care approach	What to offer	What does this involve?
Initial presentations of specific phobia with mild to moderate impairment	Explain the diagnosis	• Explain specific phobias using a CBT framework to illustrate the specific fears, physical reactions and emotions triggered by the phobic stimulus • Discuss the role of behavioural avoidance and safety behaviours in maintaining anxiety
	10 minute CBT advice about managing anxiety	• Discuss the role of graded exposure to reduce avoidance to phobic stimuli • Management of anxiety symptoms to enable the individual to remain in contact with a feared situation, leading to habituation • Applied tension for managing fainting during procedures such as injections and phlebotomy
	Signpost to self-help resources	Provide information about CBT-based books and websites for understanding and managing anxiety phobias with exposure therapy
Moderate impairment associated with specific phobia or lack of response to initial measures	First-line:	• Exposure therapy is the first-line treatment for specific phobia
	Second-line:	• Other psychological therapies such as CBT or systematic desensitisation may also be considered • Consider SSRIs in patients with marked functional impairment and a lack of response to, or refusal to engage in, psychological approaches, or those with co-morbid depression or anxiety disorders • Benzodiazepines are contraindicated in phobic states and may act as a safety behaviour in maintaining phobias, so should only be rarely considered in emergency situations
Severe or complex problem or lack of response to primary care treatment	Refer to specialist services	• Consider referral to specialist services if the person continues to experience significant symptoms after treatment with a psychological intervention • Also consider in severe cases with significant functional impairment, co-morbidity or people at high risk of self-harm or neglect

8.10 Monitoring and follow-up

The importance of monitoring in specific phobia particularly relates to its potential for predicting the development of other mental health conditions. It may therefore be helpful to review patients with phobias over time, and to monitor for the development of associated disorders.

Case example 8.2: Yasmin

Diagnosis of vomiting phobia

"I'm terrified of vomiting! It's ruining my life…"

Yasmin, a 27-year-old married office manager, presents to her GP with a fear of vomiting. She explains that thinking about the possibility of vomiting leads to overwhelming anxiety associated with a fear that she might choke and die. The phobia has been present since childhood. She recalls an experience when aged around 11 years, when she developed gastroenteritis associated with repeated vomiting. This was extremely unpleasant, and she remembers at one point feeling as if a chunk of food had stuck in her throat, causing discomfort and a sensation that she might choke.

The impact of the fear has a major effect on Yasmin's life. She says, *"I don't know when I might feel sick, so I'm constantly having to monitor and check, and rearrange my life to make sure there's no chance I will ever vomit. Even just saying the word makes me feel sick, dizzy and shaky."*

Yasmin describes constantly monitoring her body for cues that she might feel nauseous or could possibly vomit, so that she can quickly leave a situation to prevent it. She avoids eating new foods which might not agree with her, never drinks alcohol and rarely eats out at restaurants for fear of developing food poisoning. Preparing meals takes an excessive amount of time as it involves excessive handwashing and strict hygiene. She also tends to avoid people who might be ill, and therefore rarely attends the GP surgery.

Yasmin has attended surgery today because she would like to conceive a child but is fearful to do so because of the possibility of developing morning sickness, and is also fearful that having a young child might expose her to possible illnesses causing vomiting. She has therefore been continuing to take contraception despite desperately wishing for children.

Yasmin's GP carries out a thorough assessment. She rules out other causes of the anxiety such as panic disorder. The GP initially wonders if this might be a form of OCD, when she hears about the handwashing behaviours, but is able to identify that this is a localised phobia which is specific to vomiting. The GP explains to Yasmin that the condition can be treated very effectively and recommends referral to the local psychological therapies team. Yasmin feels relieved that her condition is recognised and taken seriously and agrees to undertake psychological therapy.

8.11 Summary and key points

- Specific phobia is one of the most common and treatable psychiatric conditions.
- It is an important condition to recognise as it may be an early predictor of other psychiatric conditions.
- Sufferers experience fear or anxiety in the presence of a specific object or situation.

- Severity can be judged by assessing the number of fears, the level of anxiety and the degree of impairment.
- It is important to ask about symptoms of co-morbid disorders, which are commonly associated with specific phobia.
- Psychological treatments based on exposure techniques are first-line treatment for people with significant symptoms.

8.12 Phobias resources

- Mind: *Understanding Phobias* www.mind.org.uk/media-a/2946/phobias-2017.pdf
- Royal College of Psychiatrists: *Anxiety, Panic and Phobias* leaflet www.rcpsych.ac.uk/mental-health/problems-disorders/anxiety-panic-and-phobias
- Sanders, D. *Overcoming Phobias* booklet. Oxford Cognitive Therapy Centre www.octc.co.uk/product/booklets/overcoming-phobias
- Fear of flying courses: a variety of organisations offer graded exposure for fear of flying which may use flight simulation or participation on real air flights in a group therapy format.

Chapter 9
Social anxiety

Social anxiety quick reference guide

What is social anxiety?	Fear and avoidance of social or performance situations due to fears about being observed or evaluated negatively by other people.
How common is it?	One of the most common and functionally impairing of the anxiety disorders. The lifetime prevalence rates may be as high as 12%.
Risk factors	First-degree relatives are at higher risk of social anxiety. Other risk factors include a shy or introverted temperament, experiencing stressful social events in early life, parental modelling of fear and avoidance in social situations or an over-protective parenting style.
Co-morbid conditions	There is an extremely high level of co-morbidity with other mental health problems and 70–80% of individuals experience concurrent depression, substance misuse disorder or other anxiety disorders such as GAD, PTSD or panic disorder. There is also significant co-morbidity with avoidant personality disorder.
Usual course	Generalised social anxiety disorder is associated with an earlier age of onset and a more chronic course. Treatment is most effective at early stages of the disorder. Some adolescents with social anxiety will spontaneously recover, but chances of recovery are reduced if the disorder persists into adulthood. There is a relatively high risk of relapse after discontinuation of medication, which is reduced with CBT.
Common presentations	Social anxiety is under-recognised and only around half of sufferers ever seek treatment, possibly due to feelings of shame or anxiety about the condition. Adults typically describe symptoms of anxiety in social situations, avoidance behaviour and isolation, and may also present with co-morbid depression or substance misuse. Children may present with school refusal, or with crying, freezing or non-specific 'difficult' behaviour triggered by anxiety-provoking situations.
How to make the diagnosis	Answering yes to either of the following questions suggests the need for further assessment for social anxiety disorder: • *"Do you find yourself avoiding social situations or activities?"* • *"Are you fearful or embarrassed in social situations?"* Other useful diagnostic tools include the Mini-Social Phobia Inventory (Mini-SPIN) and Liebowitz Social Anxiety Scale (LSAS). GAD-7 and HADS may also be helpful to identify general symptoms of anxiety.

What else could it be?	Differential diagnosis and possible co-morbid conditions include other anxiety disorders (e.g. panic disorder, agoraphobia, GAD), depression, physical health conditions, substance misuse and avoidant personality disorder.
Self-management strategies	There is evidence that CBT-based self-help interventions can be effective in social anxiety disorder. Important self-management strategies using 10 minute CBT include recognising and labelling negative thoughts that arise in social situations (cognitive defusion) and reducing self-focus using attention training. Other useful strategies include reducing unhelpful or safety behaviours that are maintaining anxiety, and mindfulness.
Treatment of social anxiety	First-line treatment is with individual CBT. Second-line options include SSRI medication, which may be beneficial but has lower effectiveness and a higher risk of relapse compared to CBT, or guided self-help based on CBT principles. Third-line treatments include brief psychodynamic psychotherapy, or alternative medications include SNRIs and MAOIs.
When to refer	Severe or complex social anxiety with marked functional impairment or when there are concerns about risk such as self-neglect or self-harm, or a lack of response to primary care treatment strategies.
Follow-up	Long-term monitoring and support may be needed in primary care, as social anxiety often follows a chronic course. Patients prescribed antidepressant medication will require regular review and monitoring.

9.1 Introduction

Social anxiety, also referred to as social phobia, involves a fear of social or performance situations. Despite being an extremely common anxiety disorder, and the third most common psychiatric disorder after major depression and alcohol abuse, social anxiety disorder remains under-recognised in primary care.

The disorder can be differentiated from shyness and performance anxiety by its greater severity and pervasiveness, with the level of anxiety being out of proportion to the actual threat posed by the situation. The anxiety is also associated with a high degree of distress and/or impairment of function.

9.2 What is social anxiety?

Social anxiety is characterised by persistent fear about one or more social or performance situation, associated with worries about being publicly embarrassed, or of being negatively evaluated by others. This results in considerable distress, impacts on the person's ability to function effectively in important aspects of their daily life, and is often associated with avoidance of social situations. Diagnostic criteria for social anxiety disorder are shown in *Box 9.1*.

The fears in social anxiety may be discrete and only arise in specific types of social situations, or the anxiety may be diffuse, and arise in almost all social settings.

CBT framework for social anxiety

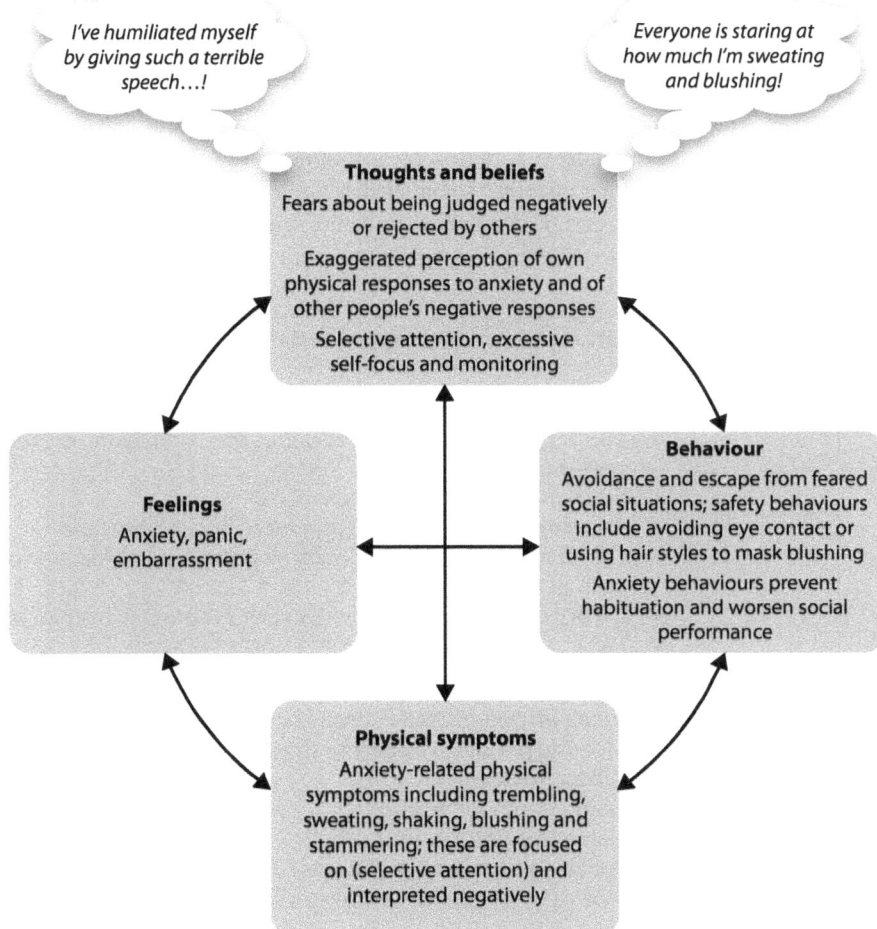

Thoughts and beliefs

Fears about being judged negatively or rejected by others

Exaggerated perception of own physical responses to anxiety and of other people's negative responses

Selective attention, excessive self-focus and monitoring

I've humiliated myself by giving such a terrible speech...!

Everyone is staring at how much I'm sweating and blushing!

Feelings

Anxiety, panic, embarrassment

Behaviour

Avoidance and escape from feared social situations; safety behaviours include avoiding eye contact or using hair styles to mask blushing

Anxiety behaviours prevent habituation and worsen social performance

Physical symptoms

Anxiety-related physical symptoms including trembling, sweating, shaking, blushing and stammering; these are focused on (selective attention) and interpreted negatively

---

Box 9.1 | **Diagnostic criteria for social anxiety**

- Marked or excessive fear about one or more social or performance situations
- The individual fears showing anxiety symptoms or acting in a way that leads to being publicly embarrassed or negatively evaluated by others
- Anxiety-provoking situations are avoided or endured with intense fear or anxiety
- Marked autonomic features often include palpitations, trembling, sweating and blushing
- Leads to considerable distress and impaired function in daily activities

Typical situations that might trigger anxiety can be broadly categorised into situations relating to performance and situations relating to social interaction (*Box 9.2*). Performance is a very broad concept, which includes carrying out everyday tasks that may be observed and potentially judged by others, as well as executing skills in controlling emotions or bodily functions, such as going to the toilet.

Social anxiety is also associated with a range of distressing physical symptoms and can affect functioning in many areas of normal life. It often leads to the avoidance of many social situations and can impact significantly on work and educational performance, interfere with social relationships and reduce quality of life. In severe cases, this may result in almost complete social isolation.

Box 9.2   **Situations which may trigger social anxiety**

Performance situations:
- Public performances such as public speaking, being on stage or giving a presentation
- Speaking in meetings or groups
- Answering questions or asking for help in a classroom
- Eating or drinking in front of other people, particularly in public areas such as restaurants
- Participating in group activities such as sports in front of others
- Playing a musical instrument in front of others
- Using public toilets

Situations involving social interaction:
- Meeting people, particularly strangers
- Talking to peers
- Going to school or work
- Going to a party or on a date
- Speaking to an authority figure, such as a boss or supervisor at work
- Asking for directions or asking a sales assistant for help in a shop

---

9.3 Epidemiology

Social anxiety is among the most common and functionally impairing of the anxiety disorders. Lifetime prevalence rates of up to 12% have been reported, and up to 7% in primary care settings. Unlike most other anxiety disorders, the prevalence of social anxiety is similar in both men and women.

The average age of onset is during late childhood and adolescence, with a median age of onset of 13 years, although it can begin as early as 7 or 8 years. Because of the young age of onset, the disorder can consequently lead to significant impairments in individuals' ability to form relationships with others and achieve important life goals.

9.4 Aetiology

No single mechanism seems to account for the development of social anxiety disorder. Its development is likely to be related to a combination of biological, psychological and environmental factors. Factors which may play a role in the development of social anxiety disorder are summarised in *Box 9.3*.

Box 9.3 **Factors associated with the development of social anxiety**

- Genetic factors: first-degree relatives are at higher risk of social anxiety
- Temperament: shyness, introversion and anxiety sensitivity
- Stressful social events in early life such as being bullied, familial abuse, public embarrassment or one's mind going blank during a public performance
- Parental modelling of fear and avoidance in social situations or an overprotective parenting style
- Behavioural factors and conditioning: learned escape, avoidance and safety behaviours act to maintain anxiety, interfere with skill development, and can lead to increasing levels of functional impairment and disability over time
- Selective attention: involves being excessively aware of and sensitive to social cues of potential negative evaluation, and internal cues supporting danger perception such as physical symptoms of anxiety.

9.5 CBT model of social anxiety

Typical thoughts in social anxiety

Socially anxious individuals experience a variety of thoughts and fears about being judged negatively by others. They worry about doing or saying something humiliating or embarrassing in front of other people, such as noticeably blushing, sweating, appearing boring or stupid, shaking, vomiting, stumbling over words, appearing incompetent or looking anxious. Direct eye-to-eye contact may be particularly stressful in some cultures.

The common theme of these fears is that the individual believes that they will behave in a way that is somehow unacceptable to others, who will judge them to be weak, foolish, stupid or crazy, and that this will lead to rejection, which is associated with a major loss of self-worth.

People with social anxiety also tend to have an exaggerated perception of other people's negative responses to them (*"He just yawned, he must think I'm so boring..."*). Unlike the fears in some other anxiety disorders, such as panic disorder or OCD, the worries in social anxiety, such as blushing or trembling, are relatively likely to actually take place. However, it is the meaning and significance of these events that is greatly exaggerated (*"I'm babbling my words so much I must look like a gibbering fool"*).

Some of the typical unhelpful thinking styles in social anxiety include:

- predicting future social interactions negatively: *"I will flush bright red, and everyone will laugh at me"*
- mind reading: *"She thinks I am totally unattractive"*
- catastrophising: *"If I mess up the presentation, I might lose my job"*
- personalisation: *"That group of people is laughing – they must be talking about me"*
- focusing on the negative: *"Stumbling over my words in the middle ruined my entire presentation"*
- *"what if...?"* statements without planning coping strategies: *"What if I can't think of anything interesting to say...?"*
- negative self-labelling: *"I'm boring and stupid".*

Physical symptoms associated with social anxiety

Social anxiety is associated with a range of anxiety-related physical symptoms, many of which are a physiological response to anxiety, including:

- sweating
- hand tremor
- blushing
- palpitations
- urgency of micturition
- nausea.

It is common for sufferers of social anxiety to have an exaggerated view of these symptoms as being more severe and noticeable to others than they really are.

Selective attention and excessive self-focus

People with social anxiety often become highly preoccupied with monitoring their own reactions to a social situation (*"I need to check how much I'm sweating..."*). This self-focus is likely to worsen the physical symptoms of anxiety as a vicious cycle. It also makes it much more difficult to pay attention to external aspects of the situation, such as listening to what other people are saying, thus making effective social interaction even more difficult.

In addition, there is a tendency to overestimate how noticeable or severe the physiological responses (e.g. *"I am trembling so badly and everyone is looking at me!"*) and to perceive their own performance as worse than it really is (*"I am stumbling over every single word in this speech – everyone must think I'm completely incompetent"*), leading to even greater levels of anxiety.

Behavioural factors in social anxiety

Behaviour in social anxiety involves avoidance of feared social interactions and performance situations. There is also a tendency to escape from situations whenever anxiety starts to arise. This tends to increase anxiety over time because people stop themselves having positive experiences that might disprove some of their fears, as well as being unable to practise and gain skills in coping with challenging situations. In addition, the longer the period of avoidance, the more daunting a social situation becomes, and it grows increasingly difficult to face.

People with social anxiety also tend to develop a range of safety behaviours, which are designed to reduce perceived risk during a social situation and to manage distressing feelings of anxiety. Examples of safety behaviours include:
- selecting a position in the situation that allows avoidance of excessive scrutiny (e.g. sitting in the back row)
- speaking softly or covering your mouth with your hand when speaking
- frequent rehearsal of what you are going to say
- avoiding eye contact or keeping your hands out of sight so others cannot see you shaking
- detaching from the situation by daydreaming
- wearing high collars or hairstyles to cover blushing
- drinking alcohol or taking drugs to lessen feelings of anxiety.

Unfortunately, safety behaviours maintain anxiety in the longer term, because the individual is unable to habituate themselves to the feared situation through exposure – instead they believe that they only coped because of the measures taken to try to control the anxiety. Some safety behaviours can also worsen performance in social situations. For example, by staying very quiet to avoid saying something 'stupid', people may appear distant or rude, and consequently experience negative reactions from others, making it harder to build effective connections with other people. Similarly, excessive internal focus associated with rehearsal of what to say stops people from engaging effectively in conversations.

9.6 Co-morbidity

There is a high level of co-morbidity between social anxiety disorder and other mental health problems, with an estimated 70–80% of individuals experiencing concurrent depression, substance use disorder or other anxiety disorders such as GAD and PTSD. There is also a high level of co-morbidity with panic disorder, and panic attacks may arise on exposure to, or on anticipation of exposure to the social situation. Behaviour such as misuse of alcohol or drugs may arise as an attempt to reduce anxiety in social situations, or to alleviate symptoms of low mood and depression. There is also a significant degree of co-morbidity between social anxiety disorder and some personality disorders, particularly avoidant personality disorder.

The presence of co-morbidity in social anxiety disorder is associated with poorer functioning and quality of life than in those with social anxiety alone. The high level of co-morbidity may also contribute to difficulties in identification of social anxiety. For example, health professionals may recognise and treat symptoms of depression, without detecting the underlying and more persistent social anxiety disorder.

9.7 Course and prognosis

Social anxiety is a common disorder which follows a chronic and debilitating course if untreated. It is often under-recognised, and access to treatment may be delayed or avoided. Generalised social anxiety disorder is associated with an earlier age of onset and a more chronic course.

A significant number of adolescents who develop social anxiety disorder will recover before reaching adulthood; however, if the disorder persists into adulthood, the chance of recovery in the absence of treatment is lower than with many other common mental health problems. Effective management therefore requires early detection and treatment.

Social anxiety can be a chronic, unremitting and long-term condition if unrecognised and untreated. However, the condition does respond to treatment with both CBT and medication, which have similar levels of efficacy. However, these may not be accessed due to lack of assessment or recognition of the disorder as a treatable condition by both patients and health professionals, as well as due to limited awareness about the availability of treatments. There is a relatively high risk of relapse after discontinuation of medication, which can be reduced by the addition of CBT. Because of this, continuation of treatment with medication for at least one year is often recommended.

9.8 Presentation of social anxiety

I'm feeling quite low because I've become so isolated I find it really hard to talk to people, so I tend to stay at home...

I just know that everyone is staring at me shaking and sweating when I'm in meetings at work. I must seem really incompetent...

Can you give me something to stop me blushing so much...? It's so embarrassing!

Adults who do present in primary care settings generally describe typical symptoms of anxiety in social situations. They may also present with avoidance behaviour and isolation, or with co-morbid mental health problems, such as depression or substance abuse.

Children and young people may present in primary care or in educational settings with symptoms arising from social anxiety. Interestingly, young people sometimes display anxiety in different ways from adults. Behaviour in socially

Case example 9.1: Khalid

How might social anxiety present?

Khalid is a 37-year-old man who attends his GP because he has been experiencing palpitations at work and is worried that he might have a cardiac problem. After a thorough assessment, he is not found to have any physical cause of his symptoms. His GP, Dr Steele, asks if he is experiencing any stress or worry and Khalid admits to experiencing significant anxiety at work. Dr Steele asks about the typical situations in which Khalid's anxiety arises.

Khalid explains that he is the manager of a small shop which was recently bought by a larger chain. He now works in a much more prominent role which involves visiting different stores and meeting management teams and customers. These visits tend to cause a lot of anxiety and worry and are associated with the physical symptoms of palpitations and chest tightness.

At this stage, the differential diagnosis remains broad, including a variety of anxiety disorders, such as generalised anxiety, panic disorder or health anxiety. Dr Steele explores further by asking questions such as: *"What makes you most anxious in this situation? What is the worst thing that might happen?"*

Khalid responds by describing fears relating to how his colleagues and the customers might perceive him. *"I just dread having to visit the other stores where I will have to talk to people. Before I set off, I keep thinking that I'm going to say or do something really stupid and they will think I'm an idiot. Until recently, I just worked in a tiny store by myself. When I'm in meetings, I get palpitations and start to feel shaky and sick. I'm sure they notice this and start staring at me. They must think that I don't know what I'm doing."*

Dr Steele then asks Khalid what he tends to focus on during meetings and how he reacts to feeling anxious. Khalid describes frequently rehearsing what he plans to say in his mind during meetings, which makes it hard to concentrate and listen to what others are saying. He also tries to hide his anxiety by saying as little as possible and not making eye contact with colleagues. Wherever possible, he tries to avoid meetings with more than one or two other people. This is causing some difficulties with carrying out his role.

This information can be summarised in a CBT framework as follows:

Thoughts	**Feelings**
I'm going to say or do something really stupid	Anxiety and worry
They will think I'm an idiot	
Everyone can see that I'm shaking	
They must think I don't know what I'm doing	

Behaviour	**Physical symptoms**
Repeated mental rehearsal of what I'm going to say	Palpitations
Not listening or focusing on what others are saying	Chest tightness
Talking as little as possible	Feel shaky and sick
Not making eye contact with colleagues	Difficulty concentrating
Avoiding meetings with large groups	

These negative thoughts about the perceptions of others, excessive self-focus, and avoidance behaviours are typical of social anxiety. The next step would be for Dr Steele to confirm the diagnosis using a diagnostic tool such as the Mini-Social Phobia Inventory (Mini-SPIN) (see *Section 9.9*), and to carry out an initial assessment of Khalid's condition.

anxious children may include crying, freezing or having tantrums in anxiety-provoking situations, in addition to avoidance. Children may therefore present with 'difficult' or challenging behaviour, as well as school refusal, which may stem from high levels of social anxiety.

9.9 Management of social anxiety

Making the diagnosis

Recognition of social anxiety disorder is extremely important in primary care, but there are significant barriers to making the diagnosis. Despite the extent of distress and impairment associated with the condition, and the fact that effective interventions are available, only about half of sufferers ever receive treatment. Of those who do receive treatment, many wait 10 years or more for it.

Having social anxiety may inhibit individuals from seeking help, as the thought of talking to a medical practitioner may trigger strong feelings of anxiety or shame, which inhibits people from disclosing their difficulties or leads to avoidance of health settings.

Social anxiety disorder should be suspected if patients present with features of persistent anxiety in social or performance situations. If suspected, the diagnosis can be confirmed using a variety of diagnostic tools.

Diagnostic and screening tools

A simple approach to identifying possible social anxiety disorder is to ask two questions:

- *"Do you find yourself avoiding social situations or activities?"*
- *"Are you fearful or embarrassed in social situations?"*

If the individual answers yes to either of these questions, it would be appropriate to carry out a more comprehensive assessment for social anxiety disorder.

Mini-Social Phobia Inventory (Mini-SPIN)

The Mini-SPIN is a very brief, three-item screening measure for generalised social anxiety symptoms which can identify up to 90% of people with generalised social anxiety disorder. It involves asking questions about fear of embarrassment and avoidance behaviour in the previous week. Its brevity and specificity make it highly suitable for use in primary care. A score of 6 or above

---

Box 9.4 | **Mini-SPIN**

Ask the person to rate the following statements using a 5-point Likert scale (0 = not at all; 1 = a little bit; 2 = somewhat; 3 = very much; 4 = extremely):

1. Fear of embarrassment causes me to avoid doing things or speaking to people
2. I avoid activities in which I am the centre of attention
3. Being embarrassed or looking stupid are among my worst fears

indicates a positive screen for social anxiety disorder and should be followed by a more comprehensive assessment for the condition.

Liebowitz Social Anxiety Scale (LSAS)

The LSAS is a 24-item self-report measure of social anxiety symptoms. Respondents rate their degree of anxiety and the extent to which they avoid performance-related and social interaction situations. An LSAS score of 80–120 indicates severe illness, 60–80 indicates moderate illness, and 40–60 indicates mild illness.

Other screening tools

As with other anxiety disorders, brief, self-report questionnaires such as GAD-7 or the anxiety questions of the HADS scale may also be helpful to assess for the presence and severity of anxiety symptoms. In combination with a clinical assessment of the nature of anxiety and the situations in which it typically arises, this may give a clear suggestion of the presence of social anxiety disorder.

Box 9.5   **Starting to talk about social anxiety**

- Does anxiety frequently arise in any specific situations? Are these situations often related to interactions with other people?
- Do you feel particularly self-conscious or concerned about how you are perceived by others?
- Can you give me an example of a time that you started feel anxious? Where were you and what were you doing?
- How did you cope with the situation or try to reduce your anxiety?
- Are you avoiding any situations in order to stop yourself becoming anxious?
- Is this having an impact on how you are able to live your life? Are you missing or avoiding any important activities because of anxiety?

Discussing symptoms of social anxiety

Social anxiety should be suspected when anxiety seems to arise mainly in social or performance situations, or if there is marked avoidance of these situations in order to prevent the individual from becoming anxious. Some useful questions for asking about symptoms of social anxiety are shown in *Box 9.5*.

What else to consider

The differential diagnosis for social anxiety disorder is shown in *Box 9.6*.

Initial assessment of social anxiety disorder

The initial assessment of social anxiety disorder should cover a range of information including the nature and severity of fear, avoidance, distress and functional impairment. It is also important to assess for co-morbid disorders, including avoidant personality disorder, alcohol and substance misuse, mood disorders, other anxiety disorders, psychosis and autism. As with all anxiety disorders, if low mood and hopelessness are prominent features, suicidal risk should be included as part of the assessment.

Box 9.6	**Differential diagnosis for social anxiety disorder**

- Panic disorder: unpredictable panic attacks arise out of the blue and not solely associated with performance situations or fear of judgement by other people
- Agoraphobia: panic attacks are associated with specific situations from which escape may be difficult
- GAD: anxiety is more diffuse with pervasive worry about multiple life areas, such as health, relationships, finances and work; anxiety is not specifically triggered by social situations or fears of negative evaluation
- Depression with anxiety: avoidance of social situations may arise due to low mood rather than social anxiety; depression may also be co-morbid or secondary to chronic social anxiety
- Physical health conditions mimicking or triggering anxiety: e.g. hyperthyroidism, caffeine
- Substance misuse: anxiety can be caused by the effects of substance use or as a result of withdrawal, or may develop secondary to chronic social anxiety
- Avoidant personality disorder (APD): pervasive pattern of social inhibition, feelings of inadequacy, and hypersensitivity to negative evaluation

The assessment includes a detailed description of the person's current social anxiety and associated problems and circumstances including:

- typical feared and avoided social situations
- what they are afraid might happen in social situations (e.g. looking anxious, blushing, sweating, trembling or appearing boring)
- anxiety symptoms
- self-perception or image in social situations
- focus of attention in social situations
- other unhelpful or safety-seeking behaviours
- occupational, educational, financial and social circumstances
- current medication, alcohol and recreational drug use
- relevant personal or family history of social anxiety and other mental health conditions.

Using a CBT framework to assess social anxiety

A CBT framework can be helpful for making a structured assessment of social anxiety in primary care. Useful questions are shown in *Box 9.7*.

Overcoming barriers to making an assessment in social anxiety disorder

Assessments of people with possible social anxiety disorder are most effective when carried out face to face. However, some individuals may find it extremely difficult or distressing to attend an initial appointment in person. If this is the case, it may be helpful to offer an initial assessment by telephone, but with the aim of seeing the person face to face for subsequent appointments and treatment.

Box 9.7   **A CBT framework for assessment of social anxiety disorder in primary care**

Thoughts
- What do you most fear might happen in the situation (e.g. looking anxious, blushing, sweating, trembling or appearing boring)?
- How do you think others see you? What might they think about you in this situation?
- How do you see yourself?
- What are you most aware of during the situation? What do you focus on (e.g. monitoring heart rate, self-checking for blushing or stammering)?

Feelings
- How do you feel in the situation?
- Do you experience panic attacks?
- How is your mood in general?

Behaviour
- What do you do when you start to feel anxious?
- Are you avoiding any places, situations or activities for fear of experiencing anxiety?
- Are you continuing to work and carry out social activities as usual?
- What do you do to try to stop people noticing that you are anxious?
- Do you have any other ways of managing your anxiety (e.g. use of alcohol or drugs)?

Physical symptoms
- What are the typical physical or bodily sensations that you experience?
- Which ones concern you the most?
- Do you feel that any physical reactions are particularly noticeable by other people?

Environmental factors and triggers
- Which particular social or performance situations tend to make you anxious?
- Are you experiencing any occupational, educational, financial and social difficulties?
- Do you have supportive friends, family and peer groups? Are you experiencing any form of bullying?
- How might your life be different if you were not experiencing this anxiety (e.g. effect on relationships, work, education, finances, etc.)?

Some other strategies for enabling an assessment of a patient with social anxiety disorder are shown in *Box 9.8*.

| Box 9.8 | **Facilitating the assessment of people with social anxiety disorder** |

- Use telephone appointments where needed to begin to establish a relationship with the patient
- Use empathetic statements and strong communication skills to build rapport
- When a person who experiences social anxiety is offered an appointment, provide information about where to go on arrival and where they can wait to be seen (written if needed)
- Offer appointments at times when the surgery is least crowded or busy
- Consider offering the use of a private waiting area or the option to wait outside to be seen
- Consider offering to meet or alert the person (for example, by text message) when their appointment is about to begin

Supporting patients in primary care

Explaining social anxiety disorder
It can be a great relief for sufferers of social anxiety to begin to gain more insight and recognition into the condition and how it is affecting them. It is important to take a non-judgemental approach and remember that patients may be highly sensitive to perceived negative evaluation by health professionals. Because of this, they may be feeling highly anxious during consultations and have difficulty concentrating or remembering verbal explanations, so it is particularly important to provide written information to support your discussion. Using a CBT framework can be helpful to illustrate and explain the patient's experiences.

Self-help strategies
Self-help strategies can be particularly helpful for people with mild to moderate social anxiety disorder. These include:
- providing written information about social anxiety and how it affects people
- highlighting relevant self-help books and websites based on CBT principles
- providing information about local and national support groups for anxiety
- lifestyle modification: physical exercise, reducing caffeine intake, smoking cessation and improving sleep habits may all be beneficial.

10 minute CBT for social anxiety
Brief interventions can be used to encourage positive self-management of social anxiety and encourage social engagement with reduced avoidance.

| Box 9.9 | **Explanation of social anxiety disorder** |

This sounds like you may be suffering from social anxiety disorder. This is a very common problem which is not the same as shyness. People sometimes don't feel confident to mention their symptoms to health professionals but it's important to do this because social anxiety can be treated effectively with psychological therapy or medication.

In social anxiety disorder, people are very sensitive to judgement by others and tend to feel very anxious in certain situations, especially if they think they will be watched or judged by others; for example, when talking to groups, eating in front of people, giving a presentation or performing in a play.

You may have **negative thoughts** that others will think badly of you, or that you will be embarrassed in public.

These thoughts lead to **feelings** of anxiety, and in turn, this creates **physical symptoms** such as shaking, sweating, stammering, blushing or feeling disorientated. You may worry that these physical reactions are very noticeable to others and will lead to negative judgements by other people. People with social anxiety are often aware these fears are a bit exaggerated, but it can be hard not to feel very anxious anyway.

This leads to **behaviour** to try to reduce or prevent anxiety. This might involve trying to hide physical reactions such as shaking or blushing. You might alter your clothing or posture, avoid eye contact so that others don't try to talk to you, or keep mentally rehearsing what you plan to say to avoid making a mistake. This can make it even harder to pay attention and join in with the conversations around you and makes it harder to involve yourself in social situations. You might also avoid social or performance situations, which tends to knock your confidence still further and increase anxiety levels in the long term.

Cognitive defusion and labelling. The process of recognising, highlighting and labelling negative thoughts can be helpful in brief settings, without necessarily proceeding to challenge the thoughts or carry out cognitive restructuring. This might involve statements such as:

- *"I'm having the thought that everyone is staring at me and this thought is making me feel anxious ..."*

"I'm having my usual worry that I'm going to stumble over my words when I start speaking, although that may not necessarily be accurate or true ..."

It can also be helpful to recognise and discuss unhelpful thinking styles which are commonly associated with social anxiety:

- Mind reading: assuming that you know what other people are thinking, and that they see you in the same negative way that you see yourself

- Fortune telling: predicting the future negatively and assuming the worst, which creates anxiety even before entering a situation
- Catastrophising: exaggerating the risks of a situation and blowing things out of proportion (*"It will be a disaster if people notice me shaking"*)
- Personalising: assuming that people are focusing on you when they may be more concerned with something completely different.

Gaining a broader perspective on negative thoughts associated with social anxiety involves:
- starting to recognise that physical symptoms of anxiety are not as noticeable to others as you fear
- accepting that people may not dislike or reject you because you are anxious
- understanding that you are not necessarily the focus of others' attention (they may be more concerned with their own worries and problems).

Reduce self-focus

Excessive self-focus and self-monitoring maintains social anxiety because it makes people become even more aware of their physical reactions and worsens anxiety as a vicious cycle. It also prevents people from fully concentrating on the people around them or maximising their own performance. Learning to switch attention from an internal to an external focus involves concentrating on the external environment and can help to reduce the impact of anxiety on the person (*Box 9.10*). Skills for reducing self-focus are also discussed in *Chapter 4* (attention training).

Other strategies

A number of other brief strategies may be helpful for people with social anxiety including:
- reducing unhelpful or safety behaviours that are reinforcing and maintaining social anxiety
- behavioural activation to increase the range of valued and meaningful life activities
- reducing hyperventilation using slow exhale, square breathing or other breathing strategies
- mindfulness to reduce the power and believability of negative thoughts during social situations.

Treatment of social anxiety disorder

Social anxiety disorder responds well to treatment, although many sufferers continue to experience some symptoms after the end of the acute treatment phase.

Psychological therapy

Individual CBT that has been specifically developed to treat social anxiety disorder is the most effective and therefore the first-line treatment for social

Box 9.10 | **Skills for reducing self-focus in social anxiety**

- Actively engage in conversation with other people: listen attentively, ask questions and try to make a connection rather than focusing on what they might be thinking about you.
- Focus on the present moment: look at other people and the surroundings. Use brief mindfulness to ground yourself – take a breath, notice your feet on the floor and keep your focus on the external environment rather than getting lost in your own thoughts.
- Accept imperfection: be kind to yourself and try to reduce the expectation that you must appear perfect or never make a mistake; instead focus on being genuine, attentive and interested.
- Remember that your anxiety is not as noticeable as you fear, and even if people do notice that you are nervous, it doesn't automatically mean they will judge or think badly of you; they may well be feeling just as anxious themselves!

Box 9.11 | **CBT in social anxiety disorder**

Individual CBT for social anxiety disorder should include elements of the following:
- Education about social anxiety disorder
- Cognitive restructuring
- Experiential exercises to demonstrate the adverse effects of self-focused attention and safety-seeking behaviours
- Graduated exposure to feared social situations
- Video feedback to correct distorted negative self-imagery
- Attention training
- Behavioural experiments to test negative beliefs
- Working with problematic memories of social trauma
- Examination and modification of core beliefs
- Modification of problematic pre- and post-event processing
- Relapse prevention

anxiety disorder in adults. Treatment should consist of up to 14 sessions of 60–90 minutes' duration over approximately 4 months. Group CBT can also be considered but is less clinically effective and less cost-effective than one-to-one therapy.

CBT-based supported self-help involves up to 9 sessions of a CBT-based self-help book over 3–4 months, with support to use the materials, either face-to-face or by telephone, for a total of 3 hours over the course of the treatment, and may be considered for mild to moderate cases. NICE recommends that this is a second-line approach for people who have declined standard CBT.

Short-term psychodynamic psychotherapy that has been specifically developed to treat social anxiety disorder also has some evidence of benefit for social anxiety disorder, although it is less clinically effective and has lower cost-effectiveness compared with CBT, self-help and pharmacological interventions. This typically involves up to 25–30 sessions of 50 minutes' duration over 6–8 months. Mindfulness may also have some benefit, but is not recommended by NICE as a sole therapeutic approach.

The effects of psychological interventions are well maintained and there is a lower risk of relapse following successful treatment than with medication.

Box 9.12

Short-term psychodynamic psychotherapy for social anxiety disorder

- Education about social anxiety disorder
- Establishing a secure positive therapeutic alliance to modify insecure attachments
- Focus on a core conflictual relationship theme associated with social anxiety symptoms
- Focus on shame
- Encouraging exposure to feared social situations outside therapy sessions
- Support to establish a self-affirming inner dialogue
- Help to improve social skills

Drug treatment

Medication is not recommended as a first-line treatment, as the evidence for drug treatment of social anxiety disorder is not as strong as that of psychological therapies. For patients who request medication in preference to CBT, the recommendation is to discuss their concerns about CBT prior to offering a pharmacological intervention.

If a patient does wish to try medication, the first-line choice would be an SSRI. Licensed options include sertraline, paroxetine and escitalopram. Guidelines for initiating and reviewing SSRI treatment are covered in *Chapter 3*.

Other choices of medication in social anxiety disorder include an SNRI. A third-line choice may be a MAOI such as phenelzine or moclobemide. There does not appear to be much difference in efficacy between different classes of medication, although there are differences in tolerability, adverse effects and risks of overdose.

Rates of relapse after discontinuation of drug therapy are relatively high. A significant proportion of people who respond to an SSRI are likely to relapse within a few months if the drug is discontinued after acute treatment. Interesting, about 25% of people who respond to SSRI treatment and continue drug treatment will also relapse within 6 months. Drug treatment should be continued for 6–12 months to reduce the risk of relapse.

Treatments to avoid in social anxiety disorder

Treatments which should not be routinely offered for the treatment of social anxiety disorder are summarised in *Box 9.13*.

Box 9.13 **Interventions that are not recommended to treat social anxiety disorder (NICE, 2013)**

- Do not routinely offer anticonvulsants, TCAs, benzodiazepines or antipsychotic medication to treat social anxiety disorder in adults
- Do not routinely offer mindfulness-based interventions
- There is no evidence for use of St John's wort or other over-the-counter preparations for anxiety to treat social anxiety disorder
- There is no good quality evidence showing benefit from botulinum toxin to treat hyperhidrosis (excessive sweating) in people with social anxiety disorder, and it may be harmful
- Similarly, there is no good evidence for endoscopic thoracic sympathectomy to treat hyperhidrosis or facial blushing in people with social anxiety disorder

---

Managing co-morbid depression

Treatment choice for patients with social anxiety disorder who are also suffering from co-morbid depression, depends on identifying which condition developed first. In primary depression, this should be treated first, as the anxiety may resolve as the mood lifts.

If social anxiety disorder preceded the onset of depression, this may indicate that the individual has become depressed as a consequence of experiencing persistent anxiety. A useful question to ask is: *"If I could give you a treatment that ensured that you were no longer anxious in social situations, would you still be depressed?"* If the person answers 'no', then the first goal is usually to treat the social anxiety.

In cases of severe depression, it is usually most effective to treat depression first, as the low mood can impair the person's ability to participate actively in the treatment for social anxiety.

Managing co-morbid substance misuse

Substance misuse is a common co-morbid problem in social anxiety disorder. As with depression, it is helpful to ascertain whether the substance misuse is primarily a consequence of social anxiety disorder or whether the anxiety has developed because of the substance misuse problem. Alcohol or drug misuse can be an attempt to reduce anxiety in social situations and should not preclude treatment for social anxiety disorder.

Where appropriate, health professionals should offer a brief intervention for hazardous alcohol or drug misuse and consider referral to a specialist service for harmful or dependent alcohol or drug misuse.

When to refer

Severe or complex cases with marked functional impairment should be referred to specialist services, or if there are concerns about risk such as self-neglect or self-harm. Also consider referring patients with persistent and marked symptoms who have not responded to primary care treatment strategies.

Treatment may involve a combination of medication and psychological therapy, although studies are small and there is no clear evidence that combination is more effective than either pharmacological or psychological therapy alone.

Summary of primary care management of social anxiety disorder

Stepped care approach	What to offer	What does this involve?
Initial presentations of mild to moderate social anxiety	General self-care	Offer advice about general self-care including regular, graded exercise and sleep hygiene
	10 minute CBT advice about managing anxiety	• Explain the diagnosis of social anxiety using a CBT framework, including how excessive self-focus and exaggerated perception of negative appraisal by others can lead to feelings and physical symptoms of anxiety as a vicious cycle • Encourage recognition and labelling of negative thoughts to reduce their power and believability (cognitive defusion) • Attention training to reduce self-focus and improve functioning during social situations • Behavioural activation to increase participation in meaningful and important life activities • Reduce unhelpful or safety behaviours during social situations
	Signpost to self-help resources	Provide information about CBT-based books and websites for understanding and managing social anxiety
Moderate anxiety or lack of response to initial measures	First-line treatment for social anxiety disorder	• Individual CBT
	Second-line treatment	• Drug treatment with SSRI (but try to resolve any concerns about psychological therapy before offering medication) continued for at least 6 months following resolution of symptoms • Guided self-help is another second-line option for people who decline individual CBT
	Third-line treatment	• Short-term psychodynamic psychotherapy specifically developed for social anxiety disorder • Alternative drug treatments include SNRIs and MAOIs (phenelzine or moclobemide)

Stepped care approach	What to offer	What does this involve?
Severe or complex problem or lack of response to primary care treatment	Refer to specialist services	• Severe or complex cases with marked functional impairment or if there are concerns about risk such as self-neglect or self-harm • Or, persistent and marked symptoms which have not responded to primary care treatment strategies

9.10 Monitoring and follow-up

Social anxiety disorder often follows a chronic course, with significant risk of relapse, particularly after discontinuation of medication. Long-term monitoring and support may therefore be needed in primary care. Patients prescribed antidepressant medication will also require regular review and monitoring.

Case example 9.2: Claire

Diagnosis and management of social anxiety

Claire is a 24-year-old student in the second year of a French language university degree. She attends her university GP surgery because she has been feeling increasingly anxious and is now finding it hard to participate in her studies. She is worried that she might fail the course.

Her GP, Dr Taylor, asks Claire to give an example of a situation that causes her anxiety. Claire explains that she copes well with written assignments but feels extremely anxious when having to demonstrate her knowledge of spoken French in the classroom environment. She is aware that she starts to feel very hot, to blush and become very shaky, and her voice starts to noticeably crack, which affects the quality of her French accent. She is very conscious that her peers and the lecturer will notice and think she is foolish and incompetent at French.

Dr Taylor asks about the thoughts that arise when Claire gets anxious, and these include negative beliefs about how she is perceived by others, and catastrophic thoughts about future negative consequences: "*Everyone will notice how nervous I am and assume it's because I'm terrible at French. They will think I am stupid and that I shouldn't be on the course at all. I'll never be able to cope in France. I will have to leave the course.*"

Dr Taylor also asks about the behaviours that Claire is carrying out to try to manage her feelings of anxiety, and the impact of the symptoms on her life. Claire reports that she has started avoiding small group spoken French classes. She also sits at the back of the class and tries to avoid eye contact with the teacher, and often mumbles to try to hide the changes in her voice. She is isolated and has made very few friends at university. She has joined the orchestra but avoids any social activities associated with the club because she fears others will find her boring. She usually goes back home to her parents at weekends. As part of her studies, she is due to participate in an exchange programme which involves living in France for 3 months with a French family and the thought of this fills her with intense fear and dread.

Case example 9.2: *contd*

Dr Taylor asks about a past history of shyness and social anxiety. Claire reports that she has always been relatively shy and introverted, and had only a few friends at school, but that this had not seemed to matter in the small and supportive school she had attended but is now a much bigger challenge in the large and busy university setting.

Dr Taylor asks Claire to complete Mini-SPIN, which scores 9, and is consistent with his clinical impression of social anxiety disorder. He explains the likely diagnosis of social anxiety disorder using a CBT framework and referring to the specific thoughts, feelings and behaviours which Claire has reported during the consultation:

Thoughts
Everyone will think I am foolish and incompetent at French
Everyone will notice how nervous I am
They will think that I shouldn't be on the course
I'll never be able to cope in France
I will have to leave the course

Feelings
Anxiety
Fear
Dread

Behaviour
Avoids small group classes
Sits at the back
Avoids eye contact with the teacher
Mumbles to hide changes in her voice
Avoids social activities at university

Physical symptoms
Feels hot, blushes
Shaky
Voice starts to crack

Environment and background
Has always been shy and had a small group of friends at school

They discuss treatment options and Dr Taylor explains that CBT is the most effective approach. Claire is extremely relieved that Dr Taylor has been so understanding, as she had been dreading attending the surgery and had put off coming for many months. She agrees to a referral for individual therapy. Dr Taylor also recommends some self-help resources relating to social anxiety and Claire agrees to look at these and return to discuss how she is coping in a future consultation.

Whilst awaiting CBT, Dr Taylor continues to review Claire and offer her support. Claire is motivated to try to overcome her symptoms and has read the self-help information that he provided. They also discuss some strategies for reducing the impact of her social anxiety on her studies including:

- making an appointment with her course tutor to discuss her anxiety and seek help with her coursework
- re-starting attendance at important small group language tutorials
- practising attention skills and using these during anxiety-provoking situations
- engaging more in social activities with the orchestra to build friendships and improve her overall wellbeing (brief behavioural activation).

9.11 Summary and key points

- Social anxiety is a common anxiety disorder which can be highly disabling for sufferers, but which remains under-recognised and undertreated in primary care.
- Sufferers experience high levels of anxiety about social or performance situations associated with fears about being publicly embarrassed, negatively evaluated or rejected by others.
- Individuals with social anxiety hold exaggerated fears that their anxiety-related somatic symptoms are noticeable by others and will lead to further negative judgements about their appearance or competence.
- Sufferers typically avoid social situations, leading to significant functional impacts on work, education and social relationships, and maintaining anxiety as a vicious cycle.
- Safety behaviours such as excessive self-focus and attempts to hide physical symptoms impair people's ability to interact socially, reduce confidence and worsen anxiety over time.
- Asking two questions can help with screening for social anxiety disorder:
  - *"Do you find yourself avoiding social situations or activities?"*
  - *"Are you fearful or embarrassed in social situations?"*
- First-line treatment for social anxiety disorder is with individual CBT, which is the most effective treatment.
- Medication is less effective; SSRIs are first-line choice when indicated, but are associated with a higher risk of relapse than CBT.

9.12 Social anxiety resources

- Centre for Clinical Interventions: www.cci.health.wa.gov.au/Resources/For-Clinicians/Social-Anxiety
- Northumberland, Tyne & Wear NHS Foundation Trust Self Help leaflets: https://web.ntw.nhs.uk/selfhelp/leaflets/Social%20Anxiety%20%20A4%20 2016%20FINAL.pdf
- Butler, G. (2016) *Overcoming Social Anxiety and Shyness: a self-help guide using cognitive behavioural techniques*, 2nd edition. Robinson.

Chapter 10
Obsessive–compulsive disorder

OCD quick reference guide

What is obsessive–compulsive disorder (OCD)?	Recurrent, highly distressing, unwanted obsessional thoughts and compulsive behavioural rituals to try to 'neutralise' the thoughts and alleviate emotional distress, which markedly interfere with the individual's daily life.
How common is it?	Fourth most common mental disorder, affecting around 2–3% of the population and with a lifetime prevalence of around 1.6%. There is an equal prevalence among males and females but men are more likely to have chronic course and a poorer response to treatment.
Risk factors	These include genetic factors and experiencing emotional abuse or neglect in childhood. Adverse life events may trigger the development of OCD symptoms in predisposed individuals. Rarely, other factors may be associated, including pregnancy or neurological conditions.
Co-morbid conditions	Depression will affect over two-thirds of people with OCD during their lifetime. Other common co-morbid conditions include social anxiety, alcohol misuse, specific phobias, GAD and BDD. People with OCD are also at increased risk of self-harm and suicide.
Usual course	The diagnosis of OCD is often delayed, and patients may experience symptoms for many years before seeking help. The untreated course of OCD is usually chronic with waxing and waning symptoms.
Common presentations	People with OCD may present with concerns about anxiety or intrusive thoughts, or with consequences of the compulsive behaviour such as dermatitis due to excessive handwashing. They may also present with functional impacts such as work or relationship problems caused by lateness due to repeated checking rituals.
How to make the diagnosis	NICE recommends asking six questions to help make the diagnosis of OCD: 1. *"Do you wash or clean a lot?"* 2. *"Do you check things a lot?"* 3. *"Is there any thought that keeps bothering you that you would like to get rid of but cannot?"* 4. *"Do your daily activities take a long time to finish?"* 5. *"Are you concerned about putting things in a special order or are you very upset by mess?"* 6. *"Do these problems trouble you?"* Other diagnostic tools include the Yale–Brown Obsessive Compulsive Scale (Y-BOCS).

What else could it be?	The differential diagnosis is broad and includes other anxiety disorders, bodily distress disorder/MUS, obsessive–compulsive personality disorder, delusional disorder, tic disorder, autism, excoriation and hoarding disorder.
Self-management strategies	General self-care including physical exercise, healthy diet and sleep hygiene are often helpful. Offer empathy and support and help patients to understand their condition by giving clear explanations of OCD. Self-management strategies using 10 minute CBT include highlighting and labelling thoughts, graded exposure, reducing compulsive behaviours, behavioural activation and mindfulness.
Treatment of OCD	Both medication and CBT involving exposure and response prevention (ERP) are effective for the treatment of OCD. Choice depends on patient preference and other factors such as availability of therapy. First-line drug therapy is with an SSRI (fluoxetine), which should be continued for at least 12 months. Doses may need to be higher than in other anxiety disorders. Alternative medications include clomipramine. In severe cases antidepressant treatment may be augmented with antipsychotic medication but this should usually only be initiated by a specialist.
When to refer	Severe symptoms associated with marked functional impairment, at risk of self-neglect, self-harm or suicide, or posing a risk to others, significant co-morbidity such as substance misuse, severe depression, anorexia nervosa, or schizophrenia or lack of response to treatment in community settings.
Follow-up	Long-term support in primary care is often required for OCD, which often has a fluctuating or episodic course. There is also a high rate of relapse after discontinuing medication for OCD, which can be improved by combining medication with CBT or continuing long-term treatment.

10.1 Introduction

Obsessive–compulsive disorder (OCD) affects around 2% of the population. It is characterised by anxiety associated with obsessional thoughts and compulsive behaviours which cause significant distress and impairment in daily functioning, interfere with relationships and have a substantial negative effect on the sufferer's quality of life.

10.2 What is OCD?

OCD is characterised by the presence of either obsessions or compulsions, but usually both. Obsessions are defined as unwanted and intrusive thoughts, images or impulses, which repeatedly enter the mind. These thoughts are typically repugnant or inconsistent with the person's values, leading to high levels of distress and anxiety. Common obsessions include fear of contamination, need for symmetry or exactness, fear of causing harm to someone, sexual obsessions, religious obsessions, fear of behaving unacceptably and fear of making a mistake (see *Box 10.1*).

The obsessional thoughts are disturbing but are recognised as originating in the person's own mind and not imposed by an external agency. The thoughts are generally recognised by the patient to be extreme or unreasonable and are only

CBT framework for OCD

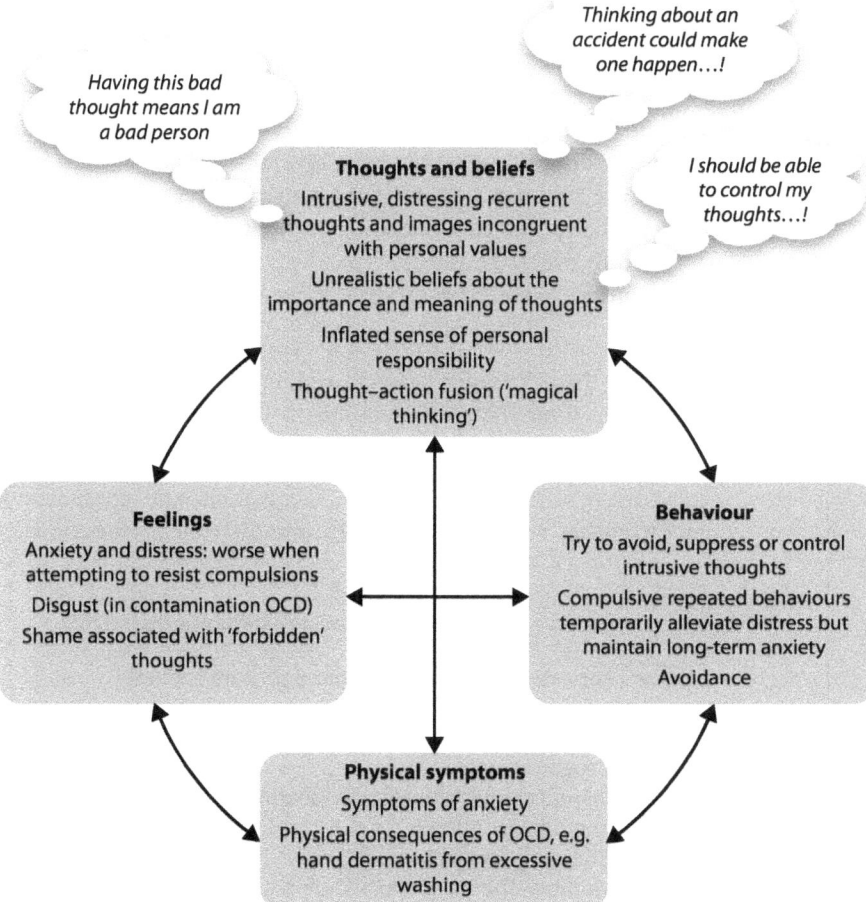

Having this bad thought means I am a bad person

Thinking about an accident could make one happen…!

I should be able to control my thoughts…!

Thoughts and beliefs
Intrusive, distressing recurrent thoughts and images incongruent with personal values
Unrealistic beliefs about the importance and meaning of thoughts
Inflated sense of personal responsibility
Thought–action fusion ('magical thinking')

Feelings
Anxiety and distress: worse when attempting to resist compulsions
Disgust (in contamination OCD)
Shame associated with 'forbidden' thoughts

Behaviour
Try to avoid, suppress or control intrusive thoughts
Compulsive repeated behaviours temporarily alleviate distress but maintain long-term anxiety
Avoidance

Physical symptoms
Symptoms of anxiety
Physical consequences of OCD, e.g. hand dermatitis from excessive washing

---

Box 10.1 **Common examples of obsessional thoughts in OCD**

- Fears about contamination from dirt, germs, bodily fluids or faeces, chemicals or other dangerous substances
- Fear of harm – e.g. that door locks are not safe, or that the oven has not been switched off
- Excessive concern with order or symmetry
- Fear of making a mistake with serious consequences
- Superstitions and fear of 'bad' numbers
- 'Forbidden' thoughts or images that violate a person's own morals or run counter to their sexual preferences (e.g. thoughts about being a paedophile, other sexual thoughts, blasphemy)
- Thoughts of violence or aggression (e.g. fears about harming others or even one's own baby)

rarely delusional in nature. The affected person often makes considerable effort to ignore or suppress these distressing thoughts or may try to 'neutralise' them by carrying out some other thought or action (i.e. by acting on a compulsion).

Compulsions are repetitive, intentional actions (e.g. checking, handwashing or ordering) or mental acts (e.g. counting, repeating words silently or praying) that the person feels compelled to perform in response to an obsessional thought, or according to rules that must be applied rigidly. These behaviours or mental acts are performed in order to prevent a feared event or to reduce distress, and usually lead to a temporary relief in feelings of anxiety. Compulsions are generally excessive and are typically not realistically connected to the event that they are designed to neutralise or prevent.

People with OCD do not find carrying out their compulsions pleasurable but do them in order to avoid the anxiety that arises if they do not perform the behaviour. This differentiates it from impulsive acts such as shopping or gambling, which are associated with immediate gratification.

To make a diagnosis of OCD, obsessions and compulsions must be time-consuming and/or cause significant distress or functional impairment. The

---

Box 10.2   **Common examples of compulsive behaviours in OCD**

- Repeated checking (e.g. that doors are locked)
- Cleaning and washing
- Ordering, symmetry, arranging or exactness
- Repeating acts
- Mental compulsions (e.g. repeating special words or prayers in a set manner, counting)
- Hoarding and collecting
- Memory checking and avoidance of triggers

Box 10.3   **Diagnostic criteria for OCD**

- Persistent obsessions or compulsions, or commonly both
- Obsessions are repetitive and persistent thoughts, images or urges that are intrusive, unwanted and usually associated with anxiety
- The individual attempts to ignore or suppress obsessions or to 'neutralise' them by carrying out compulsions
- Compulsions are repetitive behaviours or mental acts that the person feels driven to perform, including repeated mental acts
- There are usually attempts to resist a compulsion (although resistance may be minimal)
- Symptoms result in significant distress or impairment in important areas of functioning

individual typically makes unsuccessful attempts to resist both experiencing the obsessional thoughts and carrying out the compulsive behaviours, although this resistance may be very minimal in long-standing cases. ICD-10 diagnostic criteria for OCD are shown in *Box 10.3*.

10.3 Epidemiology

OCD affects around 2–3% of the population and it is estimated to be the fourth most common mental disorder, with a lifetime prevalence of around 1.6%. There is an equal prevalence among males and females. The mean age of onset is late adolescence for men and early 20s for women but it can occur at any age. Males are more likely to have chronic course and a poorer response to treatment.

The disorder appears with similar prevalence rates and symptom presentations across cultures, although there can be some cultural specificity to the content of obsessions.

10.4 Aetiology

As with most anxiety disorders, there are a number of aetiological factors which are likely to be important in the development of OCD. Risk factors for its development are shown in *Box 10.4*.

Box 10.4 | **Risk factors for the development of OCD**

- Genetic factors: first-degree relatives of people with OCD are at increased risk of developing the disorder
- Developmental factors: these include emotional, physical, and sexual abuse or neglect, social isolation, teasing and bullying
- Adverse life events and difficulties: may trigger the development of OCD in individuals who are biologically or psychologically predisposed
- Pregnancy and the postnatal period: may act as triggers for the development of obsessive–compulsive symptoms
- Neurological conditions: obsessive–compulsive symptoms can rarely present in adults as a symptom of a neurological disorder such as a brain tumour, Huntington's chorea, frontotemporal dementia or as a complication of head trauma
- Sudden onset of OCD symptoms in childhood and the presence of motor tics, hyperactivity, or choreiform movements may, extremely rarely, be associated with infectious agents and other environmental factors, including a possible autoimmune reaction to beta-haemolytic streptococci in paediatric autoimmune neuropsychiatric disorder associated with streptococcal infections (PANDAS); however, no laboratory tests are currently able to make this diagnosis

10.5 CBT model of OCD

Thoughts in OCD

The experience of intrusive, distressing thoughts and images is not limited to people suffering from OCD. This is an almost universal experience within the general population, and the content of such thoughts is indistinguishable from that of people with OCD. The difference lies in the meaning that individuals with OCD attach to the occurrence or content of the thoughts and in their reactions to them. People with OCD view such thoughts as being associated with a major risk of harm to themselves, a loved one or someone else, depending on their own response, or lack of response, to these thoughts.

'Rumination' is also common in OCD, which involves prolonged, repetitive thinking about one topic. This includes both intrusive thoughts, often in the form of doubts, worries or questions, and repeated, compulsive attempts to find an answer to these concerns.

A number of unhelpful thinking styles are typically seen in OCD. These include:
- over-importance of thoughts: unrealistic beliefs about the meaning and significance of experiencing thoughts (*"Having worries about being a paedophile means that I am dangerous and unfit to be a parent"*)
- inflated sense of personal responsibility: beliefs that the individual has a special power to cause, or the duty to prevent, negative outcomes (e.g. *"I am responsible for preventing my child from being harmed on the way to school by using mental counting"*)
- thought–action fusion ('magical thinking'): beliefs that thoughts and images can influence the external world (*"Thinking about having an accident could cause one"*) or that thinking about something is the same as carrying it out (e.g. *"Having a thought about harming my children is just as bad as actually doing it, unless I perform a 'neutralising' action"*)
- control of thoughts: beliefs that complete control over one's thoughts is both necessary and possible
- overestimation of threat: belief that negative events are highly likely and would be catastrophic in nature if they occurred
- perfectionism: belief that making mistakes and imperfection are intolerable
- intolerance of uncertainty: belief that it is necessary and possible to be completely certain that negative outcomes will not occur.

Feelings and emotions

The most common feeling associated with OCD is anxiety, although sufferers frequently go to extreme lengths to minimise experiencing this emotion. Other feelings include disgust (particularly in contamination OCD), shame associated with "forbidden" thoughts, and a distressing sense of "incompleteness" until things feel "just right".

Typical behaviour

Compulsive behaviours in OCD represent a form of safety-seeking behaviours and are attempts by the individual to either remove intrusive thoughts or to prevent any perceived future harmful consequences of the thoughts. Examples of typical compulsive behaviours seen in OCD are described in *Box 10.2*.

Compulsive behaviours are self-reinforcing as they are usually associated with a short-term decrease in anxiety and a temporary reduction in the experience of intrusive thoughts. Carrying out these actions also prevents the person from learning that their thoughts are unrealistic and strengthens the belief that carrying out the compulsion can prevent feared events from occurring. This increases the urge to perform the compulsion again, as a vicious cycle. Compulsions can also lead to an increase in unwanted thoughts by acting as a reminder of the feared outcomes (e.g. repeated handwashing leads to increased thoughts about possible contamination).

Avoidance is also a common behavioural response in OCD, which also maintains long-term anxiety as a vicious cycle. Examples include:
• avoiding touching door handles, taps or toilet seats used by others
• hiding all knives and other sharp objects
• never being left alone with a child if there are fears of being a paedophile.

Mental attempts to suppress distressing thoughts are also examples of avoidance behaviour.

The relationship between thoughts feelings and behaviour in OCD is illustrated in *Figure 10.1*.

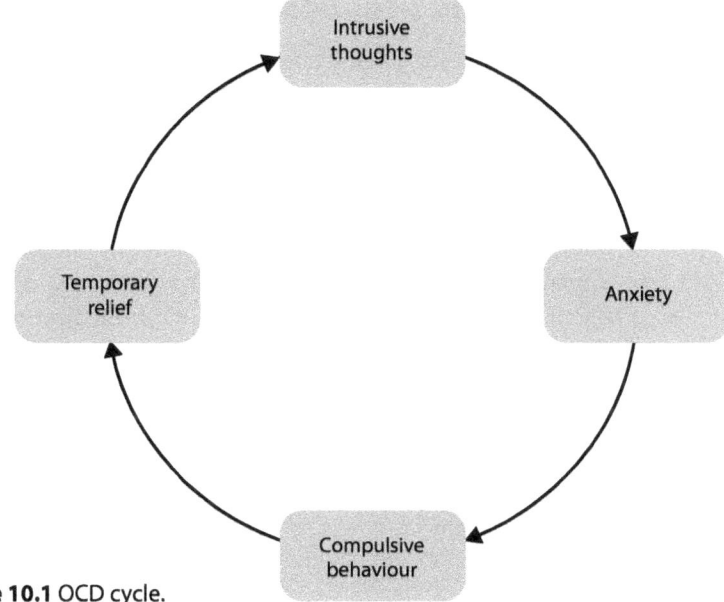

Figure 10.1 OCD cycle.

Environmental factors

The severity of OCD differs widely between individuals, and whilst some sufferers are able to hide symptoms from friends and family, it can often severely impact upon work, education, family and social relationships. Family members may become drawn into the compulsive rituals of a person with OCD. This might involve helping the individual to carry out their compulsive rituals, responding to repeated requests for reassurance or assuming responsibility for many daily activities that the person with OCD is unable to undertake, which can all act to maintain symptoms of OCD.

Behaviour patterns in OCD can cause distress and disruption for all members of the family, can lead to financial difficulties and can place a great strain on relationships. The strain of undertaking the rigid behavioural routines can lead to major family and marital difficulties, including separation or divorce. On some occasions, it may be family members who seek help on behalf of a family member.

10.6 Co-morbidity

The most common co-morbid diagnosis in people with OCD is depression, which can affect over two-thirds of people with OCD during their lifetime. People with OCD are also at increased risk of self-harm and suicide. Other common co-morbid conditions include social phobia, alcohol misuse, specific phobias, GAD and BDD. OCD is also more common in people with schizophrenia, bipolar disorder, anorexia and bulimia nervosa and Tourette's disorder.

10.7 Course and prognosis of OCD

Diagnosis of OCD is often late and patients may experience symptoms for 10–15 years or longer before seeking professional help. Patients tend to seek treatment from multiple doctors before a correct diagnosis is made.

If untreated, the course of OCD is usually chronic, often with waxing and waning symptoms. Without treatment, remission rates among adults are approximately 20%. Both medication and CBT are effective for the treatment of OCD, although a relatively high proportion of patients (40–60%) do not have a satisfactory outcome from treatment with either CBT or medication.

10.8 Presentation of OCD

Some patients will present in primary care with concerns about anxiety or intrusive thoughts and may already suspect that they are suffering from OCD. Others will attend with consequences of the compulsive behaviour such as dermatological problems due to excessive handwashing, or with general life stress arising from the demands of maintaining compulsions, such as work

> *Do you think I could be contaminated with a serious infection? Do I need a blood test...?*

> *I'm stressed because I can't get to work on time... It takes me 2 hours to leave the house...*

> *I can't get the thought out of my head that I might stab my child...*

problems caused by lateness due to repeated checking rituals carried out prior to leaving the house.

OCD should be suspected when a patient seems to be particularly concerned about the nature of their thoughts, or if they express the belief that their thoughts are somehow "bad" or dangerous. What differentiates these normal worries will also be the amount of time spent thinking about them, the level of worry or distress they cause and the extent to which people feel compelled to "get rid of them".

The diagnosis of OCD may be less obvious when the compulsions involve covert, mental acts which are not observable by others, such as mental counting or silently repeating specific phrases. Shame can also play a role in the late presentation of OCD. People with intrusive thoughts about sexuality, morality, or fears about making mistakes, may feel too ashamed and stigmatised to seek help, and may fear revealing the content of their intrusive thoughts to a health professional.

Some tips for when to suspect that a patient may be suffering from OCD are shown in *Box 10.5*.

Box 10.5 **When to suspect OCD**

- Consider OCD in patients with persistent hand dermatitis that may be secondary to excessive washing
- Consider OCD as a contributing factor in patients who report performance problems at work, such as persistent lateness
- Many people with OCD will develop depression and this may be their initial presenting symptom – OCD symptoms are likely to persist after treatment of depression and can be identified when reviewing the patient's response to treatment
- Be alert for information revealed by family members or carers about possible OCD symptoms

Case example 10.1: Angel

How might OCD present?

Angel is a 19-year-old student who attends her GP, Dr Prigo, complaining of low mood and symptoms of depression. She is assessed and is treated with SSRI medication (fluoxetine 20 mg). She returns to her GP and reports that her symptoms of low mood have improved and agrees to continue the medication for 6 months.

However, a few months later, Angel returns to see Dr Prigo, saying that she is struggling to cope with her college course. She is training as a beauty therapist but has missed many of the classes and is at risk of failing the year. She asks for a medical certificate to show her course tutor, to explain her absences.

When Dr Prigo asks the reason for the absence, Angel is initially reluctant to divulge her concerns. However, with some gentle prompting and encouragement, Angel eventually admits that she is struggling to make it to class because she feels compelled to carry out extensive checking routines.

Angel had first developed this type of behaviour in childhood. She felt compelled to cancel out any distressing thoughts, such as failing an exam, or illness or death of a family member, by pacing up and down the room whilst counting her steps and attempting to replace the 'bad' thought with a 'good' thought. She carried out these actions repeatedly until she felt better and that she had been able to neutralise the thought.

Things have become worse over the past year after starting her college course. Every morning, when she is due to leave for college, she is filled with doubts about whether she has locked the door properly, closed all the windows and whether all electrical items in the house are switched off and unplugged to prevent an electrical fire. As a result, she checks and rechecks each item, and sets off for college, but then feels compelled to return for 'one final check' to alleviate her concerns. The rituals are taking several hours each day, leading her to be late for her class or to miss it entirely.

As a result of the restriction on her lifestyle, Angel's mood had become low and she had started feeling depressed and despondent. The SSRI that she was prescribed had helped to lift her low mood but had had no noticeable effect on her checking behaviour.

This information can be summarised in a CBT framework as follows:

Thoughts	Feelings
Have I locked the door?	Low and despondent
I might have forgotten to close the window properly	Anxious (if she doesn't carry out the compulsive behaviour)
Maybe the electrical items are not switched off	
There could be a fire and it would be my fault	

Case example 10.1: *contd*

Behaviour
Repeated checking and rechecking
   rituals
Missing work and classes
Trying to replace a 'bad thought' with a
   'good thought'
Pacing up and down the room, counting
   her steps

Physical symptoms
Tense, agitated
Tired

Dr Prigo suggests to Angel that the problem may arise from OCD and Angel admits that she had suspected herself that this might be the case, but had felt too embarrassed to mention the intrusive thoughts in previous consultations.

Having recognised OCD as a possible diagnosis, the next step is for Dr Prigo to make a more detailed assessment, including confirming the diagnosis using a diagnostic tool such as the Y-BOCS and to then agree a management plan with Angel.

Case example 10.2: Marie

How might OCD present?

Marie is a 49-year-old woman who presents to her GP, Dr Fry, with marital difficulties. She says that she is worried that her husband might ask for a divorce. When Dr Fry asks for further details about some of the difficulties that the couple are facing, Marie bursts into tears and admits that much of the problem is arising from her own anxiety and compulsive need for reassurance.

Marie has never previously sought medical help, for fear that she might be labelled as 'crazy'. However, she is now so worried about her relationship with her husband that she has decided to be more open about her experiences.

Dr Fry acknowledges how difficult it can be to discuss personal emotional difficulties and congratulates Marie on being brave enough to raise the issue, and asks for more information about the problem.

Marie says she gets anxious whilst driving but seems hesitant to give more information about the issue. Dr Fry encourages Marie to give an example of a time that she has felt particularly anxious and in need of reassurance. At this stage, the differential diagnosis remains broad and includes a range of anxiety disorders and depression.

Marie gives an example during the past week where she had driven to work and then became anxious and had to return home to get reassurance from her husband. She had felt the car bump as she drove over a pothole and this

Case example 10.2: *contd*

triggered a sudden fear that she might have accidentally knocked over a pedestrian and seriously harmed them. Her distress was very high so she turned the car around and drove up and down the road several times looking for the accident victim, saying *"perhaps the body was knocked to the side, or maybe I forgot exactly where it was that I hit them. I couldn't live with myself if I hit a child and they were lying in the road suffering."*

Dr Fry asks Marie what thoughts entered her mind at this point. Marie describes frightening and distressing images of a child's body being crushed underneath her car. To try to push these thoughts out of her mind, she mentally counted to 100 and then drove her car up and down the road at least ten times, trying to find the possible accident victim. Eventually, she drove home and called her husband for reassurance that she hadn't hurt anyone. Later that evening, she also asked him repeatedly to check her car and make sure there was no sign of a collision, such as blood or clothing under her car or on her tyres.

Although she is aware that her concerns are irrational, she finds it very difficult to resist her impulses to engage in these rituals.

This information can be summarised in a CBT framework as follows:

Thoughts
Have I hit a pedestrian?
Intrusive images: a body under the car
Maybe the body was knocked to the side
Did I forget where I hit them?
I couldn't live with myself if I left a child suffering in the road

Feelings
Anxiety
Distress

Behaviour
Drove the car up and down the road to look for a possible accident
Mental counting to try to push the thoughts out of her mind
Phoned her husband for reassurance
Asked him to repeatedly check her car

Physical symptoms
Tense, agitated
Tearful

The description of intrusive thoughts about harming someone and associated compulsive behaviour is highly suggestive of OCD as a possible diagnosis. The next step is for Dr Fry to make a more detailed assessment and confirm the diagnosis.

10.9 Management of OCD

Making the diagnosis

Screening and diagnostic tools

NICE recommends asking six questions when considering the diagnosis of possible OCD (*Box* 10.6). These are very similar to a validated screening tool, the Zohar–Fineberg Obsessive Compulsive Screen (ZF-OCS). If a person responds affirmatively to one of these questions, a more formal diagnostic interview should be carried out.

Box 10.6 **Useful questions in making the diagnosis of OCD**

1. Do you wash or clean a lot?
2. Do you check things a lot?
3. Is there any thought that keeps bothering you that you would like to get rid of but cannot?
4. Do your daily activities take a long time to finish?
5. Are you concerned about putting things in a special order or are you very upset by mess?
6. Do these problems trouble you?

Diagnostic tools

The Yale–Brown Obsessive Compulsive Scale (Y-BOCS) is the most widely used measure of OCD and is designed to rate the severity and type of symptoms. It is not a diagnostic tool but is a validated self-reported measure of symptom severity, which includes both a symptom checklist and a severity rating scale. The questions in Y-BOCS include the following:

- How much of your day is occupied by obsessive thoughts or spent performing compulsive acts (mild, less than 1 hour; moderate, 1–3 hours; severe, more than 3 hours)?
- How much do your obsessive thoughts or compulsive behaviours interfere with your social or work/school functioning (including relationships)?
- How much distress do your obsessive thoughts cause you? How would you feel if prevented from performing your compulsion(s)? How anxious would you become?
- How much of an effort do you make to resist the obsessive thoughts or compulsions?
- How much control do you have over your obsessive thoughts? How strong is the drive to perform the compulsions?

Discussing OCD symptoms

If you suspect OCD, perhaps because a patient appears to be carrying out compulsive behavioural rituals, it is helpful to ask directly about the presence of intrusive or repeated thoughts. However, keep in mind that such thoughts can be very distressing and may be associated with strong feelings of shame. If they are unwilling to do so, it is not necessary to insist that a patient must reveal the exact content of their obsessive thoughts, prior to referring onwards for further assessment and treatment.

What else to consider

A relatively broad differential diagnosis should be considered when assessing symptoms associated with OCD (*Box 10.7*).

Box 10.7 **Differential diagnosis of OCD**

- Other anxiety disorders including BDD, health anxiety, social anxiety or panic disorder.
- Bodily distress disorder/MUS: excessive thoughts, feelings or behaviours related to distressing physical or somatic symptoms.
- Obsessive–compulsive personality disorder: preoccupation with orderliness, details, rules, organisation or schedules, to the degree that the point of the activity is lost, with absence of obsessions and compulsions; may involve discomfort if things are felt not to have been done completely.
- Delusional disorder: characterised by a false belief that is firmly sustained and based on incorrect inference about reality. Compulsions may be absent.
- Tic disorder: motor and vocal tics may appear similar to compulsive behaviours but involve focal uncomfortable somatic sensations which precede and are relieved by the tic. Unlike compulsions, tics are not usually performed in a particular sequence or location and are not carried out in response to an obsessional thought or intended to reduce anxiety or prevent harm.
- Autism spectrum disorder: compulsive behaviours may be confused with symptoms of excessive rigidity, stereotyped repetitive motor mannerisms and a need to maintain 'sameness' in autistic spectrum disorder. However, these behaviours are not driven by the desire to reduce anxiety, as in OCD.
- Trichotillomania (hair-pulling disorder): a diagnosis of OCD is not given if compulsive behaviour is restricted to hair-pulling.
- Excoriation (skin-picking disorder): similarly, a diagnosis of OCD is not given if compulsive behaviour is restricted to skin-picking.
- Hoarding disorder: persistent difficulty in discarding or parting with possessions, regardless of actual value, due to perceived need to save items and distress associated with discarding them.
- Substance-induced or medication-induced obsessive–compulsive disorder: OCD-type symptoms arise due to effects of medication or a drug of abuse.

Initial assessment of OCD

The initial assessment of an individual with OCD involves assessing the severity of the condition, including the level of associated distress and impact of the condition on work, school, relationships, social life and quality of life. The level of functional impairment can be assessed as mild, moderate or severe, which helps to inform the appropriate choice of treatment (*Box 10.8*). It is common for health professionals to underestimate the degree of functional impairment in OCD, as sufferers may minimise or under-report symptoms and the extent of their compulsive rituals.

It is also important to screen for co-morbid mental health disorders including depression, other anxiety disorders, alcohol or substance misuse, BDD and eating disorders.

The risk of suicide and self-harm should also be assessed in any patient experiencing marked distress, functional impairment or co-morbid depression. It is also important to assess any safeguarding concerns for children or vulnerable adults in the care of a parent or carer suffering from OCD, particularly if the obsessions or compulsions affect the individual's ability to care for the child. If there is any uncertainty, or in complex or severe cases, there should be a referral for further assessment by mental health professionals with specific expertise in the assessment and management of OCD.

The CBT framework can help to guide a structured assessment of OCD (*Box 10.8*).

Initial management in primary care

One of the most important roles in primary care is to provide support, empathy and understanding for patients with OCD, who often feel ashamed and embarrassed by their condition. Family members and carers may also need support, as OCD can have a devastating impact on their lives. Where appropriate and possible, it may be helpful to involve family members in an OCD patient's treatment plans, including advice about how not to become involved in their rituals and compulsions.

Explaining OCD
It is important to provide OCD patients with accurate information about the disorder, its likely causes, course and treatment. This can be provided both in written format and verbally during consultations.

Try to explain that distressing obsessive and intrusive thoughts are a core aspect of OCD, but that such thoughts are experienced at times by almost everybody, and are not a sign that there is something 'wrong' with the individual or with their mind.

| Box 10.8 | **A CBT framework for assessment of OCD disorder in primary care** |

Thoughts
- Do you experience any repeated thoughts that worry you or are difficult to control?
- What thoughts come into your mind? What is the most distressing or upsetting thought?
- What might happen if you did not act on the thoughts?
- How much time do you spend going over these obsessive thoughts?

Feelings
- How do you feel emotionally?
- How much do your obsessive thoughts distress you?
- What feelings arise when the unwanted thoughts enter into your mind?
- How would you feel if you were prevented from performing the compulsive behaviours?

Behaviour
- Are you repeatedly carrying out any actions to prevent something bad from happening?
- What are you doing? Are there overt actions (can be seen by others) and/or covert actions (inside the head)?
- Do you find yourself trying to resist your compulsive behaviours? How easy is this?
- How much time do you spend performing compulsive behaviours?

Physical symptoms
- What are the typical physical or bodily sensations that you experience?

Environmental factors and triggers
- What impact are the symptoms having on your work/education/relationships/quality of life?
- Did anyone in your family suffer from anxiety or OCD symptoms?
- Are there any important life stresses or problems that are affecting you?

Self-help strategies

Self-help strategies can be particularly helpful for people with mild to moderate OCD. These include:
- providing written information about OCD and how it affects people
- highlighting relevant self-help books and websites based on CBT principles

| Box 10.9 | **Explaining OCD** |

Many people with OCD experience thoughts known as obsessions. These are unwanted **thoughts**, words and images that come into the mind uninvited and are usually repugnant or horrifying, such as fears about being contaminated by germs, thoughts that something bad is going to happen to a loved one, or even that we might harm someone.

These types of thoughts are completely normal: everyone has them and they can simply be ignored. However, people with OCD find it hard to ignore these thoughts, which keep returning into the mind over and over again, leading to highly unpleasant **feelings** of anxiety and distress.

Many people with OCD develop **behaviours** known as compulsions. These are actions which are designed to neutralise or 'put right' the unwanted thoughts and get rid of any unpleasant feelings of anxiety and tension. These include repeated handwashing, tapping, checking locks, mental counting and many others. These can take up a great deal of time and interfere with many other important life activities. They also keep the focus on negative thoughts and worsen anxiety long-term.

Overcoming OCD involves learning to recognise that our thoughts are not dangerous or harmful. This can be achieved through psychological therapies which involve 'exposure' to feared thoughts, whilst learning that we do not need to carry out compulsive behaviours to prevent harm from taking place. Medication can also be helpful for people with OCD.

- providing information about local and national support groups for OCD
- general self-care and lifestyle modification: physical exercise, healthy diet, reducing caffeine intake and smoking cessation may all be beneficial.

10 *minute CBT strategies*

OCD often requires intensive one-to-one CBT due to its chronic, relapsing nature and may not respond well to brief CBT in primary care settings. However, brief interventions can be used to encourage positive self-management and encourage more helpful ways of coping with OCD symptoms, including encouraging wellbeing through promoting positive social activities and strengthening relationships with friends and family.

Highlight and label thoughts. For patients with OCD, where there can be highly distressing intrusive thoughts that trigger marked distress, shame and anxiety, it is often helpful to try not to get caught up in debating the accuracy of the content of thoughts, but simply to highlight and label the fact that the thought has arisen and is causing distress. Recognising and labelling thoughts as simply mental processes is a form of 'cognitive defusion' which may start to reduce the believability and power of negative thoughts.

However, the thoughts in OCD are very powerful and compelling, and simple defusion strategies in primary care are not designed to eliminate these negative thoughts. However, the process of describing and labelling of thoughts can help to reduce circular and repeated conversations, and offers an alternative to providing repeated reassurance (see *Box 10.10*).

Graded exposure. Patients can be encouraged to use graded exposure to gradually face feared or previously avoided situations and experiences. Patients with OCD may be unwilling to engage with exposure treatments due to the anxiety and distress that arises initially during the process. Therefore, when used as a self-help strategy, each step should be extremely small in order to maximise the chances of success.

Reducing compulsive behaviours. This should be carried out in combination with graded exposure and will help an individual with OCD to gradually learn that the feared outcome does not arise, even when the action is not carried out. The person's family should be encouraged to avoid offering excessive reassurance during this period, which can interfere with the process of habituation.

Early aims for reducing compulsions might involve reducing the number of times that a compulsive behaviour is carried out, or the length of time the behaviour is carried out for, rather than attempting to eliminate it completely.

Behavioural activation. This is one of the most important strategies for supporting patients with OCD in primary care. Rather than aiming to reduce OCD behaviours, it has a focus on increasing meaningful actions that are likely to improve overall wellbeing. This takes the pressure away from the process of exposure, which can be anxiety-provoking and exhausting. Instead, concentrate on building up 'micro-actions' that move the person toward valued areas of their life such as family, friendship, work, relaxation or physical activity. These

---

Box 10.10   **Highlight and label thoughts: what to say**

- Reflect and summarise: *"It sounds like you are having repeated thoughts that..."*
- Make an empathetic statement: *"That's a really distressing/horrifying/ frightening thought..."*
- Normalise and explain: *"Having these kinds of worry thoughts is common and normal..."*
- Highlight links with behaviour: *"So, when you have this thought, you then feel compelled to carry out a particular action...?"*
- Avoid offering repeated reassurance: *"It sounds like you are hoping for reassurance that nothing bad will happen. That's very understandable, although seeking repeated reassurance from others can undermine your own confidence and make anxiety worse in the long term..."*

actions may be very brief – perhaps only a few minutes – but can be important and meaningful ways of improving the quality of life for a person with OCD.

Mindfulness. There is currently little evidence available for the effectiveness of mindfulness in the management of OCD, although this is an area that is being researched further at present. A mindfulness-based approach may offer some benefit as an adjunct to traditional treatment approaches. Some of the core aspects of mindfulness which might be anticipated to help with managing OCD symptoms include the following:
- Mindfulness involves being in the present moment, observing internal and external experiences, whilst reducing attention paid to thoughts about past events or worries about future possibilities.
- Non-judgement of inner experience: this includes the ability to notice and label thoughts, feelings and urges without judgement.
- Mindfulness develops a recognition that the person is separate from their own thoughts and develops the capacity to notice and change automatic and habitual ways of thinking and responding to thoughts.
- Developing the capacity for non-reactivity to inner experience: the ability to reflect on thoughts and feelings without the need for action may help in resisting the urge to carry out compulsive behaviours
- Acting with awareness: this involves developing skills in paying attention to activities purposefully without being distracted.

Treatment of OCD in primary care

Both CBT and medication are effective treatments for OCD. Choice of therapy can be guided by patient preference as well as factors such as availability of psychological therapy services.

Psychological therapy
CBT is the most effective psychological treatment for OCD and usually involves exposure and response prevention (ERP). This involves the patient repeatedly testing out their fears and expectations of harm, and learning to tolerate anxiety, while being prevented from performing any compulsive or safety-seeking behaviour. The approach requires extensive counselling and discussion with the patient, as it is likely to result in an initial increase in the experience of anxiety and significant internal distress, which subsequently gradually decreases over time. The aim of ERP is for the patient to feel that they have confronted their worst fears without anything terrible happening, and thus reduce the power of the fears, whilst also learning how to reduce compulsive behaviours.

In CBT, there should be a supportive and empathetic collaborative relationship between therapist and patient, who work together to develop a shared understanding of the problem, including the experience and effects of intrusive thoughts, and how the compulsive safety behaviours undertaken to try to cope with them are likely to be counterproductive and worsen distress as a vicious cycle. This is particularly important in OCD where the therapy process can be prolonged and involve continually facing emotionally challenging experiences.

Between 60% and 85% of people report a considerable reduction in symptoms of OCD following CBT or ERP, and improvement is maintained for up to 5 years in most people who respond. However, about 30% of people refuse to engage in CBT, leave early, or do not respond to CBT and ERP. This may be because some individuals are unable to overcome fears about the consequences of not performing compulsive rituals and may also be unwilling or unable to tolerate high levels of anxiety.

The response to treatment may not be complete and up to 50% of people have some residual OCD symptoms after treatment with CBT. Factors associated with a poor response to treatment for OCD are shown in *Box 10.11*. The duration of CBT needed does not appear to be related to the length of time that people have experienced the symptom.

For people with OCD causing mild functional impairment, NICE recommends a low intensity CBT intervention involving up to 10 therapist hours of structured self-help, telephone or group CBT.

No evidence of efficacy or effectiveness exists for psychoanalysis in the treatment of OCD, and insufficient evidence is available to support the use of other psychological therapies, hypnosis or homeopathy.

Box 10.11	**Factors associated with poor response to treatment in OCD**
	<ul><li>Male gender</li><li>Early age of onset</li><li>Higher frequency of compulsions</li><li>Schizotypal personality disorder (obsessional thoughts become delusional in nature)</li><li>Concurrent tic disorder: associated with more severe OCD symptoms and greater likelihood of treatment resistance</li><li>Associated specific or diffuse brain structural abnormalities</li></ul>

Drug treatment for OCD

SSRIs. SSRIs are the first-line drug treatment of choice in OCD, and have similar effectiveness to psychological therapy. There is no evidence that any particular SSRI is more effective than another in OCD. Sertraline, fluoxetine, escitalopram, fluvoxamine and paroxetine are all licensed for the treatment of OCD in adults. Citalopram may also be prescribed, although this is an unlicensed use.

Treatment with an SSRI in OCD usually requires a higher dose than in standard doses for depression, as well as needing a longer duration of treatment for an initial response. Any trial of an SSRI should be at the highest tolerated dose for at least 12 weeks. Initiation and monitoring of drug therapy should follow recommended guidelines which are summarised in *Chapter 3*.

TCAs. Second-line medication involves the use of the TCA clomipramine, although this has a greater risk of adverse effects. For patients at significant risk of cardiovascular disease, a baseline ECG and blood pressure should be carried out before starting clomipramine. Then, commence with a small dose and titrate upwards according to response. It is also important to only prescribe small amounts of clomipramine at a time, because of its toxicity in overdose. The patient will require regular monitoring.

Antipsychotic medication. Antipsychotic drugs such as risperidone, quetiapine or olanzapine are not effective alone, but sometimes have a role in augmenting antidepressant medication where the response to an SSRI is poor or incomplete. Their use is associated with an increased risk of adverse events in the long term, and antipsychotics are less effective than offering CBT combined with antidepressant medication.

Antipsychotics are therefore recommended only in patients who are refractory to CBT plus SSRIs, and are generally only initiated by specialists in the management of OCD. When an antipsychotic is prescribed, it should be given at a low dose for a 4-week trial to determine whether it is effective.

Other medication. Novel compounds with some evidence for refractory cases include lamotrigine, topiramate, and acetylcysteine.

Risk management

Some obsessional thoughts, such as those relating to fears about committing violence to others, or of being a paedophile, can cause significant concern for health professionals who must assess whether an individual with OCD may represent a danger to others. Each case will require a through, detailed review and assessment and is likely to require specialist input.

Notably, in OCD, the fears are predominantly that the individual *might* be a paedophile, rather than actual urges or desires to carry out paedophilic actions. In fact, the likelihood of a person with OCD acting on these thoughts is extremely low. Health professionals should also remain alert for other possible risks associated with the fears, such as a mother who never picks up her baby because of fears that she might drop him.

There should also be a risk assessment in relation to the patient's mood and any risk of possible self-harm or suicide.

When to refer

Patients should be referred onwards for further assessment and treatment by specialist teams in the following circumstances:

- obsessive and compulsive symptoms are severe and associated with marked functional impairment
- at risk of self-neglect, self-harm or suicide, or posing a risk to others
- with a significant co-morbidity such as substance misuse, severe depression, anorexia nervosa or schizophrenia
- if a GP is not confident in their assessment of moderate functional impairment, or there is an inadequate response to initial treatment.

When there is specialist involvement, it is helpful to have integrated links between primary and secondary care services, enabling the provision of coordinated care. Specialist treatment options, which should only be initiated in secondary care, are shown in *Box 10.12*.

Box 10.12

Specialist treatment options for severe, complex OCD

- High intensity CBT with a specialist therapist in the treatment of OCD
- Antipsychotics to augment the effect of an SSRI, such as haloperidol, risperidone or aripiprazole
- Combination of clomipramine and citalopram
- Intensive inpatient therapy or residential/supportive care may occasionally be needed for people with chronic severe dysfunction
- Neurosurgery, such as anterior capsulotomy, is used extremely rarely for severely ill patients who do not respond to CBT and medication
- Deep brain stimulation is a new approach to treatment which may show some promise for extremely severe cases

Summary of primary care management of OCD

Stepped care approach	What to offer	What does this involve?
Initial presentations of OCD with mild functional impairment	Explain the diagnosis	• Give clear and accurate explanations of OCD • Explain and normalise the experience of intrusive thoughts • Use the CBT framework to help the patient understand their experiences and demonstrate how compulsive behaviours act to worsen anxiety and distress over the longer term
	10 minute CBT advice about managing anxiety	• Highlight and label negative thoughts, rather than engaging in discussions about their content • Use brief behavioural activation to increase participation in meaningful or enjoyable activities and improve low mood and daily functioning • Use brief graded exposure to encourage the person to reduce avoidance of feared activities in small steps • Reduce the use of compulsive behaviours • Mindfulness may be beneficial to improve recognition and coping with negative thoughts
	Signpost to self-help resources	Provide information about CBT-based books and websites for understanding and managing OCD
	Guided self-help	Low intensity CBT including ERP (up to 10 hours per person) involving structured self-help, telephone or group sessions
OCD with moderate functional impairment or lack of response to initial measures	Primary care management: CBT or medication	• First-line treatment: choice of high intensity CBT or SSRI • Second-line treatment: clomipramine – consider for patients who have had a previous good response to it or unable to tolerate SSRIs Both medication and CBT involving ERP are effective for OCD, although 40–60% of patients do not have a completely satisfactory outcome with either treatment

OCD with severe functional impairment or lack of response to primary care treatment	Consider referral to secondary care	• Combined treatment with SSRI and intensive CBT/ERP
		• Trial of an alternative SSRI or clomipramine
		• Refer to secondary care if
		  o severe symptoms with marked functional impairment
		  o risk of self-neglect, self-harm or suicide, or risk to others
		  o co-morbidity such as substance misuse, severe depression, anorexia nervosa or schizophrenia
		  o GP is not confident in their assessment of moderate functional impairment, or there is an inadequate response to initial treatment

10.10 Monitoring and follow-up

All patients who are commenced on antidepressant medication will require regular review (see *Chapter 3*). OCD can have a fluctuating or episodic course, or relapse may occur after successful treatment. Therefore, people who have been successfully treated and discharged should be seen as soon as possible with further occurrences. Long-term support in primary care is often required.

There is a high rate of relapse after discontinuing medication for OCD. This can be improved using long-term treatments (i.e. at least 12 months) and by combining with CBT, which may also be beneficial for the 40–60% of patients who do not experience complete remission of symptoms with medication.

Case example 10.3: Andrew

Diagnosis and management of OCD

Andrew is a 26-year-old man with a history of eczema. He attends his GP, Dr Johnston, with a flare-up of his hand eczema, asking for a repeat prescription of emollient and a topical steroid. Dr Johnston looks at Andrew's hands and sees that they are red, cracked and bleeding. She asks Andrew about any triggers for the problem, including asking whether he washes his hands frequently.

Andrew looks a little distressed and admits that he does wash his hands fairly often. Dr Johnston explores this in more detail, asking how often he washes his hands and what the triggers are for carrying this out.

Andrew admits that he is washing his hands as many as 20–30 times a day, in a specific, ritualised way, which involves washing each finger individually and scrubbing under each nail with a brush.

He admits that he has an intense fear of germs and experiences recurrent thoughts about contracting an illness from touching things in public places such as door handles and taps. He is particularly preoccupied about the risk of passing on germs to others and fears that he would then be responsible for making other people unwell. These thoughts lead to a high level of emotional distress, which he feels compelled to alleviate by handwashing, even though he is also aware that the risk of contracting illness through touching surfaces is quite slim.

Andrew says that he feels less anxious immediately after washing his hands, but the fear and anxiety, and thoughts about contamination rapidly return, leading to an almost irresistible compulsion to wash his hands again. He has stopped travelling into work using public transport, and avoids using public toilets, because of his symptoms.

Case example 10.3: *contd*

This information can be summarised in a CBT framework as follows:

Thoughts
I could catch an illness from touching a
   door handle or a tap
I might pass on the germs to others
I would be responsible for making other
   people ill
I couldn't live with myself

Feelings
Anxiety
Distress

Behaviour
Compulsive handwashing
Stopped using public transport
Avoids public toilets

Physical symptoms
Dry, cracked, painful
hands

Dr Johnston explains that she suspects that Andrew may be suffering from a disorder known as OCD. As well as continuing to treat the dermatitis caused by excessive handwashing, she recommends that he may also benefit from assessment and treatment of the underlying condition. Andrew is relieved to discover that his recurrent intrusive thoughts do not mean that he is "going mad" and that there may be ways to help manage the distress that is leading to his repeated handwashing behaviour.

Dr Johnston carries out a more detailed assessment and identifies that Andrew has moderate impairment of important activities due to his preoccupations and compulsive behaviour. The next steps for treatment include:

- explaining OCD and how it affects people
- use of brief self-management strategies to help Andrew reduce handwashing behaviour
- management of his hand dermatitis
- encouraging Andrew to try mindfulness to help him manage some of the intrusive thoughts
- behavioural activation: encouraging Andrew to engage in more activities that lead to a greater sense of overall wellbeing such as physical exercise and social interaction
- discussion about effective treatments for OCD and collaborative decision-making about next steps for management; Andrew does not currently wish to take medication and agrees to be referred for CBT through the local wellbeing service.

10.11 Summary and key points

- Sufferers of OCD experience obsessional thoughts and compulsive behaviours which cause emotional distress and interfere with the person's functioning in important aspects of daily life.
- Obsessions are repeated, unwanted and intrusive thoughts, images or impulses, which are usually repugnant or inconsistent with the person's values and cause high levels of distress and anxiety.
- Unhelpful thinking patterns seen in OCD include unrealistic beliefs about the significance of experiencing unwanted thoughts, an excessive sense of personal responsibility and 'thought–action fusion' (beliefs that thoughts can influence the external world).
- Compulsions are repetitive behaviours that the person believes they are compelled to perform in order to reduce emotional distress and prevent a feared outcome, although the actions are usually not connected to the feared event in a realistic way.
- Recognition of OCD can be challenging when compulsions are covert (i.e. mental acts that cannot be seen by others) or when shame about the disorder prevents its disclosure to health professionals.
- CBT which includes exposure and response prevention is the first-line psychological treatment for OCD.
- SSRIs are the medication of choice; clomipramine is a second-line option.
- A combination of psychological therapy and medication is the most effective combination for moderate to severe cases of OCD.
- Antipsychotics such as haloperidol, risperidone or aripiprazole are sometimes used in severe OCD to augment the effect of an SSRI, but should only be initiated by specialists.

10.12 OCD resources

- Northumberland, Tyne & Wear NHS Foundation Trust Self Help leaflets: https://web.ntw.nhs.uk/selfhelp/leaflets/Obsessions%20and%20Compulsions%20A4%202016%20FINAL.pdf
- Veale, D. and Willson, R. (2009) *Overcoming Obsessive Compulsive Disorder.* Robinson.

Chapter 11
Body dysmorphic disorder

BDD quick reference guide

What is body dysmorphic disorder (BDD)?	Preoccupation with an imagined flaw in physical appearance, associated with highly time-consuming behaviours such as mirror gazing, comparing with others, excessive attempts to camouflage or hide the defect, skin picking and reassurance seeking. Avoidance of social situations is common. Sufferers frequently seek cosmetic or medical treatment for the perceived defect, but this is rarely successful in alleviating distress.
How common is it?	Prevalence data for BDD is lacking compared to other anxiety disorders, but it is thought to affect about 2% of the general population. As many as 6–15% of patients attending cosmetic surgery and dermatology clinics may have BDD.
Risk factors	Risk factors for BDD include genetic factors, temperament, childhood adversity such as teasing or bullying, increased aesthetic sensitivity and a history of skin or other physical disfigurement.
Co-morbid conditions	Levels of co-morbidity are high in BDD including an increased risk of depression, social anxiety, OCD, eating disorders, substance misuse disorders, and suicidal thoughts and behaviour.
Usual course	Milder BDD symptoms in adolescence may resolve over time but those with moderate to severe symptoms often follow a chronic, lifelong course with a significant risk of relapse following successful treatment.
Common presentations	People with BDD typically attend GPs, cosmetic surgeons and dermatologists with concerns about their physical appearance and a desire to make changes to it. They are far less likely to present to mental health services, unless there are co-morbid problems such as social anxiety, depression or substance misuse. Adolescents may present with school refusal, family difficulties and social isolation.
How to make the diagnosis	NICE recommends asking five questions to assess the likelihood of BDD: "Do you worry a lot about the way you look and wish you could think about it less?" 1. *"What specific concerns do you have about your appearance?"* 2. *"On a typical day, how many hours a day is your appearance on your mind?"* *(more than 1 hour a day is considered excessive)* 3. *"What effect does it have on your life?"* 4. *"Does it make it hard to do your work or be with friends?"*

What else could it be?	Differential diagnosis and possible co-morbid conditions include OCD, social anxiety, agoraphobia and GAD, depression, eating disorders, trichotillomania, excoriation (skin picking) disorder and delusional disorders such as schizophrenia.
Self-management strategies	Useful self-management strategies using 10 minute CBT for BDD include reducing preoccupation with thoughts about appearance using attention training to focus on daily activities, mindfulness and postponing appearance preoccupation. Behavioural strategies include increasing enjoyable and meaningful activities using brief behavioural activation and reducing unhelpful behaviours such as mirror gazing and reassurance seeking.
Treatment of BDD	Both medication and CBT involving ERP are effective for the treatment of BDD. Choice depends on patient preference and other factors such as availability of therapy. First-line drug therapy is with an SSRI (fluoxetine), which should be continued for at least 12 months. Doses may need to be higher than in other anxiety disorders. Alternative medications include clomipramine. The use of antipsychotic medication is not usually recommended, even in patients with BDD beliefs of delusional intensity.
When to refer	Severe symptoms associated with marked functional impairment, at risk of self-neglect, self-harm or suicide, or posing a risk to others, significant co-morbidity such as substance misuse, severe depression, anorexia nervosa or schizophrenia, or lack of response to treatment in community settings.
Follow-up	Treatment for BDD should be continued for at least 12 months to reduce the risk of relapse and allow for further improvements. Long-term follow-up may be needed. Some individuals have chronic or episodic symptoms with relapse after successful treatment.

11.1 Introduction

People with body dysmorphic disorder (BDD) are preoccupied with worry about one or more aspects of their physical appearance, believing that these body areas look ugly, abnormal, deformed or disfigured. Such 'defects' may be objectively very minor, or may not even be apparent to others, but result in severe distress, shame and interference in the individual's life.

BDD is relatively common, but there is currently a low level of awareness about it amongst healthcare professionals. It should not be confused with body dissatisfaction, which is common but does not cause major distress or interference with life. BDD can be a highly disabling condition, often impairing sufferers even more than individuals with 'real' physical disfigurements.

Patients with BDD can consume substantial health resources, with repeated attendances at health professionals, and may undergo multiple cosmetic procedures and other treatments, often involving both NHS and private services.

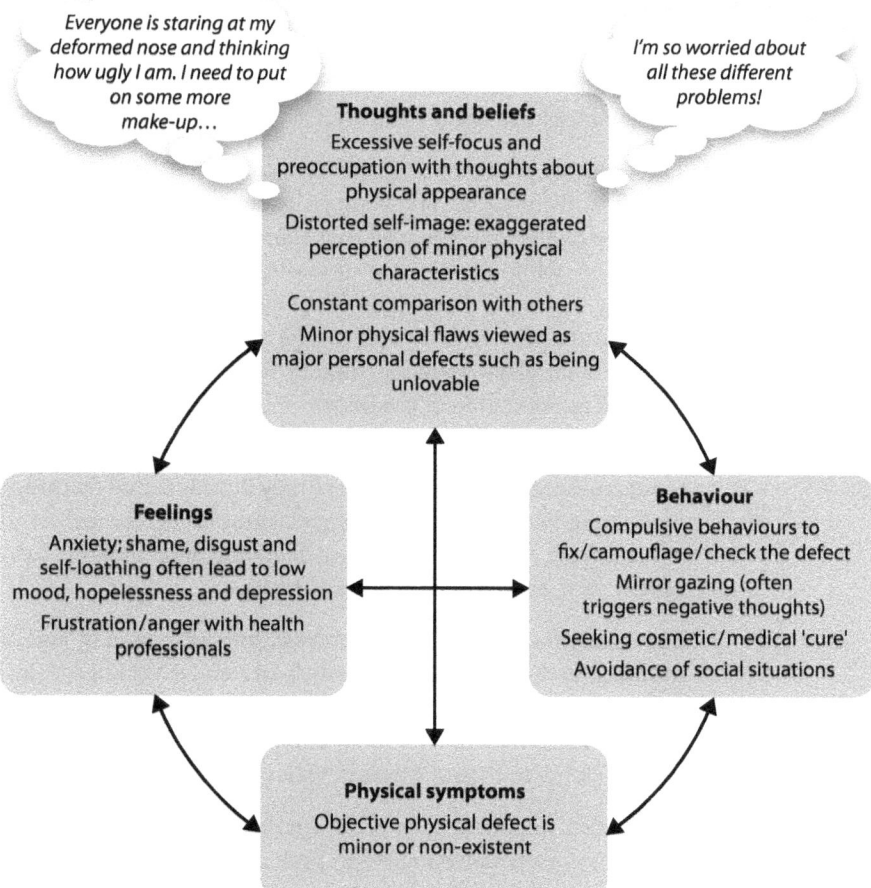

CBT framework for BDD

Everyone is staring at my deformed nose and thinking how ugly I am. I need to put on some more make-up...

I'm so worried about all these different problems!

Thoughts and beliefs
Excessive self-focus and preoccupation with thoughts about physical appearance
Distorted self-image: exaggerated perception of minor physical characteristics
Constant comparison with others
Minor physical flaws viewed as major personal defects such as being unlovable

Feelings
Anxiety; shame, disgust and self-loathing often lead to low mood, hopelessness and depression
Frustration/anger with health professionals

Behaviour
Compulsive behaviours to fix/camouflage/check the defect
Mirror gazing (often triggers negative thoughts)
Seeking cosmetic/medical 'cure'
Avoidance of social situations

Physical symptoms
Objective physical defect is minor or non-existent

11.2 What is BDD?

People with BDD experience persistent and intrusive thoughts about a perceived defect or 'ugliness' in their physical appearance. Insight in BDD is often poor, and patients are more likely to experience delusional beliefs than in related disorders, such as OCD.

The most common concerns in BDD relate to facial features, including the skin, hair, nose, eyes, eyelids, mouth, lips, jaw and chin. However, any part of the body may be involved, and the preoccupation may also be focused on several body parts simultaneously. In some cases, the complaint is extremely vague or may involve a general perception of being ugly.

The appearance preoccupations are usually difficult to resist or control and are very distressing. Common concerns in BDD involve:

- skin including concerns about acne, perceived scarring, wrinkles, blemishes or skin colour
- hair loss, or too much facial or body hair
- facial features being perceived as unattractive or not being in proportion.

The types of preoccupation in BDD can differ between the sexes. Males may be more likely to be preoccupied with their genitals, thinning hair or with muscle dysmorphia (the idea that their body build is too small or insufficiently muscular), while females are more likely to be preoccupied with hips, breasts, legs and excessive body hair. Individuals with BDD can be dissatisfied with multiple areas of the body and the nature of the preoccupation may change with time, so that after cosmetic surgery for one problem, the preoccupation often shifts to another area of the body.

The beliefs about the defect in BDD are held very strongly and are not amenable to reassurance from others. There may be delusional features, such as believing that other people are taking special notice of the defect and talking about it negatively, or that people are laughing and making fun of the sufferer's appearance, even when this is not the case.

BDD sufferers typically spend at least one hour per day, and often much longer, thinking about the disliked body part, and also engage in time-consuming, repetitive behaviours in response to their appearance concerns. These might include checking in mirrors, comparing themselves to others, excessive camouflaging to hide the defect, skin picking and reassurance seeking.

Functional impairment is often marked in BDD. Sufferers are usually highly self-conscious which can lead to problems with emotional or physical intimacy, avoidance of friends and social situations, and impairment of intimate relationships. Social situations may be endured with the use of alcohol, illegal substances or safety-seeking behaviours, similar to social anxiety.

BDD also often impacts many other areas of daily life, leading to lateness for work and social activities and impacting negatively on occupational and academic performance, and other key roles such as managing a household or caring for others. Sufferers can become unemployed, and even housebound or hospitalised in severe cases.

Developments in the classification of BDD

BDD has been previously less well understood than other anxiety disorders. In ICD-10, BDD is included as a brief term of reference within hypochondriacal disorder, rather than having its own specific diagnostic criteria. BDD symptoms are also referred to in several other diagnostic categories, including delusional

Box 11.1

Diagnostic criteria for BDD

- Persistent preoccupation with one or more perceived defects or flaws in appearance that are non-existent or very minor and may only be slightly noticeable to others
- Excessive self-consciousness, often with ideas of reference (being convinced that other people are noticing, judging or talking about the perceived defect or flaw)
- Repetitive and time-consuming behaviours including repeated checking and excessive attempts to camouflage or alter the perceived defect
- There is often marked avoidance of social situations
- Symptoms result in significant distress or impairment in important areas of functioning
- Levels of insight relating to BDD beliefs can be classified as:
  - ○ fair to good insight: the individual is mostly able to recognise that the BDD beliefs may not be accurate and is willing to accept an alternative explanation, although insight may be decreased or absent when the individual is highly anxious
  - ○ poor to absent insight: the individual is convinced that the BDD beliefs are true and cannot accept any alternative explanations

disorder and schizotypal disorder, leading to potential diagnostic confusion and inappropriate treatment. However, in ICD-11, BDD is included as a separate diagnosis, in the category of obsessive–compulsive and related disorders, which may lead to improved recognition and treatment of the condition.

11.3 Epidemiology

Data on the prevalence of BDD is lacking compared to other anxiety disorders. However, it is thought to be relatively common, with a prevalence of about 2% in the general population. As many as 6–15% of patients attending cosmetic surgery and dermatology clinics may have BDD.

BDD occurs equally in both sexes and the onset typically occurs during adolescence. There is usually a delay of up to 10 years or more before diagnosis is made. Compared with adults, adolescents who present with BDD have more severe symptoms with a higher risk of suicide and more delusional beliefs.

11.4 Aetiology

It is likely that the development of BDD is multifactorial, although data on this is currently limited. Factors involved in aetiology are shown in *Box 11.2*.

> **Box 11.2**
>
> **Factors associated with the development of BDD**
>
> - Genetic predisposition: BDD is more common in relatives of affected individuals
> - Environmental risk factors include childhood adversity, neglect, trauma and abuse, and bullying
> - Personality traits including shyness, perfectionism and anxiousness
> - A history of skin or other physical disfigurement
> - Being more aesthetically sensitive than other individuals

11.5 CBT model of BDD

Thoughts and cognitive aspects of BDD

People with BDD become preoccupied with negative thoughts and images associated with physical appearance, often for many hours of the day. The excessive self-focus and selective attention are associated with a distorted self-image, where sufferers perceive minor physical characteristics as being much more noticeable and severe than they really are. Negative thoughts about self-image are often triggered by viewing an external representation of the person's appearance, such as by looking in a mirror.

In BDD, there is a tendency to overestimate the meaning and importance of perceived physical imperfections and to misinterpret minor flaws, such as perceived asymmetry, as major personal defects (*"If my skin is not perfect, I am unlovable"*). Similar to OCD, a 'felt' body sense can become fused with reality (*"If my body doesn't feel right then I must appear terrible"*). There is also excessive focus on how the individual appears from an observer's perspective (*"I have to know what I look like to others"*).

People suffering from BDD often hold strong beliefs about the importance of appearance in terms of their personal value and sense of self-worth (*"If I looked better, then my whole life would be better"*). This may include beliefs that the individual is fundamentally flawed, inadequate, unacceptable to others, unlovable, or that they will always be alone as a result of the defect (*"If I am defective, I am completely worthless"*). Other important concepts in BDD include perfectionism, symmetry, youth and social acceptance.

BDD typically involves constant comparison of the self with others. This maintains focus on the defect and is associated with negative, self-critical thoughts which lower mood and self-esteem (*"My nose is so much more crooked than anyone else's, I will be alone all my life"*).

Feelings and emotions

Common emotions associated with BDD include shame, anxiety, frustration and anger, and a sense of disgust and self-loathing. These can lead to depression, low self-esteem and hopelessness at the person's perceived failure to reach an unrealistic aesthetic standard.

Behaviour

The preoccupations in BDD lead to repetitive behaviours that are intended to fix, hide, check or obtain reassurance about the disliked body parts, and to cope with the distressing emotional experiences that arise as a response to their perceived defects. Such behaviours are often compulsive in nature and are similar to those seen in OCD (*Box 11.3*).

| Box 11.3 | **Typical behaviours in BDD** |

- Camouflaging: trying to hide or cover up the disliked body areas with hats, heavy make-up, clothing, hair styles or sunglasses. This often involves repetitive behaviours such as repeatedly adjusting or changing clothing, brushing hair to hide disliked body parts, or constantly applying make-up.
- Mirror gazing and checking: frequently checking perceived defects in mirrors and other reflecting surfaces, such as windows or a mobile phone. The aim of mirror gazing is to repeatedly reassess the severity of the defect, to check how well efforts at camouflage have worked and may also arise from a belief that they will feel worse if they resist gazing.
- Avoidance: includes avoidance of social situations and certain types of clothing; some individuals avoid mirrors.
- Pressing, touching and measuring areas of the body: this is usually to check for possible defects or may be an attempt to improve the physical appearance (e.g. attempts to straighten a crooked nose).
- Comparing: repeatedly comparing the disliked features to those of other people, either mentally or when talking to others.
- Reassurance seeking: frequently asking others how they look, or if the perceived defect is noticeable. Some people with BDD may repeatedly insist that they look ugly or abnormal.
- Skin picking: Compulsively picking at skin to try to make it look better. The aim of skin picking is to improve appearance rather than cause self-harm, but it can lead to skin lesions and scarring.
- Excessive shopping: excessively shopping for make-up, other products or clothes to try to improve the appearance of the disliked body areas.
- Tanning: excessively tanning to darken skin that is considered too pale or as an attempt to minimise perceived skin conditions such as acne or psoriasis.
- Excessive exercise or weightlifting: this is particularly common in men with muscle dysmorphia.
- Excessive grooming and cleansing of the hair, face and skin: use of facial peelers, saunas or exercises to improve facial muscle tone, and other beauty treatments.
- Repeatedly seeking medical and cosmetic treatments for defects: this includes cosmetic surgery, dermatological treatments, or other cosmetic procedures.
- Mental acts such as rumination or constantly comparing the perceived defect with the same feature in other people.

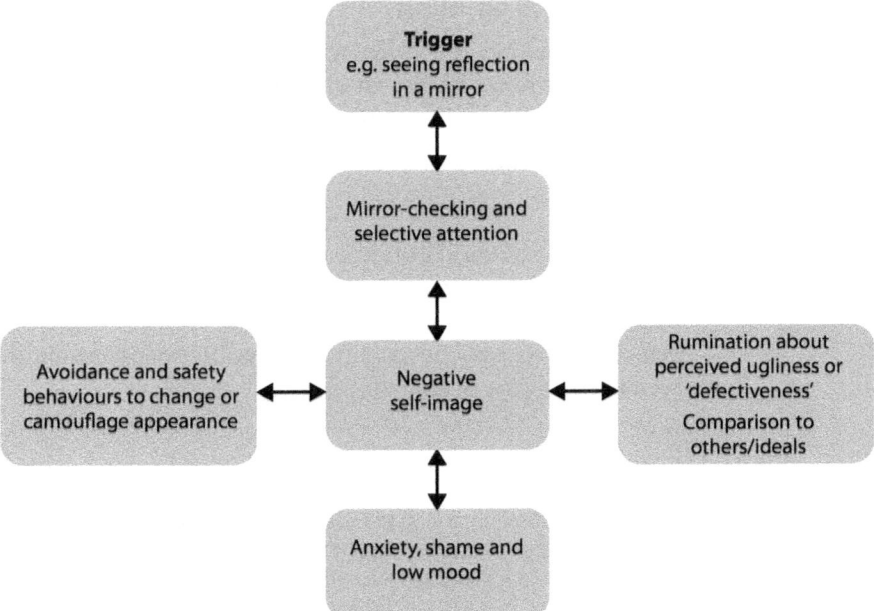

Figure 11.1 CBT model of BDD (adapted from Veale, 2001).

Compulsive behavioural rituals and avoidance usually lead to a temporary reduction in distressing emotions and are therefore negatively reinforced. This acts to maintain unhelpful beliefs and coping strategies. In the long term, these behaviours also act to heighten awareness and maintain the preoccupation with physical appearance, with a worsening of anxiety levels.

Social anxiety and avoidance are also very common in people with BDD, which may cause it to be misdiagnosed as social anxiety disorder. This can arise from fears that other people will see the perceived appearance flaws and reject, despise or ridicule the person with BDD because of how they look.

11.6 Co-morbidity

High levels of co-morbidity are reported in BDD including associations with depression, social anxiety, OCD, eating disorders and substance misuse disorders. There is also a high rate of suicidal ideation (up to 45%), suicide attempts and completed suicides. Individuals with the muscle dysmorphia form of BDD have even higher rates of suicidality and substance use disorders as well as poorer quality of life than individuals with other forms of BDD.

Co-morbid social anxiety is diagnosed if there are additional fears of acting in a way that leads to humiliation or embarrassment. Co-morbid OCD occurs when the obsessions or compulsions are not restricted to concerns about appearance; for example, if they also include repeated checking of door locks or handwashing.

11.7 Course and prognosis of BDD

BDD is often a chronic disorder which persists for many years if left untreated. Milder symptoms in adolescence may resolve over time but people with moderate to severe symptoms often follow a chronic, lifelong course characterised by increasing frequency of unsatisfactory attempts to alter the perceived defect associated with deteriorating mood and increased co-morbid mental health conditions and suicide attempts.

CBT and SSRIs are both effective treatments in reducing the severity of symptoms of BDD. However, some patients continue to experience BDD symptoms despite treatment. Relapse is also common following successful treatment and patients may need treatments to be re-initiated or referral back to specialist services.

11.8 Presentation of BDD

I'm so worried about my acne. My skin is terrible and I'm starting to feel really depressed about it...

I would like you to refer me to a plastic surgeon about my crooked nose...

I'm getting anxious in social situations and I'll never get a girlfriend because my body is so skinny and ugly...

People with BDD can present in primary care or to a wide range of specialists, including cosmetic surgeons and dermatologists, with concerns about their physical appearance and a desire to make changes to it (see *Box 11.4*). The preoccupation with the physical defect makes it rare for patients to present to mental health services unless there are marked additional difficulties such as significant depression, becoming housebound or being at risk of suicide.

Some people with BDD may avoid admitting their preoccupation to health professionals because they fear being viewed as vain or narcissistic. They may be more likely to present with symptoms of depression or social anxiety, or with drug or alcohol-related problems which have arisen as a consequence of anxiety relating to underlying BDD.

Box 11.4

Common specialties involved in patients with BDD

- Cosmetic surgery
- Dermatology
- Ear, nose and throat (ENT)
- Gynaecology
- Urology
- Maxillofacial services
- Dentists and orthodontists

Adolescents with BDD may present with school refusal, family difficulties and social isolation, rather than directly admitting concerns about their physical appearance.

Box 11.5 includes some tips for recognising possible BDD in primary care.

Box 11.5

Tips for spotting BDD

- Seeking dermatology/cosmetic surgery referral for objectively minor problems
- Severe distress and repeated attendances for objectively minor blemishes or disfigurements
- Wearing excessive make-up/hairstyles/clothing to try to hide a perceived problem
- Specific attire such as hats, scarves or sunglasses which are out of context and used to hide the feature
- Scars from skin picking
- Making poor eye contact
- Anyone describing themselves as 'ugly'

Case example 11.1: Sinead

How might BDD present?

Sinead is a 35-year-old woman who attends her GP, complaining of depressed mood. Dr Hughes is immediately struck by the heavy make-up and large dark glasses that Sinead is wearing. He discovers that over the past few years, Sinead has slowly withdrawn from her friends and often feels unable to leave the house.

Dr Hughes asks Sinead to explain what she finds most difficult about leaving the house. Sinead replies by saying: "It just worries me too much to see other people." This statement suggests that she may be feeling anxious and that the behaviour reflects avoidance, rather than simply withdrawal relating to depression or low mood.

Case example 11.1: *contd*

Dr Hughes continues to explore Sinead's thoughts about leaving the house and seeing other people, by asking: "*What would worry you most about seeing other people? What's the worst thing that might happen?*"

Sinead explains that she finds it extremely difficult to come into contact with other people because of the lines and dark circles around her eyes, which she feels are very marked and make her look much older than she really is. "*The baggy lines and dark rings under my eyes are just getting worse and worse. They make me look hideous – like an old crone.*"

Dr Hughes continues by asking how much time Sinead spends thinking or worrying about her facial appearance. Sinead admits she spends several hours each day thinking about her appearance. She frequently checks her face in the mirror and spends hours each day applying eye cream and concealer make-up. She avoids going shopping or leaving the house without wearing heavy make-up, and she has grown a long fringe to try to conceal her eyes as much as possible. When she does go out, Sinead feels extremely self-conscious, believing that others are constantly staring at her face and that they will be repulsed by her advanced ageing.

Dr Hughes asks about the impact of the symptoms on Sinead's life. The patient explains that she used to work as a receptionist in a hairdressers but now feels unable to carry out the role, which involves being seen by others, and is currently unemployed. Sinead is struggling financially because she is no longer working and has accrued debts from spending large amounts of money on expensive beauty treatments, creams and make-up.

Dr Hughes examines Sinead's face, but is unable to see the defects that the patient is so concerned about. He tells Sinead the lines under her eyes are barely noticeable, and are normal for her age, but she does not seem reassured by this, saying that Dr Hughes is "just being kind".

Sinead then asks for a referral for cosmetic surgery. She says that she is only depressed because she cannot afford the plastic surgery that she is certain would fix the problem.

Dr Hughes gently explains that Sinead would not meet the criteria for a cosmetic surgery referral. He invites her to come back to the surgery to talk about her mood and the anxiety and stress that the facial problems are causing her.

During subsequent appointments, Dr Hughes is able to carry out a more detailed assessment of Sinead's mental health and make a provisional diagnosis of BDD.

11.9 Management of BDD

Making the diagnosis

Despite its prevalence and impact, BDD often goes undiagnosed. This may be due to a number of factors, including the person's feelings of shame and embarrassment about symptoms, lack of insight into the problem and the strong desire for non-mental health treatments such as cosmetic surgery.

BDD should be considered and explicitly asked about in the following situations:
- a patient with a preoccupation with and recurrent attendances about a relatively minor problem with physical appearance
- patients who seem to view a physical feature as much more noticeable or abnormal than the health professional does
- patients seeking cosmetic or dermatological procedures for relatively mild disfigurements or blemishes
- people at a higher risk of BDD: individuals with symptoms of depression, social phobia, alcohol or substance misuse, OCD or eating disorders.

To assess the patient's level of concern about the problem, it can be helpful to ask the patient to rate how noticeable or abnormal they believe their defect is on a scale of one to ten.

Screening and diagnostic tools

NICE recommends asking five questions to further assess the likelihood of BDD (*Box 11.6*).

Other diagnostic tools include the Body Dysmorphic Disorder Questionnaire, which is a four-item measure that has high sensitivity and specificity in detecting BDD in a range of settings.

The BDD version of the Yale–Brown Obsessive Compulsive Scale (BDD-YBOCS) is a widely used 12-item semi-structured clinician-administered interview that rates the severity of BDD symptoms during the past week. This is the gold standard measure to assess the severity of BDD symptoms but is relatively

---

Box 11.6 **Useful questions to make a diagnosis of BDD**

1. Do you worry a lot about the way you look and wish you could think about it less?
2. What specific concerns do you have about your appearance?
3. On a typical day, how many hours a day is your appearance on your mind? (more than 1 hour a day is considered excessive)
4. What effect does it have on your life?
5. Does it make it hard to do your work or be with friends?

Box 11.7

Body Dysmorphic Disorder Questionnaire (BDDQ)

1. Are you worried about the way you look? Do you wish you could think less about your appearance?
2. How has this problem affected your life? Has it upset you a lot? Has it got in the way of work, social activities or relationships? Are there things you avoid because of how you look?
3. On an average day, how much time do you usually spend thinking about how you look (in total throughout the day): less than 1 hour, 1–3 hours or more than 3 hours?

Scoring: BDD likely if the person answers:
- Yes to both parts of question 1
- Yes to any of the parts of question 2
- Spends more than 1 hour per day thinking about their appearance
- Does not have an eating disorder (i.e. the preoccupation is not primarily with being too fat)

---

lengthy and requires some specialist training to use, so is unlikely to be feasible for routine use in primary care settings.

Discussing emotional symptoms in BDD

One of the major challenges in managing BDD will be to begin to discuss psychological and emotional factors with an individual who may hold very fixed, and possibly even delusional, beliefs that the problem lies in their physical appearance, and the need for medical or surgical intervention.

Box 11.8

Broadening the agenda in BDD

- Reflect back the patient's worry and anxiety about their appearance: *"Your skin condition seems to be worrying you a lot.."*
- Identify which fears are relating to the area of concern: *"What worries you most about having acne? How does this affect how you see yourself or how others might see you?"*
- Acknowledge their desire for medical treatment: *"How would this cosmetic procedure improve things for you?"*
- Ask about avoidance and the functional impact of the condition: *"How much is this affecting your life? Are you avoiding any situations because of your concerns? How would life be different if you were no longer concerned about your appearance?"*
- Tentatively explore whether they had considered the possibility of anxiety: *"Have you ever considered that anxiety or worry might be part of the problem?"*

It is helpful to avoid direct conflict or arguments about the diagnosis or the severity of the defect. Ensure that you take a thorough and complete history of the physical problem, so that the patient feels that their concerns are being taken seriously.

The next step is to begin a slow process to broaden the agenda, to include psychological and emotional factors as well as physical aspects of the problem. This process is likely to occur in a number of consultations over a period of time, and is covered in more detail in the section below, *Engaging the patient in treatment for BDD*.

What else to consider
The differential diagnosis for BDD is shown in *Box 11.9*. Note that many of these conditions may also be co-morbid with BDD in some individuals.

Box 11.9 | **Differential diagnosis of BDD**

- OCD
- Social anxiety disorder
- Agoraphobia
- GAD
- Depression
- Eating disorders: distorted beliefs about body image in eating disorders are confined to concerns about weight and body shape, and are associated with disordered eating patterns
- Trichotillomania (hair-pulling disorder) – in BDD hair tweezing, plucking and pulling is carried out in order to improve perceived defects in appearance of body or facial hair, rather than as an irresistible urge to pull out hair
- Excoriation (skin picking) disorder: similarly, skin picking in BDD is intended to improve perceived defects in the appearance of skin, versus compulsive urges to pick the skin in excoriation disorder
- Delusional disorders including schizophrenia and schizoaffective disorder; note that delusional beliefs about appearance may be common in BDD

Initial assessment

The initial assessment of an individual with BDD should involve assessing the severity of the condition, including the level of associated distress and the degree to which the condition is affecting the person's work, school, relationships, social life and quality of life. It is also important to assess for co-morbid disorders, such as depression, social anxiety or substance misuse, and any relevant psychosocial factors that may play a role in the development of the condition.

Risk assessment

All patients with BDD should also undergo an assessment for the presence of suicidal thoughts and behaviour, particularly if they are also suffering from low mood and depression. If the patient is a parent, also consider a risk assessment for child protection issues if the disorder could affect their parenting ability.

Assessing insight in BDD

One of the major challenges in working with patients with BDD is that insight is often absent or poor, and patients are convinced that they really do appear abnormal, deformed or ugly. This can make the individual reluctant to accept the diagnosis of BDD, and consequently unwilling to consider psychiatric medication or psychological treatment options, preferring to pursue cosmetic treatments.

Patients with delusional BDD beliefs should not be treated as a psychotic disorder, but follow the same treatment ladder as in non-delusional BDD (see below).

Cosmetic procedures and BDD

People with BDD commonly seek cosmetic surgery and other procedures in an attempt to improve the appearance of their perceived flaw. However, cosmetic treatment in BDD is typically associated with negative outcomes, including poor patient satisfaction, persistence or worsening of BDD symptoms, and higher levels of post-operative complications such as scarring and pain, which can worsen problems as a vicious cycle. Dissatisfaction with the cosmetic practitioner is also common.

Clinical assessment of BDD should routinely include a discussion about desires and plans for cosmetic treatments. When there is a strong suspicion of BDD, it is helpful to try to avoid making unnecessary referrals for cosmetic procedures wherever possible. Patients with suspected or diagnosed BDD should ideally be assessed by a mental health professional with specific expertise in the management of BDD before undergoing cosmetic surgery or dermatological treatment.

However, in some cases, continuing medical treatments which are relatively low risk and unlikely to lead to complications, may help to build a trusting relationship with patients with BDD, which can form a basis for encouraging them to accept a psychological explanation of the problem.

Using a CBT framework in the assessment of BDD

The CBT framework can help to guide a structured assessment of BDD (Box 11.10).

| Box 11.10 | **A CBT framework for assessment of BDD in primary care** |

Thoughts
- Are you worried about your appearance in any way? What are your main concerns?
- What is the most distressing aspect of this for you? What might it mean about you?
- How do you feel others view your appearance?
- Do you believe other people if they say that there isn't a major problem with your appearance?
- How much time per day do you find yourself thinking about your appearance a lot? Do you often compare yourself with others?

Feelings
- How do you feel emotionally?
- How much does this aspect of your appearance distress you?
- What feelings arise when you look in the mirror or check your appearance?
- How would you feel if you tried to stop checking your appearance?

Behaviour
- Are you avoiding anything because of your appearance?
- Are you trying to cover up or hide the area you are worried about? How do you do this?
- Do you often look in the mirror or check your body?
- Would you be able to stop doing this?
- How much time per day do you spend on carrying out these behaviours?

Physical symptoms
- Are there any physical symptoms or body sensations that concern you?

Environmental factors and triggers
- What impact are your concerns about your appearance having on your work/education/relationships/social life/quality of life?
- Are there any important life stresses or problems that are affecting you at the moment?

Initial management in primary care

Treatment of BDD can be initiated in primary care, particularly in mild to moderate cases. More severe cases, or those which are refractory to initial treatment strategies, may need referral to specialist services.

Engaging the patient in treatment for BDD

Building a strong and effective relationship with patients suffering from BDD will not only provide support and understanding but can also form a platform for treating the condition. This will involve use of communication skills such as expressing empathy, making eye contact, genuineness, active listening and use of open questions to explore the person's perspective of the problem. Health professionals should also try to demonstrate that they care about the problem and are attempting to act in the patient's best interests. It is also helpful to acknowledge and validate the sufferer's feelings of shame and distress and the degree to which their life is affected by the problem.

In many cases, it is helpful to acknowledge the existence of any genuine physical defect or difference in appearance, even if it is extremely mild, which may validate the person's experience and demonstrate understanding of their viewpoint. However, this may be less useful in individuals who are more concerned with an internal feeling of things being 'right' or symmetrical than with being believed or acknowledged.

Broadening the agenda: a 'two-track' approach

Some people with BDD may refuse to accept the diagnosis or consider any form of mental health treatment. Using a 'two-track' approach which combines medical approaches with psychological treatments can sometimes help patients begin to accept the diagnosis. This approach is also discussed in more detail in *Chapter 13* on health anxiety.

Box 11.11 — **Engaging a patient in treatment for BDD: what to say**

"I can see that your concerns about your acne are causing you major distress and worry. I take your concerns really seriously and I would like to do my very best to help you. I am happy to continue to try to treat your acne with any appropriate medical treatments that are not likely to cause harm.

It seems like the acne is having a major effect on your quality of life. You mentioned that you are really concerned about how others see you and that you haven't been able to go out because of it. I'm wondering if you have a recognised condition known as body dysmorphic disorder, where people get particularly worried about an aspect of their physical appearance. This can be treated effectively with both medication or a talking therapy known as CBT.

Could I suggest a 'two-track approach'? This means that as well as looking at medical treatments for your skin, we could also try to find some ways to help you cope with it, so that it has less effect on your mood and wellbeing. If you don't feel that this approach is right for you at the moment, that's absolutely fine, and I will be happy to discuss this with you again at any point in the future if you think it might be helpful."

However, in other cases, particularly if insight is very poor, it may be necessary to recognise that the individual is not yet ready to change, and to simply encourage them to return in the future. This may involve continuing some medical treatments which are unlikely to have a significant risk of side-effects or adverse consequences.

Explaining BDD

Providing clear and accurate information about BDD is important, including the prevalence, and common symptoms of the disorder. Emphasise that BDD is a recognised problem for which there is successful treatment. Building an alternative understanding of BDD involves helping patients to recognise that their problem stems from high levels of distress and anxiety associated with excessive concern about a physical feature, rather than simply being due to the presence of a physical defect.

An example of an explanation about BDD is shown in *Box 11.12*.

Box 11.12 | **Explaining BDD**

People with BDD experience repeated and often intrusive negative **thoughts** about an aspect of their physical appearance. Sufferers can spend many hours a day thinking and worrying about it. They remain convinced that the problem makes them appear unattractive to others, even when others reassure them that the problem is very minor.

These persistent worries lead to strong **feelings** of anxiety, distress and shame. To try to reduce these difficult feelings, people with BDD usually carry out repeated **behaviours** including:

- trying to hide or camouflage the body part with clothes, hair or make-up
- repeatedly checking in mirrors ('mirror gazing')
- comparing themselves to other people.

These behaviours are often 'compulsive' in nature – the person feels a strong urge to carry them out and would feel anxious or distressed if they did not do so, but they ultimately worsen the problem as a vicious cycle and can take up a great deal of time, getting in the way of other important life activities.

People often seek medical advice or surgical treatments to solve the problem. However, in BDD, these treatments rarely improve feelings of distress and may worsen the problem through complications such as scarring. BDD can also lead to people isolating themselves from others, and interfere with work, education and relationships, leading to low mood, loss of confidence and even thoughts of suicide.

It is important to recognise BDD when it is present, as it can be treated effectively with medication or psychological therapy.

Self-help strategies

Self-help strategies can be helpful for people with mild to moderate BDD. These include:

- providing written information about BDD and how it affects people
- highlighting relevant self-help books and websites based on CBT principles
- providing information about local and national support groups for BDD
- general self-care and lifestyle modification: physical exercise, healthy diet, reducing caffeine intake and smoking cessation may all be beneficial.

10 minute CBT strategies

Brief interventions can be used to encourage positive self-management and encourage more helpful ways of coping with BDD symptoms, including promoting wellbeing through encouraging important and meaningful activities and strengthening relationships with friends and family.

Attention training: focus on daily activities. Attention training can help people with BDD to reduce their focus on negative thoughts and worries and reduce their preoccupation with physical appearance. This informal type of mindfulness can be developed by learning to pay full attention to everyday tasks, such as brushing teeth, washing up, preparing meals, walking and driving, without allowing the mind to wander. Each time the mind wanders off into thought, it can be gently and kindly brought back to the task.

Box 11.13 **Attention training in BDD**

Attention training in BDD involves focusing and paying attention during daily activities rather than allowing the mind to get 'lost in thought'. This might involve paying attention to the following:

- **Physical touch**: notice how the activity feels in the hands, feet or other parts of the body. Notice the texture and temperature and how these change.
- **Movement**: notice if your body is moving as you carry out the activity; are you moving your hands, arms, legs or your whole body? How does it feel to move this way?
- **Sight**: what do you see? Notice the light, colours, shadows and how these may change.
- **Hearing**: what noises can you hear? What are the loudest and quietest sounds that you can notice? Is the task itself creating sounds or are there other sounds in the background?
- **Smell**: is the task associated with any particular smells? Which are the strongest?
- **Taste**: what flavours can you become aware of? Do these change or stay the same?

Developing the skill of focusing attention on daily tasks is likely to take time and requires regular practice. In order to develop their skills and confidence in the technique, the patient should practise regularly, several times each day, initially at times when anxiety levels are low, and without the specific aim of reducing preoccupation with appearance. They can gradually start to use the skills more widely over time.

Mindfulness. Practising mindfulness meditation may also help people to reduce their focus and preoccupation with negative thinking in BDD, although there is currently very limited evidence for this approach. However, as with OCD, mindfulness might be expected to help patients with BDD to reduce their excessive focus and preoccupation with negative thoughts about appearance.

Postponing appearance preoccupation. This is a process which is similar to the use of 'worry time' in GAD (see *Chapter 5*). This involves planning to only think and worry about appearance during a regular daily 'worry time.' The stages for this are shown in *Box 11.14*.

Behavioural strategies. Useful brief behavioural strategies in BDD include:
- brief behavioural activation to increase positive activities and lift low mood; this is likely to be one of the most effective strategies for use in primary care settings
- reducing unhelpful behaviours such as checking in mirrors, camouflaging of the perceived defect or reassurance seeking
- reducing avoidance and increasing social interaction.

Box 11.14 | **Postponing appearance preoccupation ('worry time')**

1. Plan a daily time to think or worry about your appearance. Aim for around 30 minutes daily, or alternatively gradually reduce the amount of time that you are currently spending on this activity. Don't choose just before bedtime. Pick the same place to carry this out each day.
2. When you notice thoughts arising about your appearance during the day, write them down in a journal or notebook and decide to think about them later in the day during the planned 'worry time'.
3. Use attention skills or distraction to bring your mind back to the present moment and continue with your day.
4. Repeat this process as many times as needed.
5. When 'worry time' arrives, look through your journal. Only think about the things you've written down if you still think they are important, otherwise just cross them out. If you haven't got through the list by the end of the time, postpone it until the next day.
6. At the end of 'worry time', use attention skills or distraction, or carry out some physical exercise to help you get back to your daily activities.

Treatment

Initial treatment for BDD can be initiated in primary care, and usually involves CBT, which is the first-line treatment, or antidepressant medication. Patients with more impaired functioning, higher levels of co-morbidity, or poor response to initial treatment will require care from specialist teams with greater levels of expertise and experience in the management of BDD.

Psychological therapy for BDD
CBT is the most effective psychological treatment for BDD and should be the first-line approach for most people. It typically involves 12–22 weekly sessions, and like OCD, usually involves elements of ERP.

People with mild functional impairment can be offered low intensity CBT including ERP with structured self-help materials, via the telephone or in a group format. Individuals with moderate functional impairment or persistent symptoms, are likely to need intensive individual therapy.

The initial aim of CBT is to develop and maintain the patient's engagement with a psychological explanation of the problem and to gradually shift their agenda away from the preoccupation with their physical appearance, and towards alleviating emotional distress and reducing the impact of the problem on their daily life. The focus is on building an alternative understanding of the problem and reducing self-focused attention and ruminating. This is carried out through the use of graded exposure and behavioural experiments to test out their fears.

ERP involves gradually confronting feared situations, such as looking in mirrors, bright lights or attending social situations, and resisting the urge to perform safety-seeking behaviours, such as use of excessive make-up or camouflaging strategies. The aim is to habituate the individual to these situations, resulting in a reduction in associated anxiety.

Additional CBT strategies include cognitive restructuring of unhelpful thoughts and thinking styles and perceptual and mirror retraining. Mirror retraining addresses distorted body image perception and helps patients learn to engage in healthier mirror-related behaviours, such as not getting too close to the mirror, stopping the use of magnifying mirrors and reducing mirror avoidance if present. Perceptual retraining strategies teach patients to broaden their attention from the preoccupation with their own appearance to include awareness of other aspects of the environment, such as concentrating fully on a conversation, noticing colours or sounds, or paying attention to the taste of food when eating.

Medication for BDD
SSRIs are the medication of choice for BDD, although their evidence for effectiveness is less strong than in OCD. Individuals with BDD beliefs of delusional intensity respond to SSRIs just as favourably as those without

delusional beliefs. NICE recommends fluoxetine as the initial choice of SSRI in adults with BDD, because there is more evidence for its effectiveness in BDD than other SSRIs. Initiation and monitoring of drug therapy should follow recommended guidelines, which are summarised in *Chapter 3*.

Current data suggests that effective treatment of BDD often requires SSRI doses that are higher than those required to treat depression and are similar to those required to treat OCD. Therefore, if there has not been an adequate response to a standard dose of an SSRI, and there are no significant side-effects after 4–6 weeks, a gradual increase in dose should be considered. Alternative SSRIs can be tried if there is no response to maximal doses of fluoxetine or the patient is unable to tolerate it due to side-effects.

Clomipramine is also effective in BDD and can be considered as a second-line treatment in patients who do not respond to, or are unable to tolerate SSRIs, although it has a greater risk of adverse effects. For patients with a significant risk of cardiovascular disease, a baseline ECG and blood pressure should be carried out before starting clomipramine. Then, commence with a small dose and titrate upwards according to response. It is also important to only prescribe small amounts of clomipramine at a time, because of its toxicity in overdose. The patient will require regular monitoring.

Currently there is no evidence to suggest that augmentation of SSRIs with any other medication, including antipsychotics, is likely to improve outcomes in BDD, including in patients with delusional beliefs. Antipsychotics are also not recommended as a monotherapy for treating BDD.

Other drugs that are not recommended for the treatment of BDD include:
- TCAs other than clomipramine
- SNRIs, including venlafaxine
- MAOIs
- anxiolytics (except cautiously for short periods to counter the early activation of SSRIs).

Combined treatment
In most cases, adults with BDD with severe functional impairment should be offered combined treatment with an SSRI and CBT. It may also be considered in people who do not respond to monotherapy with either psychological therapy or medication.

When to refer

Patients should be referred onwards for further assessment and treatment by specialist teams in the following circumstances:
- BDD symptoms are severe and associated with marked functional impairment

- at risk of self-neglect, self-harm or suicide, or posing a risk to others
- with a significant co-morbidity such as substance misuse, severe depression, anorexia nervosa or schizophrenia
- if a GP is not confident in their assessment of moderate functional impairment, or there is an inadequate response to initial treatment.

Secondary care treatment may involve high intensity CBT with a specialist therapist in the treatment of BDD and the addition of buspirone to an SSRI, which should only be initiated in secondary care. Intensive inpatient therapy or residential/supportive care may occasionally be needed for people with chronic severe dysfunction.

Summary of primary care management of BDD

Stepped care approach	What to offer	What does this involve?
Initial presentations of BDD with mild functional impairment	Explain the diagnosis and broaden the agenda to include emotional and physical factors	• Give clear and accurate explanations of BDD • Use the CBT framework to help the patient understand their experiences and demonstrate that compulsive behaviours such as mirror gazing act to maintain preoccupation with appearance and worsen anxiety • Broaden the agenda to include discussions about the impact of appearance preoccupation on the person's mood and wellbeing • Avoid referral for cosmetic procedures where possible
	10 minute CBT advice about managing anxiety	• Use of attention training and focusing on daily activities to reduce preoccupation with appearance • Mindfulness • Postponing appearance preoccupation ('worry time') • Reduce unhelpful behaviours such as mirror gazing, reassurance seeking and excessive camouflaging of the perceived defect • Use brief behavioural activation to increase engagement in social activities and exercise which may improve mood and quality of life
	Signpost to self-help resources	Provide information about CBT-based books and websites for understanding and managing BDD
	Guided self-help	Low intensity CBT/ERP (up to 10 hours) involving structured self-help, telephone or group sessions
BDD with moderate functional impairment or lack of response to initial measures	Primary care management: CBT or medication	• First-line treatment: choice of high intensity CBT/ERP or SSRI; fluoxetine is first-choice SSRI • Second-line treatment: clomipramine – consider for patients who have had a previous good response to it or unable to tolerate SSRIs

Stepped care approach	What to offer	What does this involve?
BDD with severe functional impairment or lack of response to primary care treatment	Consider referral to secondary care	<ul><li>Combined treatment with SSRI and intensive CBT/ERP</li><li>Trial of an alternative SSRI or clomipramine</li><li>Refer to secondary care if:<ul><li>severe symptoms with marked functional impairment</li><li>risk of self-neglect, self-harm or suicide, or risk to others</li><li>co-morbidity such as substance misuse, severe depression, anorexia nervosa or schizophrenia</li><li>GP is not confident in their assessment of moderate functional impairment, or there is an inadequate response to initial treatment</li></ul></li></ul>

11.10 Monitoring and follow-up

Regular follow-up should be carried out for all people commencing antidepressant treatment (see *Chapter 3*). More intensive monitoring is needed in patients with severe BDD causing marked distress, and those who show poor response to treatment or have refused treatment, due to the high risk of suicide.

Treatment for BDD should be continued for at least 12 months to reduce the risk of relapse and allow for further improvements.

Case example 11.2: Donald

Diagnosis of BDD

Donald is a 28-year-old man who has visited his GP on a number of occasions with concerns about hair loss and male pattern balding. He attends the surgery today wearing a cap. He has tried topical treatment from a private clinic and is hoping for a referral to see a dermatologist. Dr Tasnim examines Donald's scalp and notes that there is a very mild degree of hair loss, with some thinning at the crown of his head and a slightly receding hairline. When the GP reports these findings to Donald, the patient disagrees completely with the assessment and tells the GP that she is not taking him seriously. He believes that the hair loss is extremely noticeable and that it is causing major problems in his personal life.

Dr Tasnim makes a reflective statement about Donald's clear distress about the perceived hair loss. "This seems to be causing you a great deal of distress and worry."

Donald responds by sharing some of his concerns about his hair loss, saying: "I can't go on dates and I will never be able to get married or have a family looking like this. Who would want me? I am completely repulsive to women like this."

Dr Tasnim goes on to acknowledge that there is some hair loss and assures Donald that she takes his concerns very seriously. Due to the marked difference between her own perception and Donald's view of the problem, she asks the five questions recommended by NICE to explore the possibility of BDD:

Case example 11.2: *contd*

"Do you worry a lot about the way you look and wish you could think about it less?"	Donald agrees that he does worry a great deal about his appearance and that the preoccupation is very distressing. He tries to think about it less, but the worries feel impossible to control.
"What specific concerns do you have about your appearance?"	He describes his concerns about an abnormal and unattractive level of hair loss.
"On a typical day, how many hours a day is your appearance on your mind?"	Donald admits that it is hard to stop thinking about his hair loss, and he spends 2–3 hours per day thinking about and checking his appearance.
"What effect does it have on your life?"	Donald feels anxious in many social situations, even with close family, and has become very isolated due to avoidance.
"Does it make it hard to do your work or be with friends?"	He finds it hard to make close friendships and is not in a relationship due to his concerns. He works as an IT programmer and has begun working largely from home in an effort to avoid people at work.

Dr Tasnim finishes by asking the ways that Donald tries to check or camouflage the problem. Donald explains that he spends several hours each day checking his scalp with a magnifying mirror for further hair loss. He has grown his hair longer and uses thick hair gel to try to hide the problem. He also usually wears a hat or a cap to try to hide the problem.

Dr Tasnim also begins to assess Donald's level of insight about the problem. She asks how much Donald believes that other people are aware of or notice the hair loss. Donald replies by saying: *"I can't go out where there are other people, because they just stare at my ugly, balding head. Sometimes I can see that they are talking about me and laughing at how bad I look."*

Donald then asks Dr Tasnim to refer him to see a dermatologist for a possible hair implant or other scalp treatment. Dr Tasnim explains that despite Donald's concern, the hair loss is unlikely to be severe enough to require a hair implant. She also carries out an assessment of suicidal risk, as he has marked low mood and anxiety in response to the problem.

Dr Tasnim shares the possible diagnosis of BDD with the patient; however, Donald is not initially willing to accept any form of psychological explanation for his symptom and remains focused on needing cosmetic hair treatment. Dr Tasnim suggests a 'two-tracks' approach, to help Donald manage the distress and worry that has arisen from concerns about his hair loss alongside the physical problem. Donald is initially resistant to this idea, but over time, becomes more willing to consider the diagnosis of BDD and to participate in discussions about effective treatments such as SSRI or CBT.

11.11 Summary and key points

- BDD involves an intense preoccupation with a perceived flaw in physical appearance.
- It is not simple vanity or dissatisfaction with appearance but a highly distressing disorder which is frequently associated with depression, social anxiety and suicide attempts.
- People with BDD spend large amounts of time checking their appearance in mirrors, comparing themselves to others and trying to hide or conceal the area of concern.
- BDD can interfere with many important aspects of daily life, including work, academic performance and relationships with others.
- Many individuals with BDD will not reveal the degree of their concern to a health professional unless asked directly.
- Suspect BDD in people who view a minor problem with physical appearance as much more noticeable or abnormal than the health professional does, and those seeking cosmetic or dermatological procedures for mild disfigurements or blemishes.
- Engaging the patient in treatment for BDD can be a challenge if the individual is strongly fixated on a cosmetic solution to the perceived problem; helpful strategies include validating the patient's distress, acknowledging the existence of minor defects and discussing emotional and behavioural aspects of the problem.
- First-line treatment is with CBT/ERP; alternatively an SSRI (fluoxetine is first-line) at the highest tolerated dose may be offered.
- Delusional beliefs are common in patients with BDD; however, treatment pathways do not differ for this group, who should not be treated with antipsychotic medication.
- Patients with BDD have a high risk of suicidal thoughts and acts and need regular monitoring if experiencing high levels of distress or a lack of response to treatment.
- Many patients continue to have some residual symptoms of BDD even after successful treatment, which should be continued for at least a year due to the high risk of relapse.

11.12 BDD resources

- Centre for Clinical Interventions self-help leaflet: www.cci.health.wa.gov.au/Resources/Looking-After-Yourself/Body-Dysmorphia
- Veale, D., Willson, R. and Clarke, A. (2009) *Overcoming Body Image Problems including Body Dysmorphic Disorder.* Robinson.

Chapter 12
Post-traumatic stress disorder

PTSD quick reference guide

What is post-traumatic stress disorder (PTSD)?	PTSD may develop after being exposed to a significant traumatic event such as a severe accident, acts of violence or military action. Sufferers develop intrusive symptoms such as involuntary re-experiencing of images and other somatic experiences associated with the traumatic event in the form of flashbacks, nightmares and distressing mental imagery. Thoughts or reminders of the traumatic event trigger intense distress, leading to avoidance. Hyperarousal symptoms include hypervigilance for threat, exaggerated startle responses, irritability, difficulty in concentrating and sleep problems. Complex PTSD can arise after severe or multiple traumas and is associated with a negative self-view, difficulty regulating emotions and problems in relationships with others.
How common is it?	The prevalence of PTSD varies widely between countries and for different groups within countries, due to differing rates of exposure to potentially traumatic experiences. The lifetime prevalence of PTSD in the UK is around 6.8%.
Risk factors	Risk factors for PTSD include being in a professional group with a higher risk of experiencing a traumatic event, such as the armed forces, emergency service personnel and refugees. Risk factors for developing PTSD following a traumatic experience include the severity of the incident, low social support, multiple life stressors and a previous experience of trauma or a mental health problem.
Co-morbid conditions	As many as half of people with PTSD will also experience other mental health disorders, including depression, anxiety disorders, somatic symptom disorder, psychoses and increased risk of suicide. Drug and alcohol misuse and physical health problems such as chronic pain, somatoform disorders, cardiovascular disease and diabetes are also associated with PTSD. Adverse social consequences of PTSD include unemployment, relationship problems and poor performance at school.
Usual course	Many people will experience an acute stress reaction for up to one month following a traumatic event. Around one-third will go on to develop PTSD, although this resolves spontaneously in about half of these cases. The development of PTSD can also be delayed and may present up to a year or more after the event.

Common presentations	The most common presentation of PTSD is with re-experiencing symptoms, such as flashbacks or nightmares, following a recent traumatic event. Other presentations include depression, anxiety, panic attacks, agoraphobia, irritability, somatic symptoms, sleep problems and difficulties at work or in relationships. In a small proportion of cases, the onset of symptoms may be delayed following a traumatic experience. PTSD may also present as unexplained recurrent physical symptoms.
How to make the diagnosis	PTSD should be suspected in all individuals following a traumatic experience. It is important to ask all individuals at high risk of PTSD due to social or occupational circumstances about exposure to trauma experiences. Screening for PTSD should be carried out at one month following a major disaster or traumatic experience. Validated screening tools include the Trauma Screening Questionnaire (TSQ), which should be used no earlier than 3 weeks following exposure to a traumatic event.
What else could it be?	The differential diagnosis for PTSD includes adjustment disorder or acute stress disorder and other mental health conditions such as depression, other anxiety disorders, dissociative disorders and psychosis.
Self-management strategies	General self-care including physical exercise, healthy diet and sleep hygiene are often helpful. Offer empathy and support and help patients to understand their condition by giving clear explanations of PTSD. Self-management strategies using 10 minute CBT include reducing avoidance and encouraging social support and connection with friends and family members.
Treatment of PTSD	First-line treatment for PTSD involves psychological therapy (trauma-focused, CBT, exposure therapy or EMDR). Medication including SSRIs or SNRIs are considered second-line treatment. In severe cases, psychological therapy and medication can be combined or there may be augmentation of treatment with an antipsychotic such as risperidone, but this should only be initiated by a specialist.
When to refer	Severe symptoms associated with marked functional impairment, at risk of self-neglect, self-harm or suicide, or posing a risk to others, significant co-morbidity such as substance misuse, severe depression, anorexia nervosa, or schizophrenia or lack of response to treatment in community settings.
Follow-up	Active monitoring should take place for the first month after a traumatic event followed by review and screening for persistent symptoms of PTSD. Patients with PTSD will require regular follow-up to monitor their symptoms, functioning, and response to treatment.

12.1 Introduction

More than 70% of adults worldwide will experience a traumatic event in their lifetime such as a road traffic accident, physical assault or a natural disaster. Following stressful events or situations of an exceptionally threatening or catastrophic nature, it is common to experience feelings of distress, anxiety, irritability and insomnia, but many people demonstrate remarkable resilience and capacity to recover following exposure to trauma and these symptoms will often dissipate with time. However, for some, distressing psychological symptoms can persist after a traumatic experience, and this may involve the development of post-traumatic stress disorder.

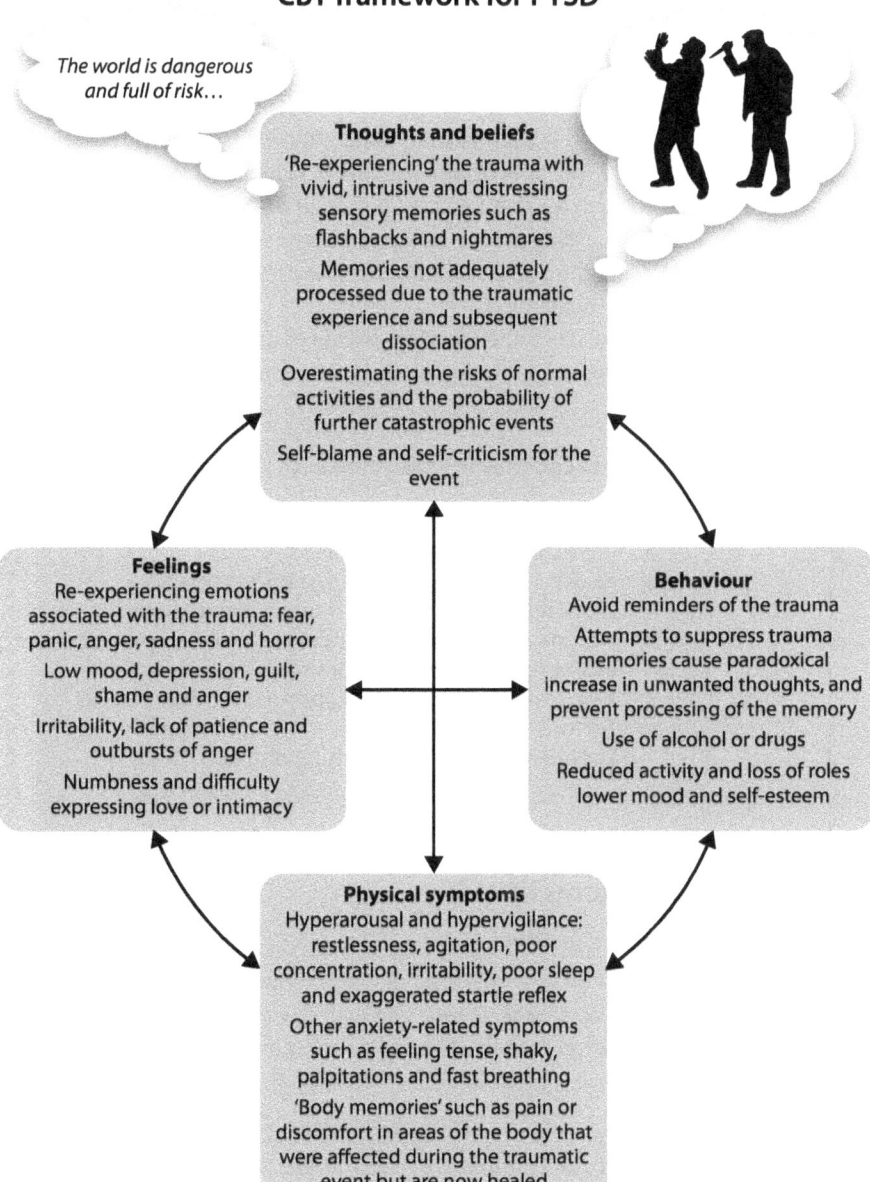

CBT framework for PTSD

The world is dangerous and full of risk…

Thoughts and beliefs
'Re-experiencing' the trauma with vivid, intrusive and distressing sensory memories such as flashbacks and nightmares

Memories not adequately processed due to the traumatic experience and subsequent dissociation

Overestimating the risks of normal activities and the probability of further catastrophic events

Self-blame and self-criticism for the event

Feelings
Re-experiencing emotions associated with the trauma: fear, panic, anger, sadness and horror

Low mood, depression, guilt, shame and anger

Irritability, lack of patience and outbursts of anger

Numbness and difficulty expressing love or intimacy

Behaviour
Avoid reminders of the trauma

Attempts to suppress trauma memories cause paradoxical increase in unwanted thoughts, and prevent processing of the memory

Use of alcohol or drugs

Reduced activity and loss of roles lower mood and self-esteem

Physical symptoms
Hyperarousal and hypervigilance: restlessness, agitation, poor concentration, irritability, poor sleep and exaggerated startle reflex

Other anxiety-related symptoms such as feeling tense, shaky, palpitations and fast breathing

'Body memories' such as pain or discomfort in areas of the body that were affected during the traumatic event but are now healed

12.2 What is PTSD?

Post-traumatic stress disorder (PTSD) is the most common major psychopathological consequence of trauma. It can be a severe and disabling condition and is characterised by flashbacks, nightmares, avoidance, numbing and hypervigilance.

PTSD can occur after a single traumatic event or from prolonged exposure to trauma, such as sexual abuse in childhood. Experiences likely to trigger PTSD typically involve feelings of intense fear, helplessness or horror. Examples of traumatic experiences that may trigger PTSD are detailed in *Box 12.1*.

To develop PTSD, an individual may experience the traumatic event themselves directly, or, according to DSM-V criteria, it can also arise following indirect exposure to a traumatic experience such as:

- witnessing an event happening to someone else
- learning about a traumatic event that has happened to a close friend or family member
- exposure to distressing details of a trauma, usually in the course of professional duties, such as first responders, police officers and medics.

Box 12.1	**Events commonly associated with the development of PTSD**

- Serious accidents and injuries
- Physical and sexual assaults
- Abuse, including childhood or domestic abuse
- Work-related exposure to trauma, including remote exposure
- Trauma related to serious health problems or childbirth experiences (for example, intensive care admission or neonatal death)
- War, conflict and combat exposure; terrorist attacks
- Torture
- Experience of a serious natural disaster

Symptoms of PTSD

People with PTSD involuntarily re-experience aspects of the traumatic event in a vivid and distressing way. Symptoms include flashbacks in which the person acts or feels as if the event is recurring, nightmares, and repetitive and distressing intrusive images or other sensory impressions from the event. These experiences lead to intense emotional distress and/or physiological reactions.

Sufferers often try to avoid people, situations or circumstances which remind them of the traumatic event and are likely to trigger these distressing internal experiences. This includes trying not to think about the event, by attempting to push memories of it out of the mind, and by avoiding thinking or talking about it in detail. Others may ruminate excessively about the problem in a way that prevents them from coming to terms with the experience.

Hyperarousal is also common, which includes hypervigilance for threat, exaggerated startle responses, difficulty in concentrating and sleep problems. Negative trauma-related emotions include fear, horror, anger, guilt or shame.

People with PTSD may also describe symptoms of emotional numbing or dissociation. This includes an inability to experience positive feelings, feeling detached and alienated from other people, giving up previously significant activities and having amnesia for significant parts of the event. The symptoms must impair function for a diagnosis to be made.

Diagnostic criteria for PTSD

Diagnostic criteria for PTSD in ICD-11 have changed in comparison to previous criteria in ICD-10, with the aim of making it easier to recognise PTSD in primary care and other non-specialist settings (*Box 12.2*). The changes also draw attention to the different levels of severity of PTSD, with a new diagnostic category of complex PTSD for more severe cases.

Box 12.2 **Diagnostic criteria for PTSD**

PTSD may develop following exposure to an extremely threatening or horrific event or series of events and is characterised by:
- re-experiencing of the traumatic event in the form of vivid intrusive memories, flashbacks, or nightmares, accompanied by strong or overwhelming emotions, particularly fear or horror, and strong physical sensations
- avoidance of thoughts and memories of the event, or activities, situations or people reminiscent of the event
- persistent perceptions of heightened current threat, such as hypervigilance or an enhanced startle reaction to stimuli such as unexpected noises
- other symptoms include sleep problems, irritability or outbursts of anger and difficulty concentrating
- symptoms persist for at least several weeks and cause significant impairment in personal, family, social, educational, occupational or other important areas of functioning

---

Complex PTSD

Complex PTSD develops in a subset of people with PTSD, after exposure to a sustained or prolonged event, or repeated events of an extremely threatening or horrific nature, from which escape is difficult or impossible. This includes situations such as torture, slavery, genocide campaigns, prolonged domestic violence and repeated childhood sexual or physical abuse.

Complex PTSD is characterised by the core symptoms of PTSD, and involves three additional groups of symptoms causing significant impairment in important areas of functioning:
- Problems in regulating emotions and behaviour

- Negative self-concept involving persistent beliefs about oneself as diminished, defeated or worthless, accompanied by deep and pervasive feelings of shame, guilt or failure related to the traumatic event
- Difficulties in sustaining relationships and in feeling close to others.

12.3 Epidemiology

In England, around 30% of adults report having experienced at least one major trauma in their lifetime, although the prevalence of PTSD seems to be much lower. The lifetime prevalence of PTSD is around 6.8%, with a 12-month prevalence ranging from 1.3% to 3.6% in the UK.

The 2014 Adult Psychiatric Morbidity Survey of Mental Health and Wellbeing found that overall prevalence was similar in men and women, but PTSD was more common in younger people, affecting 8% of those aged 16–24 years compared with 0.6% of those aged 75 and over. In females, rates of PTSD were highest in younger women and then declined sharply with age. In men, rates remained stable in most age groups, only dropping in later life after the age of 64. Approximately 1–2% of women develop PTSD postnatally.

The prevalence of PTSD varies widely in different countries, ranging from 1–12%. This is likely to be due to differences in risk of exposure to potentially traumatic events, social factors and differences in study design and methods of diagnostic assessment. Rates are doubled in populations affected by conflict and may be as high as 50% in survivors of rape. Rates of PTSD also vary within countries, with certain groups of individuals who are at a higher risk of exposure to traumatic stressors having a higher prevalence of PTSD (*Box 12.3*).

Box 12.3	**Groups of individuals at high risk of PTSD**
	- Members of the armed forces, including combat veterans and ex-service personnel
	- Members of the ambulance, police, prison and fire services, and other emergency personnel, including those no longer in service
	- Nursing and medical professionals, especially in front-line situations, such as accident and emergency or first responders
	- Journalists
	- Refugees and asylum seekers, especially from conflict zones

12.4 Aetiology

Risk factors for development of PTSD

PTSD is unique amongst the anxiety disorders, in that its development can be directly attributed to an external causative factor, which is the exposure to potentially traumatic experiences. Risk factors for the development of PTSD following exposure to a traumatic event are shown in *Box 12.4*. There is some evidence that the subjective appraisal or perception of threat is more important for the development and maintenance of PTSD than objective trauma severity.

Box 12.4 | **Risk factors for development of PTSD**

- Severity of the incident – more severe traumatic events, associated with a great perceived threat to life, have a higher chance of PTSD
- Low social support and social disadvantage is one of the strongest predictors of PTSD
- Previous experience of trauma
- Presence of multiple major life stressors
- History of a mental health disorder
- In children exposed to trauma, the risk of PTSD is reduced by good family support and when there is less parental distress
- Female sex – women experience higher rates of PTSD than men; however, this varies depending on the type of trauma and specific age group being assessed
- Younger age – among people exposed to disaster or trauma, older adults have a lower risk of developing PTSD than younger adults

---

Aetiological theories for PTSD

A number of psychological and neurobiological theories have been suggested to explain the pattern of symptoms characteristic of PTSD.

Emotional processing theory

This involves the concept of 'fear structures' as internal processes which produce cognitive, behavioural and physiological reactions when activated, designed to help the individual avoid or escape from danger. Emotional processing theory argues that in PTSD, due to difficulties in processing information about the traumatic event, fear structures become pathological. People who have experienced a traumatic event can develop negative associations arising from objectively safe reminders of the event, such as situations, people or news stories, develop altered beliefs about the world and the self, such as perceiving the world as dangerous and viewing the self as incompetent or unable to cope, and excessive or unhelpful responses, such as numbing of feelings and avoidance of safe situations.

Dual representation theory

This is based on the existence of different types of memory, including verbally accessible memory (VAM) and situationally accessible memory (SAM). Memories of a traumatic event are initially retained in SAM. These memories primarily involve sensory information, such as images, smells, sounds, feelings such as fear or horror, and physical sensations such as pain, associated with the experience. SAM is generally unconscious, but may be triggered by reminders of the experience, leading to symptoms of re-experiencing of the traumatic event. The purpose of the memory is to protect the individual from any future similar danger.

In healthy processing of a traumatic experience, these memories are subsequently processed using VAM to consciously reflect on the information, attempting to understand and integrate the different experiences. According to dual representation theory, PTSD can develop if this process does not occur. Attempts to dissociate from the event or block the memory, in order to avoid negative emotional states, can lead to the memory being retained in SAM. Cues or stimuli in the environment that are associated with the traumatic event can then activate SAM, leading to the characteristic intrusive visual images and flashbacks which occur in PTSD.

12.5 CBT model of PTSD

PTSD is classified as an anxiety disorder. From a CBT perspective, anxiety is viewed as arising from fears about a potential future threat, although in PTSD, the threat is a traumatic experience which has taken place in the past. To explain this paradox, the cognitive behavioural model suggests that persistent PTSD occurs when individuals process the traumatic event in a way which makes them perceive the threat as ongoing and current.

As with other anxiety disorders, the persistent sense of threat in PTSD leads to feelings of anxiety, anger and low mood and to a series of behavioural and cognitive responses which are intended to reduce the sense of risk and alleviate distress in the short term, but which often have the unwanted consequence of maintaining the disorder over time.

Re-experiencing the trauma

The commonest symptom of PTSD is the repeated re-experiencing of highly vivid unwanted, intrusive and distressing memories related to the trauma. These re-experiencing memories feel like they are happening in the here and now and this creates the sense of current threat that is characteristic of PTSD. Flashbacks involve sudden and vivid re-experiencing memories, lasting from a few seconds to several minutes, which feel as if the trauma is happening again. They are typically associated with powerful emotions and there can be a loss of awareness of other things that are going on around the individual. Repeated nightmares about the trauma are also common.

Re-experiencing memories tends to involve sensory impressions, rather than verbal thoughts. They are mainly visual, but also include emotions, sounds, smells, tastes and physical sensations. These can arise sporadically and in disconnected and confusing ways, almost like snapshots of a film.

Alongside the unwanted sensory intrusive memories, people with PTSD often have difficulty in intentionally retrieving a complete memory of the traumatic event, and there may be missing details and problems recalling the exact temporal order of events. According to dual representation theory, this corresponds to the memories being stored as SAM, rather than being processed and retained as VAM.

Re-experiencing memories are triggered by a wide range of stimuli and situations associated with the traumatic experience. These include physical cues such as a spatial location, the shape of a person, smells, or specific phrases said in a certain tone of voice. They may also be triggered by experiencing emotional states, such as feeling helpless or trapped, or other internal cues such as being touched on a certain part of the body, or other internal physical sensations.

Emotions in PTSD

Intrusive memories in PTSD often include experiencing distressing emotions associated with the trauma, such as fear, panic, anger, helplessness, sadness and horror. There may also be numbness associated with difficulty expressing love or intimacy following the event, which develops as a mental strategy to protect themselves from the horror of the situation.

Secondary emotions which arise as a response to the ongoing experience of PTSD include the development of low mood and depression. There may also be strong feelings of guilt, shame or anger, which may be directed at the self or others for having been unable to prevent the event from arising.

Irritability, lack of patience and outbursts of anger are also common in PTSD. These can arise rapidly and seemingly 'out of the blue', although are often linked to some kind of trigger to traumatic memories which has not been consciously recognised.

Physical sensations in PTSD

Typical physical sensations in PTSD are of hyperarousal, including feeling restless, agitated and irritable, and having poor concentration and poor sleep. There may be hypervigilance for potential danger leading to a constant sense of tension and an exaggerated startle reflex. Many other common symptoms of anxiety also arise, such as feeling tense, shaky, having a racing heart and fast breathing. Individuals with PTSD may also experience body memories of the trauma, such as pain or discomfort in areas of the body that were affected during the event, even after being physically healed.

Other cognitive aspects of PTSD

Cognitive factors in PTSD include experiencing persistent negative beliefs about the self or the world and distorted ideas of blame related to the traumatic event or its consequences. This may involve catastrophic interpretations about the meaning of symptoms such as flashbacks, lack of concentration or numbing (e.g. *"Having such vivid flashbacks must mean that I am going mad"*). There may also be fears about being permanently damaged by the experience (e.g. *"Having this disorder means I am flawed and no longer capable"*). These negative interpretations lead to increased anxiety and avoidance as a vicious cycle.

Other cognitive aspects of PTSD include:
- overestimation of the risks of many normal activities and exaggeration of the probability of further catastrophic events: *"The world is a terrible, dangerous place"*
- excessive self-blame and self-criticism for the event having taken place: *"I attract disaster"* or *"This happened to me because I deserve it"*
- negative interpretations of other people's reactions: *"I am tainted by the experience and no longer acceptable to others"*
- excessively negative interpretation of the impact of the experience on other life domains such as financial or professional consequences: *"I'll never be able to work now I feel this way"*.

Behavioural reactions in PTSD

Avoidance of reminders of the trauma, such as people, situations or circumstances resembling the event or associated with it, is a common behavioural reaction, which serves as an attempt to control or minimise distressing emotions. However, whilst avoidance may reduce anxiety in the short term, it leads to significant restriction of daily life as well as a gradual increase in anxiety in the longer term. Attempts to suppress memories and push unwanted thoughts out of the mind also typically lead to a paradoxical increase in the frequency of unwanted intrusive recollections.

Safety behaviours represent another type of avoidance which are designed to prevent or minimise potential future harm. This might involve driving more slowly, avoiding motorways or only driving during the daytime after a road traffic accident.

Other common unhelpful behavioural strategies in PTSD include the following:
- Use of alcohol or other drugs to 'self-medicate' and suppress the symptoms of PTSD leads to reduced processing of the trauma memories, reduced ability to participate fully in daily life and a loss of self-esteem.
- Reduction of meaningful activity: many individuals with PTSD give up or avoid activities that were important to them before the traumatic event,

including sports, hobbies, work or social activities. This lowers mood and self-esteem still further.

- Some behaviours used to control some of the PTSD symptoms may increase other symptoms. For example, trying to prevent nightmares by going to bed very late or reducing sleep may increase symptoms of poor concentration, irritability and low mood.
- Excessive rumination about the trauma and its consequences, how it could have been prevented, or thoughts about justice or revenge, lead to increased low mood and tension, and can prevent the person from coming to terms with the experience.

12.6 Co-morbidity

As many as 50% of cases of PTSD co-occur with other mental health disorders. These include depression, anxiety disorders, somatic symptom disorder, psychoses and increased risk of suicide. Problems with drug and alcohol use are also highly co-morbid with PTSD and may be used as a form of self-medication, acting as a coping strategy to reduce the distress associated with symptoms of PTSD. Children with PTSD may also be more likely to develop ADHD, oppositional defiant disorder and conduct disorders.

People with PTSD are also at increased risk of experiencing poor physical health including somatoform disorders, chronic pain, cardiovascular disease, hypertension, diabetes, autoimmune diseases, dementia, serious disability and premature death.

Adverse social consequences of PTSD include unemployment, problems with school performance, poverty, relationship problems with partners, peers and family members, and engagement in problematic health behaviours such as smoking.

12.7 Course and prognosis of PTSD

Many people subjected to a traumatic event will experience an acute stress reaction for up to a month afterwards. In most people, these symptoms will gradually disappear as they come to terms with the experience. However, in around one-third of people, the symptoms will persist and can develop into PTSD, although this rate varies with the type and severity of the traumatic event.

In about half of these cases, PTSD symptoms will spontaneously remit over the following year. However, for others, the condition can be severe and enduring. The severity of symptoms two weeks after trauma is a good predictor of the degree of severity in the longer term, after six months. The development of PTSD can also be delayed and present up to a year or more after the event.

Effective treatments for PTSD exist but due to the stigma associated with help-seeking and delayed recognition of symptoms, treatment is often delayed for many years. However, individuals can benefit from treatment even when the symptoms have been present for many years.

Among individuals with chronic PTSD, the severity of symptoms fluctuates over time, with periods of greater severity potentially reflecting sensitivity to co-occurring stressors. The National Comorbidity Survey in the USA found that the average duration of symptoms was 36 months in people receiving treatment and 64 months among those untreated. In more than one-third of people, symptoms never fully remitted.

12.8 Presentation of PTSD

I'm an ex-serviceman and I keep getting these headaches...

I've been getting all panicky since having a car crash and I can't drive any more...

I'm not sleeping and I'm really irritable... I guess it started when I was attacked a few months ago...

Some individuals will present with a clear history of PTSD-type symptoms following a recent traumatic event. However, others may find it difficult to disclose the details of the trauma, particularly in cases of rape or sexual abuse. In a small proportion of cases, the onset of symptoms may be delayed following the experience, and the individual may be less likely to recognise the link between their current difficulties and the traumatic event, which can present a barrier to diagnosis.

The commonest presenting symptoms of PTSD are of re-experiencing, such as flashbacks or nightmares. Other presentations include depression, anxiety, panic attacks, agoraphobia, irritability, somatic symptoms, sleep problems or functional difficulties such as problems coping at work.

In some cases, PTSD can present as recurrent, unexplained physical symptoms leading to repeated attendances at health services. It can be helpful to ask all recurrent attenders whether they have ever experienced a traumatic event.

Case example 12.1: Peter

How might PTSD present?

Peter, a 35-year-old male combat veteran, presents to his GP with headaches. The GP takes a thorough history and carries out a full examination, which is normal.

On further questioning, he also describes symptoms of poor sleep, tearfulness and nightmares. He has now left the armed forces and works as an electrical engineer but has been finding it increasingly difficult to focus on his work. He also reports that his marriage and friendships have been suffering, and he has been avoiding seeing many of his old friends from the army, because he does not want to be reminded of his past experiences.

"I often start to feel restless. I can't concentrate on anything and I get really irritable and snap at my wife and kids for no reason. That's when the headache comes on, it's like a tight band around my head. Sometimes, I get myself so worked up that I start to feel quite panicky. During those times, I can feel my heart starting to thump in my chest in the same way it did when I was in the service and it brings back the same fear I had back then."

When feeling low or agitated, Peter tends to smoke cigarettes and drink alcohol. He has tried to overcome these symptoms alone but has been unsuccessful and now recognises a need for formal help. He does not wish to take medication at this time.

Peter had not initially recognised the link between his headaches and his experiences as a combat veteran but is aware that several of his friends have undergone treatment for PTSD following their time in the army. He agrees to contact the charity Combat Stress, as several of his friends have had support from them and found it helpful.

Presentation in children

Children with PTSD may present differently to adults, and can exhibit symptoms such as:
- experiencing dreams of the trauma, which may change into nightmares of monsters
- reliving the trauma in their play
- losing interest in things that they previously enjoyed
- expressing the belief that they will not live long enough to grow up
- somatic symptoms such as abdominal pain and headaches.

12.9 Management of PTSD

Making the diagnosis

PTSD is often under-recognised, even among high-risk groups, and should be suspected in all patients following a traumatic event. Directly asking about exposure to trauma, particularly in individuals at high risk of PTSD due to social or occupational circumstances, may improve the recognition rate, keeping in mind that the event(s) may have occurred many months or years previously. Sensitive questioning is often required to elicit symptoms of PTSD, as patients may avoid disclosing details of their traumatic experience due to the emotional distress that arises when recalling the event. It may also be necessary to take active steps to overcome language and cultural barriers to making the diagnosis, for example by using interpreters. In some cases, it can be helpful to provide examples or a checklist of potentially traumatic events and common symptoms, particularly for people who find it difficult to verbalise their experiences.

Diagnostic tools for PTSD

Screening for PTSD using a validated, brief diagnostic tool should be carried out for individuals at high risk of PTSD at one month following a major disaster or traumatic experience. This can be carried out by organisations coordinating a disaster plan or may sometimes be carried out in primary care. For refugees and asylum seekers at high risk of PTSD, screening should comprise part of a comprehensive physical and mental health assessment.

Trauma Screening Questionnaire. In primary care, the Trauma Screening Questionnaire (TSQ) is a validated brief screening tool, which can be helpful to identify individuals with PTSD. It is freely available to download and only takes a few minutes to administer. It is designed to be used no earlier than three

---

Box 12.5 | **Trauma Screening Questionnaire**

Following a traumatic event, the individual is asked to identify whether they have experienced any of the following reactions at least twice in the past week:

- Upsetting thoughts or memories about the event that have come into your mind against your will
- Upsetting dreams about the event
- Acting or feeling as though the event were happening again
- Feeling upset by reminders of the event
- Bodily reactions (such as fast heartbeat, stomach churning, sweatiness, dizziness) when reminded of the event
- Difficulty falling or staying asleep
- Irritability or outbursts of anger
- Difficulty concentrating
- Heightened awareness of potential dangers to yourself and others
- Being jumpy or being startled at something unexpected

weeks following exposure to a traumatic event, to allow for natural recovery processes to occur. The questionnaire consists of 10 questions which measure re-experiencing and arousal symptoms over the past week. An individual scoring six or more positive responses to the questions is at risk of PTSD and should be referred for further detailed assessment by a specialist.

PC-PTSD. This is a brief screening tool suitable for GP settings. Answering 'yes' to three or more of the questions should warrant further questioning.

Other screening tools for PTSD. There are other screening and diagnostic tools for PTSD; however, many of these are longer and more complex or time-consuming to complete, and therefore are less suitable for use in primary care. Examples of alternative scales include:
- Impact of Events Scale-Revised: this 22-item self-report measure, answered on a scale of 0 to 4, assesses intrusion, avoidance and hyperarousal associated with traumatic events.
- PTSD Checklist for DSM-V: a 20-item self-report measure which assesses 20 symptoms of PTSD according to DSM-V criteria.
- Davidson Trauma Scale: a 17-item self-report measure which assesses symptoms of post-traumatic stress disorder based on DSM-IV.

Box 12.6 **PC-PTSD**

In your life, have you ever had any experience that was so frightening, horrible or upsetting that, in the past month, you:
- have had nightmares about it or thought about it when you did not want to?
- tried hard not to think about it or went out of your way to avoid situations that reminded you of it?
- have been constantly on guard, watchful or easily startled?
- felt numb or detached from others, activities or your surroundings?
- felt guilty or unable to stop blaming yourself or others for the event(s) or any problems the events have caused?

What else to consider

PTSD should be considered in all individuals who have experienced a traumatic event. The assessment should also include an acute stress disorder or adjustment disorder, and other mental health conditions which may be associated with trauma or co-morbid with PTSD. *Box 12.7* shows the differential diagnosis of PTSD.

Box 12.7

Differential diagnosis of PTSD

- Adjustment disorder or acute stress disorder: variable symptoms of low mood, anxiety, worry, traumatic stress symptoms, and feelings of inability to cope, plan ahead or carry on. This often arises soon after experiencing a trauma and symptoms may resolve spontaneously. Symptom intensity is usually less than with PTSD.
- Depression: low mood, lack of energy, loss of interest, suicidal thoughts.
- GAD: persistent excessive anxiety and worry about multiple events or activities, which is accompanied by additional symptoms such as restlessness, fatigue, difficulty concentrating, irritability, muscle tension or disturbed sleep.
- Panic disorder: recurrent, unexpected panic attacks, which are not triggered by stimuli that recall a specific traumatic event.
- Specific phobias: fear and avoidance restricted to certain situations.
- OCD: distressing obsessional thoughts which may arise as images, associated with repeated compulsive behaviours.
- Dissociative disorders: persistent and recurrent feelings of detachment from the self, associated with gaps in recall (dissociative amnesia). This condition is also often related to experiencing traumatic events but there is an absence of the re-experiencing and hyperarousal symptoms of PTSD.
- Psychosis: hallucinations and delusions, which may be experienced as vivid intrusive images and flashbacks, associated with perceptual and cognitive disorganisation.

Initial assessment in primary care

Assessment of people with possible PTSD in primary care involves recognition of the condition and an initial assessment of physical, psychological and social needs. If the person is exhibiting severe distress or functional impairment, co-morbid depression or another mental health disorder, or there are other concerns, it is important to assess their risk of suicide and self-harm, as well as any potential risk to other people. A risk assessment is also needed to consider an individual's risk of continued exposure to trauma-inducing environments, such as ongoing domestic violence.

Assessment should also include screening for coexisting conditions such as depression or substance misuse. Generally, treatment of PTSD is associated with an improvement in low mood. However, if depression is severe enough to make psychological treatment of the PTSD difficult, the depression should be treated first. People with co-morbid drug and alcohol misuse should not be excluded from treatment for PTSD.

A CBT framework offers a helpful structure for making the assessment of PTSD in primary care. Useful questions are shown in *Box 12.8.*

Box 12.8

A CBT framework for assessment of PTSD in primary care

Thoughts
- Do you find yourself re-experiencing a traumatic event through 'flashbacks' or nightmares?
- Do you have amnesia for any parts of the experience?
- Do you experience 'dissociation' where you feel disconnected from yourself or the world around you?
- Have you started viewing yourself more negatively, feeling diminished, defeated or worthless?

Feelings
- How is your mood?
- Are you having problems with low mood or anxiety?
- Are you more irritable or quick to anger than usual?
- Are you having difficulty managing extreme emotions?
- Do you feel emotionally numb and find it difficult to feel any positive emotions?

Behaviour
- Are you avoiding any situations or people that trigger unpleasant memories of the event?
- Do you try to avoid thinking and talking about it?
- Have you given up any activities that you previously enjoyed?
- Are you engaging in any other behaviour that might be seen by others as 'self-destructive' or reckless?

Physical symptoms
- Do you find yourself physically tense and 'on edge'?
- Are you experiencing difficulty concentrating or problems with sleep?
- Are you having any other physical symptoms that are causing concern?

Environmental factors and triggers
- Have you experienced a traumatic event within the past year?
- Did you suffer any significant traumatic experiences in your early life?
- Are you having difficulties with relationships with important others, following a traumatic experience?
- Have you recently moved to this country from abroad due to political instability or war?

Supporting patients in primary care

The provision of information and support to people with suspected and confirmed PTSD is an important primary care role. This should include:

- explanations about common reactions to traumatic events, the typical symptoms of PTSD and its usual course
- reassurance that PTSD is a treatable condition
- discussion of treatment options, including those which may be offered by a specialist
- where their care will take place
- background information about PTSD including written patient information leaflets
- information about local and national support groups.

Supporting families and carers is also important. This includes giving advice on how they can support the person in getting access to treatment and in getting better. Family and friends can be reassured that talking about the traumatic event with the victim will not make PTSD worse. In fact, avoiding talking about the event in order not to distress the victim is often a bigger problem which may be interpreted by the sufferer as a sign that others do not care, or that they think the event was partly the victim's own fault. It is also important to review the carer's own mental health and wellbeing and discuss how they are being affected personally by the individual's PTSD.

Initial management after trauma

NICE recommends a period of active monitoring for the first month after a traumatic event, which includes an explanation of the condition, as well as giving advice about self-management, including sleep hygiene, and using friends and family as support. It is often helpful to normalise the experience of PTSD-type symptoms in the first few weeks following a traumatic event, and reassure the individual that for many people, these symptoms will resolve spontaneously with time.

People with severe ongoing symptoms should be offered further assessment and treatment. Debriefing is not recommended as it is ineffective and may even worsen the problem.

Explaining PTSD

Providing an accurate explanation of PTSD and helping patients to understand and make sense of the common responses to trauma will help to reduce the downward spiral of worsening anxiety, fear and avoidance, as well as minimising the impact of PTSD symptoms on the individual's life (see *Box 12.9*).

Box 12.9

Explaining the traumatic response

Trauma forces you to suddenly confront a terrifying risk to yourself or another person, such as serious harm or death, with very little time to adjust or prepare for the experience. This can lead to feelings of extreme fear, terror and despair, both during and after the event.

Symptoms of PTSD include having involuntary, vivid flashbacks or nightmares, where **thoughts** and memories of the traumatic experience come into the mind without warning. These are often associated with strong **emotions** and **physical symptoms**. Many people also feel 'hyperarousal' where they startle easily, find it hard to concentrate and sleep, are constantly on edge and irritable, or feel numb and detached from others. You might react with **behaviour** such as avoiding situations or people that remind you of the trauma and trying not to talk about it for fear of experiencing the same distressing feelings that arose during the trauma itself.

The bodily reactions and memories that arise after a traumatic event are extremely unpleasant and scary but are part of your body's danger warning system, which has become much more sensitive, in an attempt to keep you safe in the future. These are a normal response to coming to terms with a highly traumatic experience and do not indicate that there is something 'wrong' with you. In many cases, these symptoms will settle down by themselves as you begin to process the experience over time, particularly if you try to keep up your important daily activities and stay connected to your social and family network.

In some cases, people go on to develop a longer-term problem, known as PTSD. Here, the body's warning system can start to get in the way of being able to enjoy a normal life. At this stage it becomes important to seek help, as there are effective treatments available, including psychological therapy and medication.

Self-help strategies

Self-help strategies can be particularly helpful for people during the initial period of watchful waiting in the first month after a traumatic event, and for people with mild to moderate symptoms of PTSD. These include:

- providing written information about PTSD and how it affects people
- highlighting relevant self-help books and websites based on CBT principles
- providing information about local and national support groups for PTSD
- lifestyle modification: physical exercise, reducing caffeine intake, smoking cessation and improving sleep may all be beneficial.

10 *minute CBT for PTSD*

Whilst effective treatment for PTSD involves in-depth psychological therapy from appropriately trained therapists, several brief supportive strategies can be offered in primary care to individuals with mild to moderate symptoms of PTSD.

- Overcoming avoidance: encourage positive rather than negative or unhelpful coping strategies using brief behavioural activation to promote the gradual re-adoption of important life activities, exercise, work and hobbies, which have been reduced or avoided due to PTSD. The individual can be encouraged to focus on keeping life as 'normal' as possible, following their usual routine and trying to engage in as many meaningful and valued activities as possible, and to begin activities in small 'bite-sized' and realistic pieces.
- Encouraging healthy life behaviours such as engaging in exercise and healthy eating patterns, whilst avoiding unhealthy behaviours such as excessive alcohol, smoking, caffeine or other drugs.
- Building and maintaining social support: this is a known protective factor for PTSD. Patients can be encouraged to engage in social interaction by spending time with family and friends, and to talk about the traumatic experience with someone they trust.
- Encourage the patient to minimise self-blame or self-criticism for developing PTSD, which is a very common and normal human response to a traumatic experience, rather than being a sign of 'weakness'.
- Signposting to mindfulness, relaxation and self-compassion activities: these can aid with sleep, self-soothing and reduce physical tension.

Treatment of PTSD

Management depends on the severity of PTSD, which is assessed as being mild, moderate or severe, according to the level of emotional distress and functional impairment, including the impact on work or school, relationships, social life and quality of life.

Active monitoring

For individuals with mild or sub-clinical PTSD symptoms, particularly following a recent trauma, consider active monitoring and arrange follow-up to review within a month of the initial trauma.

Psychological therapy

Trauma-focused psychological therapies are the most effective treatments for PTSD, and should be offered if symptoms are severe at presentation, or persist for longer than one month. Importantly, psychological therapy can be effective many years after the event, so can be offered even years after the trauma. Effective therapies include trauma-focused CBT, exposure therapy and EMDR.

Trauma-focused CBT. This typically consists of a combination of exposure therapy and trauma-focused cognitive therapy. Therapy typically involves up to

12 sessions, but may involve more if clinically indicated; for example, in complex PTSD following multiple traumatic experiences. The components of trauma-focused CBT include:

- psychoeducation about reactions to trauma
- strategies for managing arousal and flashbacks
- reliving and processing of the trauma memories
- processing trauma-related emotions, including shame, guilt, loss and anger
- restructuring trauma-related meanings, including the use of imagery techniques to overcome avoidance
- behavioural strategies to promote adaptive functioning; for example, reducing avoidance and re-establishing work and social relationships
- preparation for the end of treatment include planning booster sessions, particularly in relation to significant dates such as trauma anniversaries.

Exposure therapy. This teaches individuals with PTSD to gradually confront trauma-related memories, feelings and situations that they have been avoiding, or which evoke fear, but which are now safe. This might involve driving a car down a road where an accident occurred or verbally recounting the details of a painful traumatic memory. With repeated exposure and habituation to feared experiences, the distressing emotional responses are likely to gradually reduce, and the individual will be able to learn that:

- memories and reminders of the trauma are not dangerous and can be experienced without significant distress
- any distress that does arise will pass with time
- internal physical responses to anxiety, such as a racing heart, are not dangerous
- the individual is able to cope with negative affect.

Eye movement desensitisation and reprocessing (EMDR). EMDR is one of the most effective psychological treatment options for PTSD, but should only be used for non-combat-related trauma, as the evidence suggests non-significant effects for those who have experienced military combat-related trauma. It usually involves 8–12 sessions but may need more for people who have experienced complex or multiple traumas.

EMDR uses bilateral stimulation (eye movements, taps and tones) while the person focuses on trauma-related memories and associations, particularly visual images, until the memories are no longer distressing. This process is thought to help the brain process flashbacks and to make sense of the traumatic experience. It also includes teaching self-calming techniques and strategies for coping when flashbacks arise, and developing alternative positive beliefs about the self.

EMDR is described in more detail in *Chapter 3.*

Additional psychological strategies. Further psychological strategies which may be used in PTSD include:

- supported trauma-focused computerised CBT for mild to moderate symptoms in individuals who are not considered to be at high risk
- CBT interventions targeted at specific symptoms such as sleep disturbance or anger
- compassion-focused therapy can be used to strengthen the soothing and affiliative system through the cultivation of self-compassion; this can be helpful for people who are experiencing high levels of shame and self-criticism following the traumatic event(s), and may be of particular benefit in complex PTSD
- mindfulness may lead to some improvements in PTSD symptomatology.

Drug treatment of PTSD in adults

There is less evidence of the efficacy of drug therapies compared to psychological therapies in the treatment of PTSD, so it is usually a second-line approach. However, medication can be an appropriate strategy in adults with PTSD who decline referral for psychological therapies and would prefer to try drug treatment, or for people with co-morbidity such as significant depression, which may prevent them from engaging effectively with psychological therapies.

Decisions about medication are often made by specialist services, but in some cases, it is appropriate to initiate treatment in primary care, particularly if the time for referral is likely to be significantly delayed. Drug treatments should not be offered to children and young people aged under 18 years.

Antidepressants. Antidepressants with evidence of efficacy in PTSD include SSRIs and venlafaxine. There is evidence for the use of fluoxetine, paroxetine and sertraline, although only paroxetine and sertraline are licensed in the UK for the treatment of PTSD. Paroxetine is more likely to be associated with discontinuation symptoms. There is weaker evidence that amitriptyline, mirtazapine and phenelzine may have some benefit in reducing the symptoms of PTSD.

Guidelines for initiating and reviewing antidepressant treatment are covered in *Chapter 3*.

Antipsychotic medication. Antipsychotics such as risperidone are sometimes used to augment other treatment approaches in adults who have a poor response to psychological therapies or antidepressants. This should be initiated and monitored under specialist mental health supervision only.

Prevention of PTSD

NICE recommends a stepped approach to supporting individuals after a traumatic experience, which includes a process of active monitoring for the first month after the event. People with severe ongoing symptoms should then be offered formal assessment and intervention if the disorder is not improving.

Brief, trauma-focused, cognitive behavioural interventions (*Box 12.10*) are effective to reduce the severity of early symptoms of PTSD and should be offered to individuals with clinically significant symptoms of PTSD or an acute stress disorder. Non-targeted interventions such as psychoeducation, psychological debriefing, individual and group counselling are largely ineffective and are therefore not recommended following a traumatic event. Drug treatments, including benzodiazepines, are also not known to be effective and should be avoided.

There is no current evidence to support routine intervention after traumatic events involving multiple people, such as natural disasters or terrorist attacks. However, high levels of social support may be protective, and social interaction can be encouraged by health professionals.

Box 12.10

Trauma-focused CBT interventions

- Cognitive processing therapy
- Cognitive therapy for PTSD
- Narrative exposure therapy
- Prolonged exposure therapy

When to refer

People with clinically important PTSD symptoms should be referred to a specialist mental health service with appropriate expertise in the management of PTSD to confirm the diagnosis and to formulate a management plan involving psychological therapy and/or drug treatment. Availability and arrangements for accessing trauma-focused psychological treatments may vary locally, and there may sometimes be a significant delay before treatment begins.

If there is difficulty finding a specialist locally, the UK Psychological Trauma Society website (www.ukpts.co.uk) lists trauma centres that provide a specialist mental health service with expertise in managing PTSD. The diagnosis of PTSD may also be confirmed in primary care by a GP with appropriate training and experience.

Armed forces veterans with service-related PTSD can be referred to secondary care more rapidly than civilians under the veterans' priority scheme. There are also charities which offer support for veterans experiencing PTSD, such as Combat Stress.

Care for people with PTSD and complex needs

Patients with complex PTSD should receive specialist multidisciplinary care and may benefit from a combination of psychosocial therapy and medication. For people with complex PTSD or additional needs:

- There may be a need for an increase in duration or number of therapy sessions to allow extra time to develop a trusting relationship with the individual.
- Consider the safety and stability of the person's personal circumstances (for example, their housing situation) and how this might affect engagement with and success of treatment. Liaison with other agencies such as social services, health visitors or occupational health services may be needed.
- Support the person to manage any issues that might be a barrier to engaging with trauma-focused therapies, such as substance misuse, dissociation, emotional dysregulation, interpersonal difficulties or negative self-perception.
- Plan any ongoing support they will need after the end of treatment; for example, to manage any residual PTSD symptoms or co-morbidities, or to cope with practical difficulties such as developing return to work plans.

Summary of primary care management of PTSD

Stepped care approach	What to offer	What does this involve?
First month following a traumatic event	Active monitoring	• Give advice about self-management, including sleep hygiene, peer support and using friends and family as support; do not offer debriefing • Review within one month and screen for PTSD; offer further assessment and treatment for people with ongoing significant symptoms • Consider offering brief, trauma-focused CBT interventions for people with significant early symptoms of PTSD or an acute stress disorder
Initial presentations of mild to moderate PTSD	General self-care	Offer advice about general self-care including regular, graded exercise and sleep hygiene
	10 minute CBT advice about managing anxiety	• Reduce avoidance and increase positive coping strategies using brief behavioural activation • Encouraging healthy life behaviours such as exercise, healthy eating, and avoiding excessive alcohol, smoking, caffeine and other drugs • Building and maintaining social support • Minimise self-blame or self-criticism • Mindfulness, relaxation and self-compassion to help with sleep, self-soothing and reduce physical tension
	Signpost to self-help resources	• Provide information about CBT-based books and websites for understanding and managing PTSD • Signpost to relevant local and national PTSD support groups and charities

PTSD with moderate impairment or lack of response to initial measures	First-line treatment for PTSD	• Trauma-focused CBT, exposure therapy or EMDR • EMDR should not be offered for trauma in combat veterans
	Second-line treatment	• Drug treatment: SSRI or SNRI
	Third-line treatment	• Alternative drug treatments include amitriptyline, mirtazapine and phenelzine
Severe or complex problem or lack of response to primary care treatment	When to refer to specialist services	• Severe or complex cases with marked functional impairment or if there are concerns about risk such as self-neglect or self-harm • Persistent and marked symptoms which have not responded to primary care treatment strategies
	Treatment options	• Increase in duration or number of psychological therapy sessions • Combined treatment with psychological therapy and medication • Antipsychotics such as risperidone to augment other treatment approaches in adults who have a poor response to psychological therapies or antidepressants • Management of co-morbid problems or barriers to engaging with trauma-focused therapies, such as substance misuse, dissociation, emotional dysregulation, interpersonal difficulties or negative self-perception

12.10 Monitoring and follow-up

Patients with PTSD will require regular follow-up to monitor their symptoms, functioning and response to treatment. If management is shared between primary and secondary care, there should be a written agreement confirming which party is responsible for monitoring. Any such decisions should also involve the person and, if appropriate, their family or carers.

Case example 12.2: John

Diagnosis and treatment of PTSD

John is a 35-year-old salesman who attends his GP, Dr Gokaraju, with his wife. They are worried about his health and their relationship, which is under strain.

John was involved in a minor car accident three months previously when he was hit from the rear at low speed. However, since the accident, he has become very irritable, with mood swings and angry outbursts directed at his wife and family with the slightest provocation.

His sleep is disturbed by distressing nightmares, and he is increasingly tired and having difficulty concentrating during the day. He finds it hard to get the accident out of his mind and tries to keep himself busy to distract himself from the memory.

Case example 12.2: *contd*

"There are times that I just don't want to go to sleep for fear of my nightmares. In my dreams, I relive the accident over and over again. The dreams seem so real that when I wake up, it takes a long time for me to be sure that it's not really happening to me again."

He has resumed driving for work purposes but avoids any other driving wherever possible. He feels very anxious, jumpy and low in mood. He also reports some odd sensations in his body, including numbness in his face and arms, blurred vision, vertigo and tinnitus. His alcohol consumption has escalated, and he admits to drinking in an attempt to blot out his nightmares.

Dr Gokaraju asks whether he has ever experienced anything similar in the past. John explains that aged 22, he had suffered similar symptoms. On this occasion, he had stopped at a car crash on a motorway and had witnessed the death and mutilation of a mother and child. On this past occasion, his symptoms had mostly resolved after about four weeks.

Dr Gokaraju suspects PTSD based on the history and asks John to complete the trauma screening questionnaire. This asks the patient to report which of the following symptoms have occurred at least twice in the past week:

Symptom	Present at least twice in the past week?
• Upsetting thoughts or memories about the event that have come into your mind against your will	Yes
• Upsetting dreams about the event	Yes
• Acting or feeling as though the event were happening again	Yes
• Feeling upset by reminders of the event	Yes
• Bodily reactions (such as fast heartbeat, stomach churning, sweatiness, dizziness) when reminded of the event	Yes
• Difficulty falling or staying asleep	No
• Irritability or outbursts of anger	Yes
• Difficulty concentrating	Yes
• Heightened awareness of potential dangers to yourself and others	No
• Being jumpy or being startled at something unexpected	Yes

The score for the TSQ is 8. As this lies above the cut-off level of 6, this supports the possible diagnosis of PTSD. Dr Gokaraju explains the diagnosis to John and reassures him that there are effective treatments available.

Case example 12.2: *contd*

They discuss the treatment options. The waiting list for trauma-focused CBT is over a year in this area, so John decides to have a trial of sertraline whilst waiting for the referral for psychological therapy to take place.

Dr Gokaraju also encourages John to improve his self-care by:

- reducing alcohol intake and restarting regular exercise
- improving sleep patterns using sleep hygiene and mindfulness
- increasing social support by spending time with his wife and other important friends and family members
- talking about the experience with trusted individuals.

12.11 Summary and key points

- PTSD may develop following exposure to a major traumatic event of an exceptionally threatening or catastrophic nature such as road traffic accident, physical or sexual assault or a natural disaster.
- It is common to experience temporary feelings of distress, anxiety, irritability and insomnia following a traumatic experience, and for many people these symptoms will resolve spontaneously with time.
- Lack of social support, isolation and social disadvantage are associated with the development of PTSD after a traumatic event.
- Common symptoms of PTSD include intrusive thoughts such as flashbacks and nightmares, avoidance, numbing and a persistent sense of threat, with hyperarousal and hypervigilance.
- Complex PTSD can arise after prolonged or repeated traumatic events, with additional symptoms including negative self-beliefs, difficulty regulating emotions and behaviour, and relationship problems.
- PTSD is frequently co-morbid with other problems such as depression, anxiety, anger, substance misuse and multiple physical health problems.
- Ask about a history of trauma in a patient who presents repeatedly to primary care with unexplained physical health problems.
- Management of patients with PTSD is ideally carried out by specialist PTSD services; however, the provision of services is variable and waiting lists may be long in some areas.
- Trauma-focused psychological therapy is the treatment of choice for PTSD, although drugs and other forms of psychological treatment may also help in some cases.
- Patient choice and availability of psychological therapy will influence the treatment given.

12.12 PTSD resources

PTSD self-help resources

- National Centre for Mental Health: http://ncmh.info/conditions/post-traumatic-stress-disorder-ptsd
- Northumberland, Tyne & Wear NHS Foundation Trust Self Help leaflets: https://web.ntw.nhs.uk/selfhelp/
- Royal College of Psychiatrists: www.rcpsych.ac.uk/expertadvice/problemsdisorders/posttraumaticstressdisorder.aspx
- Herbert, C. (2017) *Overcoming Traumatic Stress: a self-help guide using cognitive behavioural techniques*, 2nd edition. Robinson.
- van der Kolk, B. (2015) *The Body Keeps the Score: mind, brain and body in the transformation of trauma*. Penguin.

PTSD support groups and charities

- Anxiety UK – a UK charity providing fact sheets for anxiety disorders (including PTSD) (www.anxietyuk.org.uk/)
- Combat Stress – a military charity which specialises in the welfare of ex-servicemen and -women who suffer from psychiatric disabilities. It offers a national service, including brief bespoke residential treatments (www.combatstress.org.uk/)
- Cruse – a UK charity providing support and offering information, advice, education, and training services for people who have experienced a bereavement (including traumatic bereavement) (www.cruse.org.uk/)
- Rape Crisis England and Wales – a UK charity which provides a range of specialist services for women and girls who have been raped or who have experienced another form of sexual violence (whether as adults or children) (https://rapecrisis.org.uk/)
- Veterans UK – provides support services to both military personnel and the armed forces veterans community (www.gov.uk/government/organisations/veterans-uk)
- Victim Support – free and confidential help for the victims of crime, witnesses of crime, and their families, friends and anyone else affected (www.victimsupport.org.uk/)

Chapter 13
Health anxiety

Health anxiety quick reference guide

What is health anxiety?	Intense fear and preoccupation with having a serious illness, which persists despite appropriate medical evaluation and being reassured that no medical condition is present. Repeated behaviours are compulsive in nature and include body checking, internet browsing and frequent attendance at medical clinics seeking investigation and referrals, and reassurance seeking.
How common is it?	Lifetime prevalence is between 1% and 5% of the general population and is much higher in medical settings, affecting around 10% of attenders in primary care and up to 20% in medical outpatients.
Risk factors	There is uncertainty about the aetiology of health anxiety, but risk factors may include a past history of a serious childhood illness or a parent with a serious illness, being raised by an overprotective parent, childhood abuse, a family history of health anxiety, experiencing stressful life events and anxiety-prone personality traits.
Co-morbid conditions	Common co-morbid mental health conditions include depression, panic disorder, GAD and OCD, and it is also more common in patients with physical health conditions, including cancer.
Usual course	Health anxiety often follows a prolonged course where symptoms wax and wane over time and acute exacerbations of anxiety are typically triggered by specific health-related stressors. A worse prognosis is associated with more severe presentations and when individuals are highly harm-avoidant or less cooperative with medical approaches.
Common presentations	People with health anxiety who typically present repeatedly to multiple health professionals seeking investigations and assessment for feared symptoms, are unlikely to perceive the condition as a mental health problem. This can cause frustration on both sides and may lead to a breakdown of relationships with health professionals, as well as leading to unnecessary investigations, referrals and treatments, and the consequent risk of iatrogenic harm.
How to make the diagnosis	The diagnosis of health anxiety is often clinical. The health anxiety inventory is a validated tool for assessing levels of health anxiety. GAD-2, GAD-7 and HADS can also be used to measure background levels of anxiety.

What else could it be?	The differential diagnosis for health anxiety includes underlying physical health conditions causing persistent symptoms, somatic disorders causing distressing symptoms such as chronic pain and chronic fatigue syndrome, GAD and other anxiety disorders including BDD and OCD, depression, drug-seeking behaviour and factitious disorders.
Self-management strategies	General self-care including physical exercise, healthy diet and sleep hygiene are often helpful. Offer empathy and support and help patients to understand their condition by giving clear and credible explanations for physical symptoms and explaining the vicious cycle of self-focus, preoccupation with health and unhelpful behaviours such as reassurance seeking and internet searching in maintaining health anxiety. Use a 'two-tracks' approach to broaden the agenda to include both physical and psychological factors affecting health. Self-management strategies using 10 minute CBT include highlighting and labelling thoughts, reduction in safety behaviours and behavioural activation.
Treatment of health anxiety	Both CBT and SSRIs are effective treatments for health anxiety, although both treatments may have low acceptability. Choice can be guided by patient preference, as well as other factors including the availability of psychological therapy services. Medication should be started at low doses as many health-anxious patients are at particularly high risk of experiencing increased anxiety associated with side-effects when starting antidepressant medication.
When to refer	Severe symptoms associated with marked functional impairment, at risk of self-neglect, self-harm or suicide, or posing a risk to others, significant co-morbidity such as substance misuse, severe depression, anorexia nervosa or schizophrenia, or lack of response to treatment in community settings.
Follow-up	The prolonged and intermittent course means that long-term support and follow-up are needed for many health-anxious patients in primary care, who may present on multiple occasions associated with new symptoms or other triggers for increased anxiety.

13.1 Introduction

Health anxiety is an important condition in which sufferers are preoccupied by the belief that they may be physically unwell, despite appropriate medical evaluation and reassurance that no medical condition is present. Health anxiety is very common in primary care and may be growing more prevalent due to increased use of the internet to seek knowledge about illness. It is associated with persistent fear or distress and can have a debilitating effect on sufferers' quality of life, social and occupational functioning.

Health anxiety is an important disorder to recognise and treat in clinical practice. It has a major impact on healthcare resource utilisation, with sufferers tending to consult medical professionals unnecessarily and frequently, placing a major burden on primary healthcare services. This can also lead to excessive, unnecessary investigations and treatments, with the risk of iatrogenic harm.

Despite the importance of this topic, there are no current guidelines for management of health anxiety in primary care. This chapter has drawn

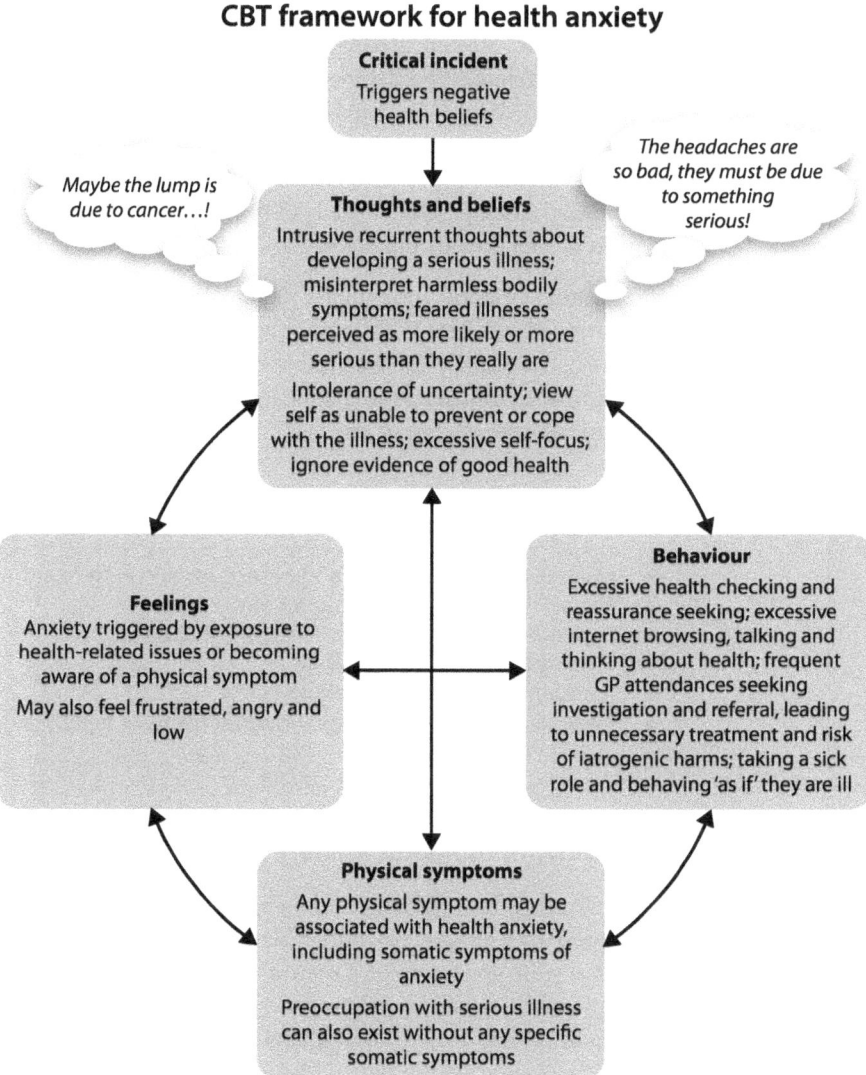

CBT framework for health anxiety

Critical incident
Triggers negative health beliefs

Maybe the lump is due to cancer…!

The headaches are so bad, they must be due to something serious!

Thoughts and beliefs
Intrusive recurrent thoughts about developing a serious illness; misinterpret harmless bodily symptoms; feared illnesses perceived as more likely or more serious than they really are

Intolerance of uncertainty; view self as unable to prevent or cope with the illness; excessive self-focus; ignore evidence of good health

Feelings
Anxiety triggered by exposure to health-related issues or becoming aware of a physical symptom

May also feel frustrated, angry and low

Behaviour
Excessive health checking and reassurance seeking; excessive internet browsing, talking and thinking about health; frequent GP attendances seeking investigation and referral, leading to unnecessary treatment and risk of iatrogenic harms; taking a sick role and behaving 'as if' they are ill

Physical symptoms
Any physical symptom may be associated with health anxiety, including somatic symptoms of anxiety

Preoccupation with serious illness can also exist without any specific somatic symptoms

information from a variety of sources, including adapting guidelines for the management of medically unexplained symptoms.

13.2 What is health anxiety?

Overview of health anxiety

Health anxiety is characterised by an excessive fear of having or developing a serious illness. Sufferers misinterpret harmless somatic sensations as evidence of a serious health problem and are convinced that their anxiety can be alleviated by being told that the disease they fear is not actually present.

As a result of their anxiety, people with health anxiety constantly check for signs of illness, and repeatedly seek reassurance that nothing serious is wrong by talking to friends or relatives, and consulting multiple health professionals seeking investigations, referrals and medical reassurance. A great effort is often expended to convince others that symptoms are real and that there is a yet to be discovered medical explanation for the physical symptoms. These checking and reassurance-seeking behaviours lead to a temporary reduction in distress, but the relief is short-lived, and anxiety recurs and worsens over time.

Some health-anxious individuals try to control their anxiety by avoiding information about illness and reducing contact with health professionals. This group is consequently far less likely to present in primary care and this can lead to unnecessary delays in diagnosis of actual diseases. The main features of health anxiety are shown in *Box 13.1*.

Box 13.1 **Features of health anxiety**

- Excessive worrying about and preoccupation with health
- Fear of having or developing a serious illness
- Repeated checking of body for signs of disease
- Constant need for reassurance
- Frequent medical consultations
- Excessive internet browsing and other forms of health checking

---

The spectrum of health anxiety

Health anxiety is a serious and debilitating condition that is often poorly understood by the general public as well as by the medical community. It refers to a wide spectrum of patients with anxiety about their physical health, ranging from mild and transient illness-related concerns and worries to severe preoccupation and fear in individuals whose thoughts and actions are centred around the overestimated risk of having or developing a serious, life-threatening illness.

There is significant overlap between the concepts of health anxiety and the older term, hypochondriasis. However, this latter term may be perceived as pejorative and judgemental, and has therefore been avoided where possible. Interestingly, DSM-V has now replaced the term with a new category of Illness Anxiety Disorder.

It is also important to recognise that patients with milder or 'sub-clinical' forms of health anxiety have been shown to experience just as much functional impairment in terms of occupational role, physical impairment and health perception as those who fully meet diagnostic criteria. Sub-clinical health anxiety is also associated with high levels of psychological distress, lower quality of life and elevated healthcare utilisation.

Developments in the classification of health anxiety

Based on recent research, the classification of health anxiety has been recently changed in ICD-11, and now forms part of the group of obsessive–compulsive and related disorders. This reflects the considerable overlap between health anxiety and OCD. The ruminations and preoccupations in health anxiety are similar to obsessions in their intrusiveness, persistence and ability to increase feelings of anxiety. Safety behaviours associated with health anxiety, including recurrent checking and monitoring of health and repeated reassurance seeking, are also similar to compulsive rituals in OCD.

Other changes in the diagnostic criteria for ICD-11 reflect the recognition that the presence of a physical symptom is not necessary for the diagnosis of health anxiety, and in many cases a preoccupation with or fear for a serious illness can exist without somatic symptoms. The absence of physical illness is also no longer necessary for the diagnosis. This is important, as many patients with health anxiety may also experience coexisting physical health disorders, and rates of health anxiety have been shown to be higher in people with physical health problems. In some cases, the onset of a physical disorder can act as a trigger for the onset of health anxiety.

Box 13.2

Diagnostic criteria for health anxiety

- Persistent preoccupation with the fear of having a serious, progressive or life-threatening disease
- Catastrophic misinterpretation of the meaning of harmless physical symptoms or bodily signs, including the somatic symptoms of anxiety
- Repetitive and excessive health-related behaviours or avoidance
- The preoccupation persists or re-occurs despite appropriate medical evaluation and reassurance
- The symptoms result in significant distress or significant impairment in important areas of functioning
- Levels of insight are classified as:
  - fair to good insight: the individual is mostly able to recognise that the health beliefs may not be accurate and is willing to accept an alternative explanation, although insight may be decreased or absent when the individual is highly anxious
  - poor to absent insight: the individual is convinced that the health beliefs are true and cannot accept any alternative explanations

Health anxiety and somatic disorders

Health anxiety is often viewed as being similar to conditions such as medically unexplained symptoms and somatisation, but there are some key differences between the two groups of conditions. In health anxiety, sufferers are focused on freeing themselves from crippling anxiety that their symptoms indicate a serious undiagnosed illness, by finding reassurance that there is nothing really serious wrong. They will often feel initially better after medical reassurance such as a negative test result, even though this relief is not maintained over time. Somatic symptoms are often absent or mild, and if present, the interference with daily functioning does not result from the symptoms themselves but is a consequence of fears about the meaning of symptoms and the associated behaviour.

In somatic conditions such as bodily distress disorder, patients experience highly distressing, persistent symptoms which affect function and quality of life. Here, distress tends to arise as a direct consequence of symptoms such as pain and fatigue, and the search for a diagnosis is in order to relieve the discomfort and distress by alleviating the symptoms.

13.3 Epidemiology

Health anxiety is common and may be increasing in prevalence. The reported prevalence varies, which reflects the changing rates of the disorder as well as the varying definitions used in different studies. The lifetime prevalence of health anxiety is between 1% and 5% of the general population. However, the prevalence is much higher in medical settings, with rates of around 10% of all attenders in primary care and up to 20% in medical outpatients. Some studies suggest that women and older people have a higher risk of health anxiety.

13.4 Aetiology

There is a great deal of uncertainty and some conflicting results about the aetiology of health anxiety. A number of risk factors for health anxiety have been suggested (*Box 13.3*), although there is no current definitive consensus and further research is needed. There does not appear to be a genetic basis for the condition.

Box 13.3	**Possible risk factors for health anxiety**

- History of a serious childhood illness or a parent with a serious illness
- Being raised by an overprotective parent with an excessive focus on minor health concerns
- Family history of health anxiety
- Experiencing stressful life events
- Experiencing the threat of a serious illness that turns out not to be serious
- History of abuse as a child
- Personality traits, such as having a tendency toward being a worrier
- Excessive health-related internet use

13.5 CBT model of health anxiety

In a CBT model, health anxiety develops in vulnerable individuals when a critical incident activates underlying negative beliefs about health, developed from past experiences (*Figure 13.1*). These beliefs include:

- viewing themselves as highly vulnerable to illness: *"My immune system is weak so I'm constantly getting ill"*
- fears about the experience of illness or death: *"Having cancer would mean an agonising death"*
- loss of self-esteem due to changing roles associated with ill health: *"I'm a complete failure if I can't work because of illness"*.

Thoughts and thinking styles in health anxiety

Unhelpful thinking styles which may be associated with health anxiety include:

- beliefs that particular illnesses are more likely or more serious than they really are (*"The lump must be due to cancer"*)
- excessive attention and awareness of physical symptoms (*"I don't feel quite right... could it be something serious?"*)
- viewing themselves as being at high risk of developing a rare and serious illness (*"I'm bound to be the one in a million who gets this illness"*)
- misinterpreting the meaning of harmless bodily symptoms and sensations as indicating serious underlying illness (*"The fatigue in my legs could mean that I have multiple sclerosis"*)
- intolerance of uncertainty – having an unrealistic desire for absolute certainty about health issues (*"I must be 100% certain there is nothing wrong, to feel OK"*)
- viewing themselves as unable to prevent or cope with the illness if it did occur (*"Being in a wheelchair would ruin my life!"*)
- focusing on information that confirms their fears whilst ignoring evidence of good health; this is a common cause of misunderstandings in medical communications (*"I think the doctor said it might be something serious"*).

Feelings in health anxiety

Patients suffering from health anxiety experience a great deal of anxiety, which may be triggered by health-related information, such as watching a television programme about health-related topics, receiving news that a family friend has experienced a heart attack or becoming aware of a physical symptom such as tinnitus or pain. Chronic anxiety often leads to low mood and depression. Feelings of anger and frustration are also common, and may be directed towards health professionals, who are perceived as ignoring or failing to diagnose a severe underlying medical condition.

Behaviour in health anxiety

Common behaviours in health-anxious individuals include the following:

Reassurance seeking: seeking constant reassurance from health professionals, family and friends leads to a temporary reduction in anxiety but is associated with a longer-term increase in anxiety and the desire for further reassurance as a vicious cycle.

Excessive monitoring and checking for 'danger' symptoms and signs of disease. Repeated prodding and self-examination can cause new symptoms such as pain, redness or swelling which are also interpreted negatively. They may also be more likely to notice normal variations in bodily functions and interpret these as evidence of serious ill health.

Frequent attendance at health services with requests for tests and referrals to confirm the diagnosis. Negative results from medical investigations may temporarily reassure the patient but ultimately increase anxiety in the long term (*"The doctor must think it is something serious"*) and reinforce beliefs about the need for medical tests to investigate symptoms.

Seeking medical information: health-anxious patients typically spend excessive amounts of time researching their symptoms in books and magazines and on the internet. This worsens anxiety as they learn about other potentially serious medical problems that might account for their symptoms.

Continual talking and thinking about health increases the preoccupation with illness and worsens anxiety. Health-anxious individuals are often highly talkative about their symptoms during consultations with medical professionals, which can reflect the underlying belief that if they could only be clearer or more thorough, then a solution to their difficulties would be found. It may also represent a strategy to try to suppress underlying terrifying thoughts and fears about the possible illness and what it might mean if they did develop it.

Taking a 'sick role' or behaving 'as if' they are ill: this may involve reducing activity, using unnecessary medication, using a wheelchair, stopping work or taking an illness role in family life. Family, friends and colleagues may reinforce these behaviours by taking on their responsibilities and encouraging the reduction in activity levels, which leads to a loss of self-confidence and self-esteem, a reduction in mood and increased time spent preoccupied by health worries. The avoidance of strenuous activities can also lead to physical deconditioning, which produces further body symptoms.

Avoidance: some health-anxious individuals tend to try to suppress their fears by avoiding information that is concerned with illness, especially serious conditions such as cancer. They avoid consulting health professionals and are consequently rarely seen in health settings. Unfortunately, attempts at thought suppression often result in a paradoxical increase in unwanted thoughts, with a consequent increase in anxiety over time.

Physical symptoms and bodily reactions

Health-anxious patients may misinterpret the meaning of physical symptoms associated with minor or benign conditions, as well as somatic symptoms of anxiety, normal variations in body sensation, or symptoms of a coexisting physical health problem. These are believed to indicate a severe undiagnosed health problem, leading to increased anxiety and further symptoms.

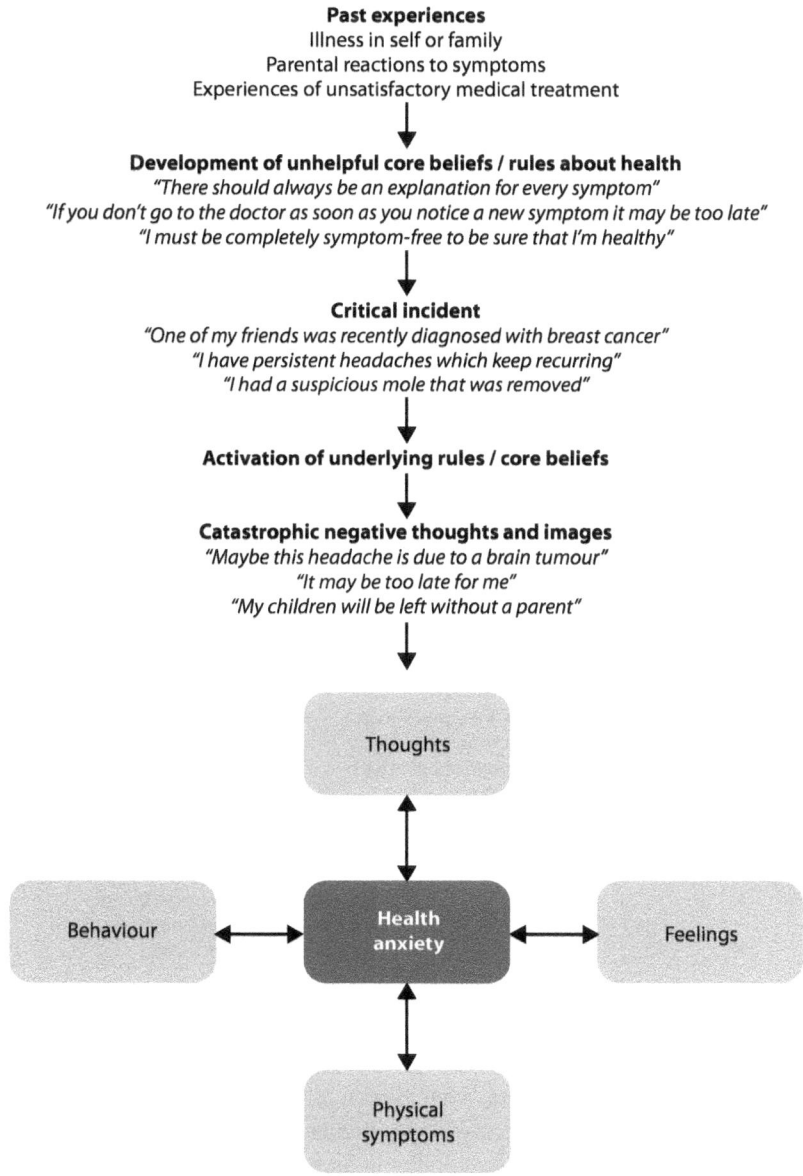

Figure 13.1 CBT model of health anxiety.

13.6 Co-morbidity

Coexisting mental health conditions, including depression, panic disorder, GAD and OCD are common in patients with health anxiety. Higher rates of health anxiety have also been shown in patients with physical health conditions, including cancer.

13.7 Course and prognosis of health anxiety

Health anxiety can be a persistent condition with a prolonged course where symptoms wax and wane over time. Many health-anxious patients will have had the condition for many years before it is diagnosed. Acute exacerbations of anxiety are typically triggered by specific stressors, such as the death of a family member, developing a physical symptom or illness, or in response to health-related items in the mass media.

Health anxiety can be effectively treated with CBT and medication. There are relatively few studies of long-term outcomes; however, some evidence suggests that this benefit is retained and that treatment can lead to long-term remission in a substantial proportion of patients.

In some, the condition may improve spontaneously, although many individuals continue to experience significant symptoms five years after diagnosis. A worse prognosis is associated with having a more serious condition at first presentation, and with personality factors such as being highly harm-avoidant and being less cooperative with medical approaches.

13.8 Presentation of health anxiety

I'm really worried about these lumps in my neck, even though the scan was normal...!

I really think I need a referral to another specialist to investigate my headaches – it's not normal they are so severe and are not going away!

I was looking on the internet and I'm worried it might be cancer...

Most patients with health anxiety will present to primary and secondary health services seeking medical investigations and assessment and are unlikely to perceive the condition as a mental health problem. There may be repeated attendances for the same symptom, and health-anxious individuals will often seek opinions from multiple health professionals to try to confirm the diagnosis ('doctor-shopping'). This can result in varying opinions being expressed by different doctors, which leads to a loss of faith in the knowledge and competence of medical professionals and reduces still further the reassurance value of the results of negative tests. It can also lead to frustration on both sides and may result in a breakdown of relationships with health professionals.

The consequence of repeated presentations to medical settings is that health-anxious patients often undergo frequent medical investigations and multiple referrals to various specialists, and receive multiple treatments, which may lead to side-effects and iatrogenic harm. Undergoing frequent investigations can also lead to the discovery of mildly abnormal results, which tends to increase levels of uncertainty and to reinforce beliefs about there being a medical cause for the problem.

Case example 13.1: Olivia

How might health anxiety present?

Olivia, a 48-year-old woman, attends the surgery for a routine health check and is found to have a moderately raised blood pressure. Her GP, Dr Sood, gives her lifestyle advice and suggests that they repeat the test in a few months.

However, after the consultation, Olivia finds it increasingly difficult to stop thinking about her raised blood pressure. She buys herself a home monitor and checks it repeatedly at home. She also starts to notice other symptoms that she begins to worry about. She feels dizzy and wonders if this is a sign that her blood pressure is likely to cause more serious problems. When she starts thinking about her blood pressure, she sometimes also notices that her heart starts racing and this is also a source of worry. She has cut out a number of her usual social activities because she is so worried about her health.

Olivia returns to see Dr Sood on several occasions, with questions and concerns about her blood pressure. He notices that Olivia appears to be highly anxious about her blood pressure and that this may be making the readings higher when she attends the surgery. He also notes that Olivia repeatedly asks for reassurance, but that this does not seem to have a lasting impact on her anxiety.

He explores the problem in more detail using questions from *Box 13.4* below:

Question	Response by patient
Have you been worrying a lot about your blood pressure?	Yes, I'm really worried about it. I know you said it wasn't that high, but I keep thinking it might have gone up even higher!
What's your biggest fear?	I keep thinking that I'm going to have a stroke. I might end up paralysed like my grandmother was.

Case example 13.1: *contd*

Are you someone who tends to worry about their health?	Well, I've always been a worrier, and health is probably my biggest concern. I'm very quick to think there might be something wrong with me!
If you notice a sensation in your body, are you likely to worry about it?	Oh yes, I get really worried if I have any new aches or pains, or if I'm not feeling right.
Do you find it hard to stop thinking about your blood pressure?	Yes, I can't seem to get it out of my mind, so I just keep checking, to make sure it's not too high.
If you read or hear about an illness, do you ever experience similar symptoms?	Well, yes, I know it's silly but I read about cancer the other week and I was sure after that I might have a lump in my breast.

Dr Sood then goes on to complete a CBT framework, focusing on an occasion when Olivia was feeling particularly anxious about her blood pressure in the past few days:

Thoughts
What if my blood pressure goes even higher?
I might have a stroke
Does the dizziness mean something serious?

Feelings
Anxious, worried
Tense

Behaviour
Repeatedly checking blood pressure
Looking on the internet for the causes of dizziness
Lying down to rest to try to "bring down" the blood pressure
Not seeing friends and has cut down on social activities

Physical symptoms
Dizzy, tired
Poor sleep
Palpitations
Muscle aches

With this history, Dr Sood has identified that Olivia's anxiety may be a symptom of health anxiety and goes on to carry out a more thorough assessment with this condition in mind.

13.9 Management of health anxiety

Making the diagnosis

Recognition of health anxiety

Most GPs will be very familiar with the most health-anxious patients on their list, who frequently attend the surgery seeking reassurance about a range of health concerns, although a formal diagnosis of health anxiety may not be made. However, its variable presentation can also make health anxiety more challenging to recognise in some individuals. Health professionals can also get drawn into the patient's preoccupation and desire for medical reassurance, by focusing on medical issues, rather than addressing the underlying anxiety and distress.

Some of the challenging behaviours of health-anxious patients can lead to high levels of frustration and stress amongst health professionals, and such patients may be perceived as 'difficult' or 'heartsink' rather than as suffering from a diagnosable and treatable mental health condition. This is compounded by the fact that such patients may be highly resistant to non-medical approaches to the condition.

Some useful questions that can help to explore and identify the presence of health anxiety are shown in *Box 13.4.*

Box 13.4 **Useful questions when you suspect health anxiety**

- *"Have you been worrying a lot about this symptom/problem?"*
- *"What's your biggest fear? What's the worst thing that this could be?"*
- *"Do you tend to worry about your health in general?"*
- *"Have you ever felt that the problem is more serious than the doctors have found?"*
- *"If you notice a sensation in your body, are you likely to worry about it?"*
- *"Do you find it hard to stop thinking about possible illness?"*
- *"If you read or hear about an illness, do you experience similar symptoms?"*
- *Empathetic statement: "That must be very difficult..."*

Ruling out medical causes for symptoms

In primary care, the diagnosis of health anxiety is usually made after ruling out possible medical causes for symptoms. This can be a very challenging process, and often involves 'grey areas' which may not be easily accepted by health-anxious patients who are seeking absolute certainty about their health.

However, the diagnosis of health anxiety can be made irrespective of whether a patient has a coexisting physical health condition, and the two conditions can be managed independently. Managing an individual's preoccupation with, and anxiety about their health does not require an unrealistic level of certainty that there is no underlying physical health problem. It is never possible to give 100% certainty about the absence of physical disease, as many illnesses develop slowly over time and some conditions are difficult to diagnose. For reasons of clinical safety, it is therefore important to remain open to the possibility of physical health conditions, whilst concurrently addressing psychological aspects of health.

Screening and diagnostic tools

The diagnosis of health anxiety is often a clinical one. However, the health anxiety inventory is a validated tool for assessing levels of health anxiety (*Box 13.5*). The first section asks about symptoms of health anxiety, such as level of worry about health and beliefs about how awful it would be if they were to develop a particular illness. However, this is a relatively long questionnaire which is only of limited use in usual primary care settings.

Brief screening for anxiety can be carried out with the use of GAD-2 and a more general assessment of anxiety can be carried out using HADS or GAD-7.

Box 13.5 | **Health anxiety inventory**

The short version of the health anxiety inventory involves 14 questions asking the patient to choose which of four statements most closely applies to them (never, occasionally, much of the time, most of the time), including questions such as:
- How much time do you spend worrying about your health?
- How often do you notice aches and pains compared to other people of the same age?
- How aware are you of bodily sensations and changes?
- Are you able to resist thoughts about illness?
- How often are you afraid that you have a serious illness?
- Do you often have images or pictures of yourself as unwell?
- Do you find it difficult to take your mind off thoughts about your health?
- If your doctor tells you there is nothing wrong, do you feel relieved? How long does the relief last for?
- If you hear about an illness, do you ever think that you have it yourself?
- How high do you think your risk is of developing a serious illness?
- Do your family/friends think you worry too much about your health?

What else to consider

The differential diagnosis for health anxiety is shown in *Box 13.6*.

Box 13.6

Differential diagnosis of health anxiety

- Underlying physical health conditions causing persistent symptoms
- Somatic disorders causing distressing symptoms such as bodily distress disorder/persistent physical symptoms, chronic pain and chronic fatigue syndrome
- GAD
- BDD
- OCD
- Delusional disorder
- Depression
- PTSD
- Drug-seeking
- Factitious disorders

Initial assessment of health anxiety

Review the medical history

It is often helpful to take some time to review and summarise a health-anxious patient's medical record in advance, which can provide invaluable information about patterns of symptoms in previous attendances, results of investigations and details of letters from specialists. If possible, create a brief summary and timeline for important medical and psychosocial events such as life events, medical investigations, hospital assessments and important diagnoses. This may save time in the long run and can be invaluable in aiding clinical decision-making (*Box 13.7*).

You can reflect this information back at a later stage when seeing the patient:

> "I've taken some time to review your notes so that I am better able to understand your case. It sounds like the pain got a lot worse last year after your sister was diagnosed with breast cancer...?"

Box 13.7

Summarising a patient's medical record – what to include

- Previous illnesses and dates
- Key information from hospital letters and discharge summaries
- Previous investigations and results
- History of mental health problems and triggers
- External stresses and life events (including dates) which may trigger episodes of anxiety

Carry out an assessment of physical health

In primary care, where clinicians carry responsibility for both physical and mental health problems, it is important to make a thorough assessment of a health-anxious patient's physical health. This is important for excluding physical causes of symptoms and will demonstrate to the patient that a health professional is taking the problem seriously. It is also important to keep an open mind and be willing to review the clinical picture if symptoms change or any further clinical doubt arises about the cause of symptoms.

If possible, offer one or two longer appointments to review a complex patient's medical history and physical health. This removes time pressure and may act as an 'investment' which saves time in the longer term. Try to use this session as a 'fact-finding mission' to learn about the person's symptoms and concerns, rather than attempting to make any early diagnoses or suggestions for management. Therefore just make a list of the important symptoms without offering any explanations or possible diagnoses, which may trigger a lengthy discussion and possible disagreement:

> *"I'd like to make a list of your symptoms and the issues you are concerned about. OK, you've mentioned numbness in the hands and a feeling of dizziness. Is there anything else to add...?"*

Investigate or refer only if clinically indicated

Appropriate investigations and referrals should be carried out if there is any clinical doubt about the cause or nature of symptoms, and it is important to remain clinically safe and thorough. It is also important to avoid over-investigating or making multiple referrals for the same problem or carrying out tests or referrals 'for reassurance', which is likely to increase the patient's anxiety in the long term.

Predicting negative results in advance (*"I'm expecting the result to be normal..."*) may reduce subsequent anxiety. If a referral is necessary, be clear in the letter that you suspect health anxiety. Important information to include in a referral letter to secondary care is shown in *Box 13.8*.

Box 13.8 **Information to include in referral letters for health-anxious patients**

- Inform the specialist that you suspect the patient may be experiencing health anxiety
- Be clear what you are asking them (e.g. to rule out a specific illness)
- Include details of any relevant psychosocial factors
- Provide a detailed history of past physical and mental health problems

Use a CBT framework to broaden the discussion

After discussing the physical symptoms, the consultation can naturally progress to asking relevant questions about any underlying thoughts and fears, and the person's behavioural reactions. A CBT framework offers a useful structure for guiding this discussion (*Box 13.9*).

Box 13.9 **Exploring a CBT framework in a health-anxious patient**

Physical symptoms
- Which symptoms are bothering you the most…?
- Are there any other important symptoms that you are concerned about…?

Thoughts
- What goes through your mind when you notice the symptoms?
- What's the biggest concern or fear that you have? What's the worst thing that this might mean?
- Do you often worry about your health?
- What is it about the thought of [e.g. cancer] that scares you so much? What do you imagine happening?
- Do you find it hard to stop thinking about your health?

Behaviour
- Do you frequently test or check your health in any way?
- Are you finding that you need to ask others for reassurance? Does this help? How long do you feel better for?
- Are you looking up your symptoms in books or on medical websites? What have you found out?
- Is there anything you have stopped doing because of your concerns about your health?

Feelings
- How are you feeling at the moment?
- How does it affect you to have this symptom?
- You seem quite anxious about this. Is it worrying you a lot?
- How is your mood? Has worrying about your health led to you becoming low or demoralised about the future?

Environmental factors
- Is anything else going on in your life that is causing you stress or worry?
- Did anyone in your past experience any serious or unexpected illness? Or did they worry about their health?
- Has anything happened recently which has made you more concerned about your health?
- Is worrying about your health having a negative effect on any other areas of your life, such as family, social life or work?

Initial management in primary care

The aim of primary care management for people with health anxiety is to provide optimal care for both physical and mental health, in partnership with the patient. There are a number of strategies and communication skills that can make this process more effective.

Build the relationship

Building strong, trusting relationships with health-anxious patients is an essential platform for effective management. This can be achieved by expressing warmth, respect and concern, using non-judgemental language and non-verbal communication such as making eye contact to build a connection. Exploring the patient's perspective using active listening and open questions is also important.

You may also benefit from getting to know more about the patient as an individual:

> *"Tell me more about yourself. Who is supporting you at home? Are you working? Do you have any pets? What are your hobbies? What's important to you as a person?"*

It is possible to show empathy for the high levels of anxiety experienced by a health-anxious patient, without agreeing with the extreme or unrealistic thinking that is leading to the distress, by making empathetic statements such as:

> *"It sounds as though you are really worried about your health, and perhaps not feeling that your concerns are being taken seriously. That must be very distressing..."*

It can also be helpful to acknowledge the person's past experiences of unsuccessfully trying to seek help for the problem, and the frustration and despair that can arise as a consequence. This can also be used to support the rationale for taking a new approach:

> *"It seems like you've seen a lot of different doctors about this problem, but nothing seems to have helped so far. It might be quite difficult to find a straightforward medical solution so I'm wondering if a different approach might help...?"*

Provide explanations for key symptoms

Giving clear, concrete and credible explanations of symptoms is essential to help health-anxious people understand their experiences. For a patient with mild anxiety and good insight, this may be enough to help them gain perspective and cope with their fears more effectively. Individuals with more severe and pervasive anxiety are unlikely to be reassured by this alone, or may be initially reassured, but find that their anxiety quickly returns. This response can be used to help gauge the severity of the problem.

Begin by explicitly acknowledging that the patient's symptoms are real and a source of major concern and distress. Tell the person what you think the problem is, rather than what it isn't. Avoid using jargon and give clear, concrete and credible explanations of symptoms which address the person's underlying fears and beliefs. If there is no easy medical explanation, then give clear reasons why the symptoms do not fit with a more serious explanation. Include written information where possible.

"I believe that the cause of your symptoms is... This can cause some very distressing and powerful physical symptoms..."

Box 13.10 **Explanations that promote understanding of the person's experiences**

- Stress and worry can cause physical tension in muscles, which leads to pain and stiffness
- Thinking about symptoms makes you more aware of them and can make them feel more unpleasant and distressing
- Excessive touching or checking an area of the body can cause pain and swelling which can then cause additional concern
- Constantly thinking and reading about the cause of symptoms is likely to increase anxiety levels and gets in the way of living everyday life
- Severe symptoms such as strong pain do not necessarily have a serious underlying cause

Share the risk

Be honest and clear about the existence of any uncertainty or risk, which is an aspect of life which cannot be completely avoided. It may be helpful to stress that you will be willing to reassess in future if needed. However, try not to reassure the patient unnecessarily or repeatedly as this can pull you into a vicious cycle which encourages repeated attendances and maintains their anxiety. Be honest and acknowledge that there is no absolute answer, and that the continual search for complete certainty can have a highly negative impact on people's lives. Remind the person that continually thinking about the worst-case scenario does not reduce the risk of illness and simply fills life with increasing stress and anxiety. Worry about future illness should not prevent people from living a full and enjoyable life.

Some strategies for coping with uncertainty are also covered in *Chapter 4*.

Broaden the agenda to include psychological aspects of the problem

The next step involves broadening the patient's perspective to consider the idea that their problem is not purely an undiagnosed physical health condition, and to begin to address emotional wellbeing as well as physical health. This involves stepping back from investigating the cause of symptoms and moving towards finding ways to live a fulfilling and meaningful life despite the presence or absence of physical symptoms.

Use a 'two-tracks' approach to avoid black and white perspectives of a problem being either medical or psychological in nature. Reassure the patient that you will continue to take their physical symptoms seriously and that discussing emotional aspects of the problem does not mean that you will assume that their symptoms are 'all in their mind':

> *"It seems that worry and stress about your symptoms are causing as much difficulty as the symptoms themselves..."*

> *"I take your health concerns very seriously and will always be willing to review the diagnosis..."*

> *"It is important that anxiety and fear of future illness do not prevent you from living a full and enjoyable life. Could we also look at some ways to help you manage this distressing anxiety and worry...?"*

Explaining health anxiety

After clearly explaining the patient's symptoms, the next step is to say that you think the person may be suffering from health anxiety. Giving an accurate description of the disorder which resonates with the person's own experiences may help them to accept the diagnosis more readily. *Box 13.11* provides an example of an explanation of health anxiety using a CBT framework.

Check the patient's understanding

Finish each consultation by checking what the patient has understood from the discussion. Because of the tendency to catastrophise and misconstrue medical information, it would not be unusual for a health-anxious individual to perceive that you said they have a serious medical illness. If this is the case, respond calmly and compassionately to clarify that it was not your intention to give this message and repeat your original explanation.

> *"I think it is unlikely that your abdominal symptoms are due to bowel cancer, but are due to a very unpleasant but less serious condition known as irritable bowel syndrome..."*

Involve the whole primary healthcare team

Where possible, encourage patients with health anxiety to see one lead health professional in the team regularly, who can get to know them and their history, including typical patterns of presenting symptoms and whether these have changed from previous attendances. This could be any relevant member of the nursing or medical staff. Ideally, health-anxious patients are balanced across all members of the team to avoid undue stress in any one health professional.

Regular team meetings are invaluable to offer emotional and practical support, particularly when a patient is experiencing an acute flare in anxiety and may be

Box 13.11 | **Explaining health anxiety**

Health anxiety is a common and distressing condition which is a type of anxiety disorder. People with health anxiety are usually extremely concerned that they are suffering from a serious health problem which hasn't been diagnosed properly. It's normal to worry about health at times, but health anxiety becomes a problem if the level of worry is out of proportion to the risk of having the illness and when anxiety starts to get in the way of other important life activities.

People with health anxiety tend to **think** negatively and worry excessively about health, assume the worst or 'catastrophise' about the causes of symptoms, and wish for an impossible degree of certainty that nothing is wrong. Negative **feelings** such as anxiety, low mood and frustration are common.

Behaviour often involves reassurance seeking from family and friends, repeatedly checking the internet and visiting health professionals for advice, tests and referrals. Repeated body checking for lumps and other signs of illness can lead to pain, bruising and swelling, which causes even more worry. After being reassured, health-anxious people usually feel better for a while, but in the long term the anxiety returns and grows even stronger.

Health anxiety can interfere with relationships with family and friends, work, finances and hobbies. People can spend so much time thinking about their health that there is no time left for the things that really matter. They may start behaving 'as if' they are ill, even before this is confirmed. This all leads to a worsening spiral of feeling anxious and depressed.

Health anxiety can be triggered by a new **physical symptom** or by a health scare in the media. Many health-anxious people also have physical health problems and talking about your anxiety does not mean your physical health will be ignored. Health anxiety can be effectively treated alongside caring for your physical health. This can involve talking less about the cause of the symptoms and thinking more about how you are responding to or coping with the symptoms or condition.

Health anxiety can be effectively treated, and this can continue alongside caring for your physical health. Treatments include psychological therapy such as CBT or antidepressant medication.

displaying a variety of challenging health behaviours. Keeping clear, accurate medical records, and ensuring effective communication between primary and secondary care are also important.

10 *minute CBT strategies in primary care*
Highlight and label thoughts. Try not to get caught up in debating the accuracy of the content of negative thoughts in health anxiety, which can lead to endless

discussions about the possible causes of symptoms. Instead try to highlight and label the fact that the thought has arisen and is causing distress. This is a process of 'cognitive defusion' which may start to reduce the believability and power of negative thoughts.

Remember that the thoughts in health anxiety are very powerful and compelling, and that simple defusion strategies in primary care are unlikely to be effective in leading to lasting changes in such thoughts. However, the strategy can be very effective to reduce circular and repeated conversations, and as an alternative to providing repeated reassurance, by avoiding engaging in the content of the thought.

Behavioural activation. Increasing wellbeing through setting goals for small behavioural actions that are likely to improve overall quality of life may be one of the most useful and effective strategies for people with health anxiety. This can also move the discussion away from repetitive discussions about symptoms and their meaning. Graded exercise, social interaction and relaxation activities can be particularly beneficial. Some suggested questions to use when identifying potential behavioural changes are shown in *Box 13.12*.

Reduce unhelpful behaviours. It may also be helpful to set small bite-sized goals to reduce unhelpful behaviour that is maintaining health anxiety as a vicious cycle. Examples include the following:

- Reduce reassurance seeking: setting limits on offering repeated reassurance to health-anxious patients is often important in primary care. This may involve giving patients a written explanation and asking them to refer to this in future presentations for the same problem. This might also be discussed with families and carers who may be asked for repeated reassurance at home.
- Reduce internet browsing for health-related information.

Box 13.12   **Questions to encourage behavioural activation**

- Is there anything you are no longer doing because of worries about your health?
- What types of activity would you do more of if you felt less anxious about your health?
- Who and what is most important in your life? What are your core values? e.g. family, pets, education, work, physical exercise, gardening... What activities might relate to these?
- It is important that we try not to allow worrying about health to dominate life and to prevent us from carrying out meaningful and enjoyable activities. What tiny steps or actions could you take that relate to these important areas in your life?

- Reduce self-monitoring and body-checking: this might include agreeing a reasonable frequency for checking blood pressure or looking for lumps in the body.
- Reduce or minimise repeated presentations to health settings triggered by anxiety: this involves encouraging patients to wait until regular, planned appointments for review of symptoms that are unchanged from previous attendances.
- Reduce illness behaviour: encourage the patient to stop behaving 'as if' they are already ill.

Other useful self-help strategies. Additional useful brief strategies that may be beneficial in health anxiety include:
- distraction from negative thoughts or rumination about health
- developing attention skills on daily tasks to reduce the focus on negative thoughts and reduce preoccupation with health
- mindfulness and relaxation exercises
- postponing worries (see *Chapter 11*).

Treatment of health anxiety in primary care

Both CBT and medication are effective treatments for health anxiety, although both treatments may have low acceptability. Choice can be guided by patient preference, as well as other factors including the availability of psychological therapy services.

Psychological treatment

CBT. CBT is the most effective psychological treatment for health anxiety and improves symptoms of health anxiety, overall distress and role functioning. It may also reduce attendances in health settings and overall healthcare costs. It is usually offered as one-to-one therapy but may sometimes be offered in alternative formats such as group or internet-based CBT.

CBT is also effective for patients with health anxiety and coexisting physical health conditions, and for older adults. It is effective for a wide range of severity of health anxiety, including people without a formal diagnosis. This highlights the importance of offering CBT to all individuals experiencing significant distress and decreased quality of life associated with worry about their health, even if they do not meet full diagnostic criteria for health anxiety.

However, the acceptability of psychological treatments may be low for some health-anxious patients, who may not perceive the condition as a mental health problem and regard their anxiety as a sign of likely physical disease. In some studies, only 30% of eligible participants agreed to participate in psychological treatments, with high dropout rates of 25–30%.

One of the major tasks in treatment for health anxiety is to work with the patient to help them recognise that their health worries, ruminations, obsessional thinking and illness behaviours are the major cause of their distress and impaired function, rather than being due to an undiagnosed medical illness. The strength of the therapeutic alliance and therapist competence have been demonstrated to be important factors in the effectiveness of psychological treatments for health anxiety, and this supports the importance for GPs of working on the doctor–patient relationship prior to attempting any strategies to make change.

Some of the components of a CBT approach to health anxiety include:
- developing a shared understanding of the problem using a CBT formulation
- cognitive restructuring and the use of behavioural experiments to test out more adaptive beliefs about health
- reduction in unhelpful health behaviours such as internet surfing, medical reassurance seeking, self-monitoring and hypervigilance
- ERP – this exposes patients to anxiety-provoking triggers, whilst discouraging them from carrying out safety behaviours or rituals; this disconfirms beliefs that a catastrophic result will occur if they face a feared situation without these safety behaviours, and allows the person to habituate to their distress over time.

Other psychological treatments for health anxiety. Additional psychological approaches which may be effective for health anxiety include:
- mindfulness: limited evidence suggests that mindfulness-based approaches may be beneficial in the management of health anxiety
- acceptance and commitment therapy
- behavioural stress management.

Drug treatment
There have only been limited studies looking at drug treatment for health anxiety, but SSRIs appear to be as effective as CBT, although the benefits are not as pronounced as in other anxiety disorders and occur late in treatment, after 8–12 weeks. As many as 50% of patients may continue to have significant symptoms despite treatment.

Like psychological approaches, antidepressant treatment may not be acceptable to a significant proportion of patients with health anxiety. Drug therapy may also have problems with tolerability, as health-anxious individuals are frequently highly sensitive to adverse effects of medication, which can trigger high levels of distress and worry. Health-anxious patients may therefore be at a higher risk of experiencing an increase in anxiety at the initiation of SSRI treatment and may not continue treatment long enough or reach high enough doses to benefit from it. To reduce this risk, it can be helpful to start medication at extremely low doses, possibly initially at sub-therapeutic levels, and build up very gradually.

There is currently no evidence regarding the use of any drugs other than SSRIs in health anxiety.

Combined treatments

Combined treatment with both CBT and SSRI has been shown to be more beneficial than either approach alone and should be considered in severe or refractory cases.

When to refer

Consider referral to specialist services for further assessment and treatment for patients with:

- severe symptoms and marked functional impairment, risk of self-neglect, self-harm or suicide, or risk to others
- co-morbidity such as substance misuse, severe depression, anorexia nervosa or schizophrenia
- an inadequate response to initial treatment.

Summary of primary care management of health anxiety

Stepped care approach	What to offer	What does this involve?
Initial presentations of health anxiety with mild functional impairment	Initial management in primary care	• Review the medical history and carry out a physical health assessment • Provide clear medical explanations of all physical symptoms • Avoid unnecessary investigation and referrals • Use communication skills to build a relationship with the patient • Broaden the agenda to include psychological and physical aspects of health • Explore the problem using a CBT framework to highlight links between negative thoughts and unhelpful behaviours • Explain the diagnosis and common features of health anxiety
	10 minute CBT advice about managing anxiety	• Highlight and label negative thoughts, rather than engaging in discussions about their content • Use brief behavioural activation to increase participation in meaningful or enjoyable activities and improve low mood and daily functioning • Gradually reduce unhelpful behaviours such as reassurance seeking, internet browsing about health, and body checking. • Other strategies include distraction, attention skills and mindfulness to reduce engagement with negative thoughts about health and illness
	Signpost to self-help resources	Provide information about CBT-based books and websites for understanding and managing health anxiety
	Guided self-help	Low intensity CBT involving structured self-help, telephone or group sessions

Stepped care approach	What to offer	What does this involve?

Health anxiety with moderate functional impairment or lack of response to initial measures	Primary care management: CBT or medication	• First-line treatment: high intensity CBT or SSRI
		• Second-line treatment:
		  o Combined treatment with SSRI and intensive CBT
		  o Trial of an alternative SSRI

Health anxiety with severe functional impairment or lack of response to primary care treatment	Consider referral to secondary care	• Refer to secondary care if
		  o severe symptoms with marked functional impairment
		  o risk of self-neglect, self-harm or suicide, or risk to others
		  o co-morbidity such as substance misuse, severe depression, anorexia nervosa or schizophrenia
		  o there is an inadequate response to initial treatment

13.10 Monitoring and follow-up

Patients with health anxiety should undergo regular review in primary care. Appointments are ideally scheduled in advance, rather than prompted by the patient's anxiety. These can be more frequent in the early stages of treatment and reduced over time, and then increased if a patient experiences an acute flare-up of anxiety symptoms. Telephone appointments as well as face-to-face appointments can be helpful for some individuals. All patients who are prescribed antidepressants will require regular follow-up (see *Chapter 3*).

Case example 13.2: Ines

Diagnosis and management of health anxiety

Ines is a 30-year-old healthcare assistant who attends surgery with a lump in her neck. She is initially reassured that it feels like a benign lymph node and after a few weeks it seems to resolve. A few weeks later, Ines is quite run down and develops a series of colds and sore throats, and notices that the lump, or a similar lump, seems to have returned. She starts to feel quite anxious and checks it several times a day by pressing hard against her neck. Eventually her neck starts to feel quite painful and this worries her even more. She makes an appointment to see her GP who agrees to arrange blood tests and an ultrasound scan. These are normal.

Ines initially feels better after the negative test results, but she can't help checking to see if the lump has definitely gone. She's not sure but she thinks it may still be present, so she starts looking on the internet for possible causes of lumps in the neck and discovers some frightening possibilities such as cancer. She often asks her husband to feel her neck too. He says it feels fine – and this sometimes helps for a short while, but the anxiety always comes back

Case example 13.2: *contd*

and she feels compelled to check her neck once more. She just wants to be absolutely certain that there is nothing wrong.

Ines also makes numerous appointments at her GP surgery, but feels frustrated that no one seems to take her concerns very seriously. During appointments, she talks a lot, trying to give as much information as possible to help make the diagnosis, and also in an attempt to block out the terrifying thoughts and images that pop into her mind whenever she thinks about the lumps. She imagines herself dying in pain from cancer and her children being left without a mother to care for them. Memories arise from Ines' childhood about the devastating effect of the unexpected death of her aunt on the whole family. She could not bear that to happen to her own children.

She is referred to see an ENT specialist, who examines her quickly, looks at her scan results and tells her there is nothing wrong. Ines feels that he didn't really take enough time and finds it hard to trust the surgeon's assessment. She goes back to her GP but there seems to be nothing they can do either. She begins to feel depressed and hopeless.

Ines starts finding it difficult to concentrate at work because she is so preoccupied by thoughts about having a possible serious illness. She is surrounded by continual reminders about health at her workplace in a hospital and sometimes feels unable to go to work at all due to the severity of her anxiety. Her relationship with her husband is starting to become strained, as he is getting irritated with her repeated requests for reassurance, and she has stopped seeing friends or doing exercise because of her level of anxiety.

One day Ines attends her GP again who suggests that they book a longer appointment to review and discuss her concerns about her health. Ines feels relieved that someone seems interested in listening. The GP takes a careful history of the physical problem and has also reviewed her medical record and letters from the consultant. He provides Ines with a clear written explanation of the cause of each symptom that she is concerned about. He offers Ines a follow-up appointment arranged in advance and encourages her not to contact the surgery in between booked appointments.

Her GP also suggests that it might be helpful to look for a way to manage the stress and anxiety that is associated with worries about health. Ines is initially reluctant, but the GP assures her that he will not ignore her physical health and suggests a 'two-tracks' approach to simultaneously managing both physical and emotional aspects of health.

Over time, Ines slowly begins to recognise that her anxiety about health is as much of a problem as the health concern itself. Whilst remaining very anxious that a health condition might still be present, she also agrees to be referred to the local CBT service and finds significant benefit from undergoing therapy.

Over time, Ines develops increasing insight into her tendency to worry about her health. She continues to experience catastrophic thoughts and high levels of anxiety when faced by any new or unexpected physical symptom

> **Case example 13.2:** *contd*
>
> *or becomes aware of a health scare in the media, but her strong relationship with her GP means that she feels able to discuss these concerns with him and feels confident that he will take her physical symptoms seriously. He also encourages her to take a realistic view of the problem and not to get overly caught up in a spiral of anxiety about her health. This is extremely helpful for supporting her and maintaining her wellbeing and her ability to participate in important aspects of her life.*

13.11 Summary and key points

- Health anxiety is an important and treatable condition in which sufferers are preoccupied by obsessional thoughts that they may be suffering from a serious, progressive or life-threatening illness.
- People with health anxiety 'catastrophise' about the causes of symptoms, overestimate the risk of serious problems, underestimate their ability to cope if they become ill and are highly intolerant of uncertainty.
- Compulsive behaviour includes frequent health checking, internet searches and consulting multiple health professionals seeking investigations and referrals for symptoms.
- Reassurance alleviates anxiety in the short term but leads to a longer-term increase in anxiety and desire for further investigations.
- Rates of health anxiety are higher in patients with coexistent chronic physical health conditions, and it should be considered in patients who present frequently to medical services.
- Patients with health anxiety benefit from establishing a relationship with one lead health professional in the primary care team.
- Offering one or two longer appointments to review the person's medical history and physical health may help the patient feel that their concerns are being taken seriously and provides a platform for moving towards psychological aspects of the problem.
- Explicitly acknowledge that the patient's symptoms are real and a source of major concern and distress.
- Provide clear, concrete and credible explanations of symptoms, which address health-anxious individuals' specific underlying beliefs and fears about the possible cause.
- A 'two-tracks' approach involves reassuring the patient that looking at emotional and psychological aspects of the problem does not mean ignoring or dismissing physical health.

- Because of the high risk of catastrophising and misunderstanding of medical communication, it is helpful to routinely check what a health-anxious patient has understood from any discussion.
- First-line treatment of health anxiety involves CBT; SSRIs may be used but should be started at low doses due to the high risk of increased anxiety associated with side-effects of medication.

13.12 Health anxiety resources

- Anxiety UK — a UK charity providing fact sheets for anxiety disorders including health anxiety (www.anxietyuk.org.uk/)
- Centre for Clinical Interventions: www.cci.health.wa.gov.au/Resources/Looking-After-Yourself/Health-Anxiety
- Northumberland, Tyne and Wear NHS Foundation Trust Self Help leaflet: www.nhs.uk/conditions/hypochondria/Documents/Health%20Anxiety%20A4%20%202010.pdf
- Pennine Care NHS Foundation Trust Self Help leaflet: www.selfhelpguides.ntw.nhs.uk/penninecare/leaflets/selfhelp/Health%20Anxiety.pdf
- Willson, R. and Veale, D. (2009) *Overcoming Health Anxiety*. Robinson.

References and further reading

Text references are shown in **bold**.

Chapter 1

Baldwin, D.S., Anderson, I.M., Nutt, D.J. *et al.* (2014) Evidence-based pharmacological treatment of anxiety disorders, post-traumatic stress disorder and obsessive-compulsive disorder: a revision of the 2005 guidelines from the British Association for Psychopharmacology. *Journal of Psychopharmacology,* **28**(5): 403–439. British Association for Psychopharmacology guidelines, available at: https://www.bap.org.uk/pdfs/BAP_Guidelines-Anxiety.pdf

Boschen, M.J. and Oei, T.P. (2008) A cognitive behavioral case formulation framework for treatment planning in anxiety disorders. *Depression and Anxiety,* **25**(10): 811–823.

Katzman, M.A., Bleau, P., Blier, P. *et al.* (2014) Canadian clinical practice guidelines for the management of anxiety, posttraumatic stress and obsessive-compulsive disorders. *BMC Psychiatry,* **14**(S1): S1.

National Collaborating Centre for Mental Health (UK) (2011) *Generalised anxiety disorder in adults: management in primary, secondary and community care.* NICE.

National Institute for Health and Care Excellence (2011) *CG123: Common mental health problems: identification and pathways to care.* NICE.

Chapter 2

Baldwin, D.S., Anderson, I.M., Nutt, D.J. *et al.* (2014) Evidence-based pharmacological treatment of anxiety disorders, post-traumatic stress disorder and obsessive-compulsive disorder: a revision of the 2005 guidelines from the British Association for Psychopharmacology. *Journal of Psychopharmacology,* **28**(5): 403–439. British Association for Psychopharmacology guidelines, available at: https://www.bap.org.uk/pdfs/BAP_Guidelines-Anxiety.pdf

Kroenke, K., Spitzer, R.L., Williams, J.B. *et al.* (2007) Anxiety disorders in primary care: prevalence, impairment, comorbidity, and detection. *Annals of Internal Medicine,* **146**(5): 317–325.

National Institute for Health and Care Excellence (2011) *CG123: Common mental health problems: identification and pathways to care.* NICE.

Spitzer, R.L., Kroenke, K., Williams, J.B. *et al.* (2006) A brief measure for assessing generalized anxiety disorder: the GAD-7. *Archives of Internal Medicine,* **166**(10): 1092–1097.

Zigmond, A.S. and Snaith, R.P. (1983) The Hospital Anxiety and Depression Scale. *Acta Psychiatrica Scandinavica,* **67**(6): 361–370.

Chapter 3

Baldwin, D.S., Anderson, I.M., Nutt, D.J. *et al.* (2014) Evidence-based pharmacological treatment of anxiety disorders, post-traumatic stress disorder and obsessive-compulsive disorder: a revision of the 2005 guidelines from the British Association for Psychopharmacology. *Journal of Psychopharmacology,* **28**(5): 403–439. British Association for Psychopharmacology guidelines, available at: https://www.bap.org.uk/pdfs/BAP_Guidelines-Anxiety.pdf

BNF 77 (2019) *British National Formulary.* 77th edition. British Medical Association and Royal Pharmaceutical Society.

Bower, P. and Gilbody, S. (2005) Stepped care in psychological therapies: access, effectiveness and efficiency. *British Journal of Psychiatry,* **186**: 11–17.

David, L. (2013) *Using CBT in General Practice: the 10-minute CBT handbook,* 2nd edition. Scion Publishing.

Department of Health (2001) *Treatment Choice in Psychological Therapies and Counselling: evidence based clinical practice guideline.* DH.

Gilbert, P. (2009) Introducing compassion-focused therapy. *Advances in Psychiatric Treatment,* **15**(3): 199–208.

Goyal, M., Singh, S., Sibinga, E.M. *et al.* (2014) Meditation programs for psychological stress and well-being: a systematic review and meta-analysis. *JAMA Intern Med,* **174**(3): 357–368.

Hofmann, S.G., Sawyer, A.T., Witt, A.A. and Oh, D. (2010) The effect of mindfulness-based therapy on anxiety and depression: a meta-analytic review. *J Consult Clin Psychol,* **78**(2): 169–183.

Medicines and Healthcare products Regulatory Agency (2014) *Selective Serotonin Reuptake Inhibitors (SSRIs) and Serotonin and Noradrenaline Reuptake Inhibitors (SNRIs): use and safety.* MHRA.

National Institute for Health and Care Excellence (2011) *CG113: Generalised Anxiety Disorder and Panic Disorder in Adults: management.* NICE.

National Institute for Health and Care Excellence (2011) *CG123: Common Mental Health Problems: identification and pathways to care.* NICE.

Persons, J.B. (2008) *The Case Formulation Approach to Cognitive-Behavior Therapy.* Guilford Press.

Public Health England/NHS England guidance (2014) *Pregabalin and Gabapentin: advice for prescribers on the risk of misuse.* PHE/NHS England.

Shapiro, F. (1989) Eye movement desensitization: a new treatment for post-traumatic stress disorder. *J. Behav. Ther. Exp. Psychiatry,* **20:** 211–217.

Valiente-Gómez, A., Moreno-Alcázar, A., Treen, D. *et al.* (2017) EMDR beyond PTSD: a systematic literature review. *Front Psychol,* **8:** 1668.

Williams, C. and Garland, A. (2002) A cognitive-behavioural therapy assessment model for use in everyday clinical practice. *Advances in Psychiatric Treatment,* **8(3):** 172–179.

Chapter 4

Ekers, D., Webster, L., van Straten, A. *et al.* (2017) Behavioural activation for depression; an update of meta-analysis of effectiveness and sub group analysis. *PLoS One,* **9(6):** e100100.

National Institute for Health and Care Excellence (2015) *Insomnia.* Available at https://cks.nice.org.uk/insomnia

Veale, D. (2008) Behavioural activation for depression. *Advances in Psychiatric Treatment,* **14(1):** 29–36.

Chapter 5

American Psychiatric Association (2013) *Diagnostic and Statistical Manual of Mental Disorders,* 5th Edition. APA.

Baldwin, D.S., Anderson, I.M., Nutt, D.J. *et al.* (2014) Evidence-based pharmacological treatment of anxiety disorders, post-traumatic stress disorder and obsessive-compulsive disorder: a revision of the 2005 guidelines from the British Association for Psychopharmacology. *Journal of Psychopharmacology,* **28(5):** 403–439. British Association for Psychopharmacology guidelines, available at: https://www.bap.org.uk/pdfs/BAP_Guidelines-Anxiety.pdf

Cuijpers, P., Sijbrandij, M., Koole, S. *et al.* (2014) Psychological treatment of generalized anxiety disorder: a meta-analysis. *Clin Psychol Rev,* **34:** 130–140.

Dugas, M.J. and Koerner, N. (2005) The cognitive-behavioral treatment for generalized anxiety disorder: current status and future directions. *Journal of Cognitive Psychotherapy,* **19:** 61–81.

Fisher, P. and Wells, A. (2011) Conceptual models of generalized anxiety disorder. *Psychiatric Annals*, **41:** 127–132.

Hoge, E.A. and Fricchione, G.L. (2012) Generalized anxiety disorder: diagnosis and treatment. *BMJ*, **345:** e7500.

McManus, S., Meltzer, H., Brugha, T. *et al.* (2009) *Adult Psychiatric Morbidity in England, 2007: results of a household survey.* NHS Information Centre for Health and Social Care.

National Institute for Health and Care Excellence (2011, updated 2019) *CG113: Generalised Anxiety Disorder and Panic Disorder (with or without agoraphobia) in Adults: management in primary, secondary and community care.* NICE.

National Institute for Health and Care Excellence (2017) *Generalized anxiety disorder.* **NICE. Available at: https://cks.nice.org.uk/generalized-anxiety-disorder#!backgroundSub:1**

Nepon, J., Belik, S.L., Bolton, J. and Sareen, J. (2010) The relationship between anxiety disorders and suicide attempts: findings from the National Epidemiologic Survey on Alcohol and Related Conditions. *Depression Anxiety*, **27:** 791–798.

World Health Organization (1992) *The ICD-10 Classification of Mental and Behavioural Disorders: clinical descriptions and diagnostic guidelines.* WHO.

World Health Organization (2018) *International Statistical Classification of Diseases and Related Health Problems*, 11th revision. Retrieved from https://icd.who.int/browse11/l-m/en

Chapter 6

Austin, D., Blashki, G., Barton, D. and Klein, B. (2005) Managing panic disorder in general practice. *Australian Family Physician*, **34**(7): 563–571.

Baldwin, D.S., Anderson, I.M., Nutt, D.J. *et al.* (2014) Evidence-based pharmacological treatment of anxiety disorders, post-traumatic stress disorder and obsessive-compulsive disorder: a revision of the 2005 guidelines from the British Association for Psychopharmacology. *Journal of Psychopharmacology*, **28**(5): 403–439. British Association for Psychopharmacology guidelines, available at: https://www.bap.org.uk/pdfs/BAP_Guidelines-Anxiety.pdf

Brown, T.A. and Barlow, D.H. (1995) Long-term outcome in cognitive behavioral treatment of panic disorder: clinical predictors and alternative strategies for assessment. *J Consul Clin Psychol*, **63:** 754–765.

Clark, D.M. (1986) A cognitive approach to panic. *Behav Res Ther*, **24:** 461–470.

David, L. (2013) *Using CBT in General Practice: the 10 minute CBT handbook*, 2nd edition. Scion Publishing.

de Jonge, P., Roest, A., Lim, C. *et al.* (2016) Cross-national epidemiology of panic disorder and panic attacks in the world mental health surveys. *Depression and Anxiety*, (online) Oct 24. doi: 10.1002/da.22572.

Dow, M.G., Kenardy, J.A., Johnston, D.W. *et al.* (2007) Prognostic indices with brief and standard CBT for panic disorder: I. Predictors of outcome. *Psychol Med*, **37**: 1493–1502.

Hayes-Skelton, S.A., Roemer, L., Orsillo, S.M. and Borkovec, T.D. (2013) A contemporary view of applied relaxation for generalized anxiety disorder. *Cogn Behav Ther*, **42**(4): 292–302.

Kessler, R.C., Ruscio, A.M., Shear, K. *et al.* (2010) Epidemiology of anxiety disorders. *Curr Top Behav Neurosci*, **2**: 21–35.

National Institute for Health and Care Excellence (2011, updated 2019) *CG113: Generalised anxiety disorder and panic disorder: management.* NICE.

Pompoli, A., Furukawa, T.A., Efthimiou, O. *et al.* (2018) Dismantling cognitive-behaviour therapy for panic disorder: a systematic review and component network meta-analysis. *Psychol Med*, **48**(12): 1945–1953.

Schmidt, N.B. and Telch, M.J. (1997) Nonpsychiatric medical comorbidity, health perceptions, and treatment outcome in patients with panic disorder. *Health Psychol*, **16**: 114–122.

Shear, M.K., Brown, T.A., Barlow, D.H. *et al.* (1997) Multicenter collaborative Panic Disorder Severity Scale. *American Journal of Psychiatry*, 154: 1571–1575.

Skapinakis, P., Lewis, G., Davies, S. *et al.* (2011) Panic disorder and subthreshold panic in the UK general population: epidemiology, comorbidity and functional limitation. *Eur Psychiatry*, **26**(6): 354–362.

Chapter 7

Baldwin, D.S., Anderson, I.M., Nutt, D.J. *et al.* (2014) Evidence-based pharmacological treatment of anxiety disorders, post-traumatic stress disorder and obsessive-compulsive disorder: a revision of the 2005 guidelines from the British Association for Psychopharmacology. *Journal of Psychopharmacology*, **28**(5): 403–439. British Association for Psychopharmacology guidelines, available at: https://www.bap.org.uk/pdfs/BAP_Guidelines-Anxiety.pdf

Katzman, M.A., Bleau, P., Blier, P. *et al.* (2014) Canadian clinical practice guidelines for the management of anxiety, posttraumatic stress and obsessive-compulsive disorders. *BMC Psychiatry*, **14**: S1.

Kessler, R.C., Chiu, W.T., Jin, R. *et al.* (2006) The epidemiology of panic attacks, panic disorder, and agoraphobia in the National Comorbidity Survey Replication. *Arch Gen Psychiatry*, **63**: 415–424.

Michael, T., Zetsche, U. and Margraf, J. (2007) Epidemiology of anxiety disorders. *Epidemiology and Psychopharmacology*, **136**: 142.

National Institute for Health and Care Excellence (2011, updated 2019) *CG113: Generalised anxiety disorder and panic disorder: management*. NICE.

National Institute for Health and Care Excellence (2019) *Benzodiazepine and Z-drug Withdrawal* (CKS). NICE. Available at https://cks.nice.org.uk/benzodiazepine-and-z-drug-withdrawal#!topicSummary

World Health Organization (1992) *The ICD-10 Classification of Mental and Behavioural Disorders: clinical descriptions and diagnostic guidelines*. WHO.

World Health Organization (2018) *International Statistical Classification of Diseases and Related Health Problems*, 11th revision. Retrieved from https://icd.who.int/browse11/l-m/en

Chapter 8

Alamy, S., Wei, Z., Varia, I. *et al.* (2008) Escitalopram in specific phobia: results of a placebo-controlled pilot trial. *J Psychopharmacol*, **22**: 157–161.

Baldwin, D.S., Anderson, I.M., Nutt, D.J. *et al.* (2014) Evidence-based pharmacological treatment of anxiety disorders, post-traumatic stress disorder and obsessive-compulsive disorder: a revision of the 2005 guidelines from the British Association for Psychopharmacology. *Journal of Psychopharmacology*, **28(5)**: 403–439. British Association for Psychopharmacology guidelines, available at: https://www.bap.org.uk/pdfs/BAP_Guidelines-Anxiety.pdf

Benjamin, J., Ben-Zion, I., Karbofsky, E. and Dannon, P. (2000) Double-blind placebo-controlled pilot study of paroxetine for specific phobia. *Psychopharmacology (Berl)*, **149**: 194–196.

Eaton, W., Bienvenu, O. and Miloyan, B. (2018) Specific phobias. *Lancet Psychiatry*, **5**: 678–686.

Katzman, M.A., Bleau, P., Blier, P. *et al.* (2014) Canadian clinical practice guidelines for the management of anxiety, posttraumatic stress and obsessive-compulsive disorders. *BMC Psychiatry*, **14**: S1.

Kessler, R.C., Chiu, W.T., Demler, O. *et al.* (2005) Prevalence, severity, and comorbidity of 12-month DSM-IV disorders in the National Comorbidity Survey Replication. *Arch Gen Psychiatry*, **62**: 617–627.

National Institute for Health and Care Excellence (2011) *CG123: Common Mental Health Disorders: identification and pathways to care*. NICE.

Wardenaar, K.J., Lim, C.C., Al-Hamzawi, A.O. *et al.* (2017) The cross-national epidemiology of specific phobia in the World Mental Health Surveys. *Psychological Medicine*, **47(10)**: 1744–1760.

Wittchen, H.U., Jacobi, F., Rehm, J. *et al.* (2011) The size and burden of mental disorders and other disorders of the brain in Europe 2010. *European Neuropsychopharmacology*, **21**(**9**): 655–679.

Wolitzky-Taylor, K.B., Horowitz, J.D., Powers, M.B. *et al.* (2008) Psychological approaches in the treatment of specific phobias: a meta-analysis. *Clin Psychol Rev*, **28**: 1021–1037.

Chapter 9

Baldwin, D.S., Anderson, I.M., Nutt, D.J. *et al.* (2014) Evidence-based pharmacological treatment of anxiety disorders, post-traumatic stress disorder and obsessive-compulsive disorder: a revision of the 2005 guidelines from the British Association for Psychopharmacology. *Journal of Psychopharmacology*, **28**(**5**): 403–439. British Association for Psychopharmacology guidelines, available at: https://www.bap.org.uk/pdfs/BAP_Guidelines-Anxiety.pdf

Brook, C.A. and Schmidt, L.A. (2008) Social anxiety disorder: a review of environmental risk factors. *Neuropsychiatr Dis Treat*, **4**(**1**): 123–143.

Connor, K., Kobak, K.A., Churchill, E. *et al.* (2001) Mini-SPIN: a brief screening assessment for generalized social anxiety disorder. *Depress Anxiety*, **14**: 137–140.

Heimburg, R.G. and Becker, R.E. (2002) *Cognitive-Behavioral Group Therapy for Social Phobia*. Guilford Press.

Mayo-Wilson, E., Dias, S., Mavranezouli, I. *et al.* (2014) Psychological and pharmacological interventions for social anxiety disorder in adults: a systematic review and network meta-analysis. *Lancet Psychiatry*, **1**(**5**): 368–376.

Mennin, D.S., Fresco, D.M., Heimberg, R.G. *et al.* (2002) Screening for social anxiety disorder in the clinical setting: the Liebowitz Social Anxiety Scale. *J Anxiety Disord*, **16**: 661–673.

National Institute for Health and Care Excellence (2011) *CG115: Alcohol-Use Disorders: diagnosis, assessment and management of harmful drinking (high-risk drinking) and alcohol dependence*. NICE.

National Institute for Health and Care Excellence (2013) *CG159: Social Anxiety Disorder: recognition, assessment and treatment*. **NICE.**

Stein, M.B. and Stein, D.J. (2008) Social anxiety disorder. *Lancet*, **371**(**9618**): 1115–1125.

Williams, T., Hattingh, C.J., Kariuki, C.M. *et al.* (2017) Pharmacotherapy for social anxiety disorder (SAnD). *Cochrane Database Sys Rev*, (**10**): CD001206.

World Health Organization (1992) *The ICD-10 Classification of Mental and Behavioural Disorders: clinical descriptions and diagnostic guidelines*. WHO.

World Health Organization (2018) *International Statistical Classification of Diseases and Related Health Problems*, 11th revision. Retrieved from https://icd.who.int/browse11/l-m/en

Chapter 10

Muller, I. and Yardley, L. (2011) Telephone-delivered cognitive behavioural therapy: a systematic review and meta-analysis. *J Telemed Telecare*, **17**(**4**): 177–184.

National Institute for Clinical Excellence (2005) *Obsessive-compulsive disorder: core interventions in the treatment of obsessive-compulsive disorder and body dysmorphic disorder.* NICE.

National Institute for Health and Care Excellence (2018) *Obsessive Compulsive Disorder*: CKS. Available at: https://cks.nice.org.uk/obsessive-compulsive-disorder#!topicSummary

Olatunji, B.O., Davis, M.L., Powers, M.B. and Smits, J.A. (2013) Cognitive-behavioral therapy for obsessive-compulsive disorder: a meta-analysis of treatment outcome and moderators. *J Psychiatr Res*, **47**: 33–41.

Russell, E.J., Fawcett, J.M. and Mazmanian, D. (2013) Risk of obsessive-compulsive disorder in pregnant and postpartum women: a meta-analysis. *J Clin Psychiatry*, **74**: 377–385.

Singer, H.S., Gilbert, D.L., Wolf, D.S. *et al.* (2012) Moving from PANDAS to CANS. *J Pediatr*, **160**: 725–731.

Snider, L.A. and Swedo, S.E. (2004) PANDAS: current status and directions for research. *Mol Psychiatry*, **9**: 900–907.

Soomro, G.M., Altman, D., Rajagopal, S. *et al.* (2008) Selective serotonin re-uptake inhibitors (SSRIs) versus placebo for obsessive compulsive disorder (OCD). *Cochrane Database Syst Rev*, **23**(**1**): CD001765.

Steketee, G., Frost, R. and Bogart, K. (1996) The Yale-Brown Obsessive Compulsive Scale: interview versus self-report. *Behav Res Ther*, **34**(**8**): 675–684.

Taylor, S., Abramowitz, J. and Mckay, D. (2007) Cognitive-behavioral models of obsessive-compulsive disorder. In: *Psychological Treatment of OCD: fundamentals and beyond* (eds M.A. Antony, C. Purdon and L.J. Summerfeldt), pp. 9–29.

Veale, D. (2007) Cognitive–behavioural therapy for obsessive–compulsive disorder. *Advances in Psychiatric Treatment*, **13**: 438–446.

Veale, D. and Roberts, A. (2014) Obsessive-compulsive disorder. *BMJ*, **348**: g2183.

World Health Organization (2018) *International Statistical Classification of Diseases and Related Health Problems*, 11th revision. Retrieved from https://icd.who.int/browse11/l-m/en

Chapter 11

American Psychiatric Association (2013) *Diagnostic and Statistical Manual of Mental Disorders*, 5th edition. APA.

Aouizerate, B., Pujol, H., Grabot, D. *et al.* (2003) Body dysmorphic disorder in a sample of cosmetic surgery applicants. *Eur Psychiatry*, **18**(7): 365–368.

Bowyer, L., Krebs, G., Mataix-Cols, D. *et al.* (2016) A critical review of cosmetic treatment outcomes in body dysmorphic disorder. *Body Image*, **19**: 1–8.

Brohede, S., Wingren, G., Wijma, B. *et al.* (2013) Validation of the Body Dysmorphic Disorder Questionnaire in a community sample of Swedish women. *Psychiatry Res*, **210**: 647–652.

Crerand, C.E., Menard, W. and Phillips, K.A. (2010) Surgical and minimally invasive cosmetic procedures among persons with body dysmorphic disorder. *Ann Plastic Surgery*, **65**: 11–16.

Krebs, G., Fernández de la Cruz, L. and Mataix-Cols, D. (2017) Recent advances in understanding and managing body dysmorphic disorder. *Evidence-Based Mental Health*, **20**: 71–75.

National Institute for Health and Care Excellence (2005) *CG31: Obsessive-Compulsive Disorder and Body Dysmorphic Disorder: treatment*. NICE.

Phillips, K.A., Hollander, E., Rasmussen, S.A. *et al.* (1997) A severity rating scale for body dysmorphic disorder: development, reliability, and validity of a modified version of the Yale-Brown Obsessive Compulsive Scale. *Psychopharmacol Bull*, **33**: 17–22.

Veale, D. (2001) Cognitive–behavioural therapy for body dysmorphic disorder. *Advances in Psychiatric Treatment*, 7(2): 125–132.

Veale, D. (2007) Cognitive–behavioural therapy for obsessive–compulsive disorder. *Advances in Psychiatric Treatment*, **13**: 438–446.

Veale, D. and Bewley, A. (2015) Body dysmorphic disorder. *BMJ*, **350**: h2278.

World Health Organization (2010) *International Statistical Classification of Diseases and Related Health Problems*, 10th revision.

World Health Organization (2018) *International Statistical Classification of Diseases and Related Health Problems*, 11th revision. Retrieved from https://icd.who.int/browse11/l-m/en

Chapter 12

American Psychiatric Association (2013) *Diagnostic and Statistical Manual of Mental Disorders*, 5th edition. APA.

Benedek, D.M., Friedman, M.J., Zatzick, D. *et al.* (2009) Guideline watch (March 2009): Practice guideline for the treatment of patients with acute stress disorder and posttraumatic stress disorder. *Focus*, **7(2):** 1–9.

Benjet, C., Bromet, E., Karam, E.G. *et al.* (2016) The epidemiology of traumatic event exposure worldwide: results from the World Mental Health Survey Consortium. *Psychol Med*, **46:** 327–343.

Bisson, J.I., Cosgrove, S., Lewis, C. and Roberts N.P. (2015) Post-traumatic stress disorder. *British Medical Journal*, **351:** h6161.

BMJ Best Practice (2018) *Post-traumatic Stress Disorder.* BMJ Publishing Group.

Brewin, C.R., Dalgleish, T. and Joseph, S. (1996) A dual representation theory of posttraumatic stress disorder. *Psychol Rev*, **103(4):** 670–686.

Brewin, C.R., Rose, S., Andrews. B. *et al.* (2002) Brief screening instrument for post-traumatic stress disorder. *British Journal of Psychiatry*, **181(2):** 158–162.

Davidson, J.R., Book, S.W., Colket, J.T. et al. (1997) Assessment of a new self-rating scale for post-traumatic stress disorder. *Psychol Med*, **27(1):** 153–160.

Ehlers, A. and Clarke, D.M. (2000) A cognitive model of posttraumatic stress disorder. *Behaviour Research and Therapy*, **38:** 319–345.

Gupta, M.A. (2013) Review of somatic symptoms in post-traumatic stress disorder. *Int Rev Psychiatry*, **25:** 86–99.

Kessler, R.C., Sonneha, A., Bromet, E. *et al.* (1995) Posttraumatic stress disorder in the National Comorbity Survey. *Archives of General Psychiatry*, **52(12):** 1048–1060.

National Institute for Health and Care Excellence (2018) *NG116: Post-traumatic Stress Disorder.* NICE.

Prins, A., Bovin, M.J., Kimerling, R. *et al.* (2015) *Primary Care PTSD Screen for DSM-5 (PC-PTSD-5).* Available from www.ptsd.va.gov/professional/assessment/screens/pc-ptsd.asp

Roberts, N.P., Kitchiner, N.J., Kenardy, J. and Bisson, J.I. (2010) Early psychological interventions to treat acute traumatic stress symptoms. *Cochrane Database Syst Rev*, **3:** CD007944.

Royal College of Psychiatrists (2015) *Post-traumatic Stress Disorder.* Royal College of Psychiatrists.

Schnurr, P.P., Green, B.L. and Kaltman, S. (2007) Trauma exposure and physical health. In: *Handbook of PTSD: science and practice* (eds M.J. Friedman, T.M. Keane and P.A. Resick). Guilford Press.

Shalev, A., Liberzon, I. and Marmar, C. (2017) Post-traumatic stress disorder. *New Engl J Med*, **376(25):** 2459–2469.

Spoont, M.R., Williams, J.W., Kehle-Forbes, S.M. *et al.* (2015) does this patient have posttraumatic stress disorder? Rational clinical examination systematic review. *JAMA*, **314(5):** 501–510.

Steel, Z., Chey, T., Silove, D. et al. (2009) Association of torture and other potentially traumatic events with mental health outcomes among populations exposed to mass conflict and displacement: a systematic review and meta-analysis. *JAMA*, **302:** 537–549.

World Health Organization (2010) *International Statistical Classification of Diseases and Related Health Problems*, 10th revision.

World Health Organization (2018) *International Statistical Classification of Diseases and Related Health Problems*, 11th revision. Retrieved from https://icd.who.int/browse11/l-m/en

Chapter 13

Baldwin, D.S., Anderson, I.M., Nutt, D.J. *et al.* (2014) Evidence-based pharmacological treatment of anxiety disorders, post-traumatic stress disorder and obsessive-compulsive disorder: a revision of the 2005 guidelines from the British Association for Psychopharmacology. *Journal of Psychopharmacology*, **28(5):** 403–439. British Association for Psychopharmacology guidelines, available at: https://www.bap.org.uk/pdfs/BAP_Guidelines-Anxiety.pdf

Barsky, A.J. and Ahern, D.K. (2004) Cognitive behaviour therapy for hypochondriasis. A randomized trial. *JAMA*, **291:** 1464–1470.

Barsky, A.J., Ahern, D.K., Bauer, M.R. *et al.* (2013) A randomized trial of treatments for high-utilizing somatizing patients. *J Gen Intern Med*, **28:** 1396.

Bass, C. and Pearce, S. (2016) Severe and enduring somatoform disorders: recognition and management. *BJPsych Advances*, **22:** 87–96.

Cooper, K., Gregory, J., Walker, I. *et al.* (2017) Cognitive behaviour therapy for health anxiety: a systematic review and meta-analysis. *Behavioural and Cognitive Psychotherapy*, **45(2):** 110–123.

David, L. (2013) *Using CBT in General Practice: the 10 minute CBT handbook*, 2nd edition. Scion Publishing.

den Boeft, M., Claassen-van Dessel, N. and van der Wouden, J.C. (2017) How should we manage adults with persistent unexplained physical symptoms? *BMJ*, **356:** j268. Available at: https://doi.org/10.1136/bmj.j268

Eilenberg, T., Fink, P., Jensen, J.S. *et al.* (2016) Acceptance and commitment group therapy (ACT-G) for health anxiety: a randomised controlled trial. *Psychological Medicine*, **46:** 103–115.

Fallon, B.A., Ahern, D.K., Pavlicova, M. *et al.* (2017) A randomized controlled trial of medication and cognitive-behavioural therapy for hypochondriasis. *American Journal of Psychiatry*, **174:** 756–764.

Greeven, A., van Balkom, A.J., Visser, S. *et al.* (2007) Cognitive behaviour therapy and paroxetine in the treatment of hypochondriasis: a randomized controlled trial. *American Journal of Psychiatry*, **164:** 91–99.

Hedman, E., Andersson, E., Ljótsson, B. *et al.* (2016) Cost effectiveness of internet-based cognitive behaviour therapy and behavioural stress management for severe health anxiety. *BMJ Open*, **6:** e009327.

Hedman-Lagerlöf, E., Tyrer, P., Hague, J. and Tyrer, H. (2019) Health anxiety. *BMJ*, **364:** l774.

McManus, F., Surawy, C., Muse, K. *et al.* (2012) A randomized clinical trial of mindfulness-based cognitive therapy versus unrestricted services for health anxiety (hypochondriasis). *Journal of Consulting and Clinical Psychology*, **80:** 817–828.

olde Hartman, T., Rosendal, M., Aamland, A. *et al.* (2017) What do guidelines and systematic reviews tell us about the management of medically unexplained symptoms in primary care? *BJGP Open*, **1(3):** 17X101061.

Petrie, K.J., Müller, J.T., Schirmbeck, F. *et al.* (2007) Effect of providing information about normal test results on patients' reassurance: randomised controlled trial. *BMJ*, **334:** 352.

Salkovskis, P.M., Rimes, K.A., Warwick, H.M. and Clark, D.M (2002) The Health Anxiety Inventory: development and validation of scales for the measurement of health anxiety and hypochondriasis. *Psychological Medicine*, **32:** 843–853.

Schweitzer, P.J., Zafar, U., Pavlicova, M. and Fallon, B.A. (2011) Long-term follow-up of hypochondriasis after selective serotonin reuptake inhibitor treatment. *J Clin Psychopharmacol*, **31(3):** 365–368.

Thomson, A.B. and Page, L.A. (2007) Psychotherapies for hypochondriasis. *Cochrane Database of Systematic Reviews*, **4:** CD006520.

Tyrer, H., Ali, L., Cooper, F. *et al.* (2013) The Schedule for Evaluating Persistent Symptoms (SEPS): a new method of recording medically unexplained symptoms. *International Journal of Social Psychiatry*, **59:** 281–287.

Tyrer, P. and Tyrer, H. (2018) Health anxiety: detection and treatment. *BJPsych Advances*, **24(1):** 66–72.

Tyrer, P., Cooper, S., Crawford, M. *et al.* (2011) Prevalence of health anxiety problems in medical clinics. *J Psychosom Res*, **71:** 392–394.

Tyrer, P., Cooper, S., Tyrer, H. *et al.* (2013) Clinical and cost-effectiveness of cognitive behaviour therapy for health anxiety in medical patients: a multicentre randomised controlled trial. *Lancet*, **383**(**9913**): 219–225.

Tyrer, P., Eilenberg, T., Fink, P. *et al.* (2016) Health anxiety: the silent disabling epidemic. *BMJ*, **353**: i2250.

Weck, F., Richtberg, S. and Neng, J.M. (2014) Epidemiology of hypochondriasis and health anxiety: comparison of different diagnostic criteria. *Current Psychiatry Reviews*, **10**(**1**): 14–23.

Weck, F., Richtberg, S., Jakob, M. *et al.* (2015) Therapist competence and therapeutic alliance are important in the treatment of health anxiety (hypochondriasis). *Psychiatry Research*, **228**: 53–58.

Wells, A. (1997) *Cognitive Therapy of Anxiety Disorders*. John Wiley and Sons.

World Health Organization (2010) *International Statistical Classification of Diseases and Related Health Problems*, 10th revision.

World Health Organization (2018) *International Statistical Classification of Diseases and Related Health Problems*, 11th revision. Retrieved from https://icd.who.int/browse11/l-m/en

Index